Clinical Handbook

Medical Surgical Nursing

Critical Thinking in Client Care

SECOND EDITION

PRISCILLA LEMONE, RN, DSN, FAAN
Associate Professor
Sinclair School of Nursing
University of Missouri–Columbia
Columbia, MO

KAREN M. BURKE, RN, MS
Director of Health Occupations
Clatsop Community College
Astoria, OR

PRENTICE HALL HEALTH
Upper Saddle River, New Jersey 07458

Library of Congress Cataloging-in-Publication Data

LeMone, Priscilla.
    Clinical handbook for medical-surgical nursing : critical
thinking in client care / Priscilla LeMone, Karen M. Burke.—2nd
ed.
    p. cm.
    Rev. ed. of: Clinical handbook for medical surgical nursing /
Susan P. Gauthier. c1996.
    Includes bibliographical references and index.
    ISBN 0-8053-8126-0
1. Nursing Handbooks, manuals, etc. 2. Surgical nursing
Handbooks, manuals, etc. I. Burke, Karen M. II. Gauthier, Susan P.
Clinical handbook for medical surgical nursing. III. Title.
    RT51 .G38 2000
    610.73'677—dc21
                                                    99-34472
                                                        CIP

Editor-in-Chief: Cheryl L. Mehalik
Project Editors: Virginia Simione Jutson, Grace Wong
Managing Editor: Wendy Earl
Associate Editor: Stephanie Kellogg
Publishing Assistants: Susan Tehan, Peggy Hammett
Production Supervisor: David Novak
Production Coordinator: Bettina Borer
Director of Manufacturing and Production: Bruce Johnson
Manufacturing Buyer: Ilene Sanford
Text Designer: Terri Wright
Cover Designer: Yvo Riezebos Design
Compositor: Marian Hartsough Associates
Printer/Binder: Banta Book Group
Cover Illustration: The quilt is entitled *Color Blocks #35*,
    ©1993 Nancy Crow. 34 x 1/2" x 36 1/2";
    Photo by J Kevin Fitzsimons

Previously published by Addison-Wesley Nursing,
A Division of the Benjamin/Cummings Publishing Company, Inc.
Menlo Park, California 94025

©2000 by Prentice-Hall, Inc.
Upper Saddle River, New Jersey 07458

Printed in the United States of America.
10 9 8 7 6 5 4 3 2 1
ISBN 0-8053-8126-0

Prentice-Hall International (UK) Limited, London
Prentice-Hall of Australia Pty. Limited, Sydney
Prentice-Hall Canada Inc., Toronto
Prentice-Hall Hispanoamericana, S.A., Mexico
'rentice-Hall of India Private Limited, New Delhi
 ntice-Hall of Japan, Inc., Tokyo

Preface

The *Clinical Handbook for Medical-Surgical Nursing* is a handy, pocket-sized reference for the conditions most frequently encountered in clinical situations. While primarily developed as a supplement to the second edition of *Medical-Surgical Nursing: Critical Thinking in Client Care*, to which it is cross-referenced, the *Clinical Handbook* may also be used as a stand-alone reference text. It provides nursing students in the clinical area essential information in an easy-to-follow format, allowing them to respond quickly when a client's condition changes or when they are assigned to a new client.

Organization

The *Clinical Handbook* covers 163 of the most common conditions nursing students are likely to encounter in medical-surgical nursing. The conditions appear in alphabetical order for quick retrieval of the most vital information.

Key Features

The *Clinical Handbook* presents varying amounts of information about each condition according to its prevalence and/or seriousness. Basic definitions, as well as epidemiologic, pathophysiologic, and nursing information are provided in the following format:

- *Overview* includes the definition of the condition, as well as its classification within other categories, incidence, and basic pathophysiologic mechanisms.
- *Causes* lists actual causes, when known, or provides a risk-factor assessment when appropriate.
- *Signs & Symptoms* appear in order of those most characteristic of the condition to those less frequently encountered.

- *Diagnostics* includes the most frequently used laboratory tests, diagnostic imaging tests, and/or other testing methods, as well as the significance of abnormal results.
- *Medical Interventions* lists the interventions most commonly associated with each condition.
- *Nursing Diagnoses* lists the nursing diagnoses of high priority, along with related *Nursing Interventions, Client Teaching*, and *Home Care Considerations*.
- Cross-references guide students to more detailed information available in *Medical-Surgical Nursing: Critical Thinking in Client Care*.

Every effort has been made to ensure that the *Clinical Handbook* is as accurate, current, and practical as possible so that nursing students can find ready answers to clinical problems.

Acknowledgments

Our thanks to the editorial staff at Addison Wesley Longman, especially Ginnie Simione Jutson and Grace Wong, for their guidance in the revision of the second edition of *The Clinical Handbook for Medical-Surgical Nursing*. We are grateful to the students who use the book to provide safe and knowledgeable client care and to the faculty who have found it to be a useful teaching–learning tool in the clinical setting. In memorium, we dedicate this book to Susan P. Gauthier, RN, PhD.

Priscilla LeMone, RN, DSN, FAAN
Associate Professor
Sinclair School of Nursing
University of Missouri–Columbia
Columbia, MO

Karen M. Burke, RN, MS
Director of Health Occupations
Clatsop Community College
Astoria, OR

Contributors to the First Edition

Contributors: Barbara K. Rideout, RN, MSN, Temple University; Marguerite Carty Gripton, RNC, MSN, Temple University .
Consultant: Joanne M. Johnson, RNC, MSN, Cincinnati State Technical College

iv

Contents

Acid–Base Disorders

Respiratory Acidosis
Respiratory Alkalosis
Metabolic Acidosis
Metabolic Alkalosis

OVERVIEW

- To function normally, all human cells require a precise balance between acids and bases.
- The correct concentration of hydrogen ions is critical for normal metabolic function within cells.
- The arterial hydrogen ion concentration is a reflection of the total body concentration and can be measured by way of an arterial blood gas (ABG) sample.
- The balance between the body's acids and bases can be indirectly calculated from the ABG values for partial pressure of carbon dioxide ($Paco_2$), an acid-forming gas, and the body stores of bicarbonate (HCO_3), a base.
- The ratio of base to acid is reported as a unitless number known as pH. The lower the pH, the higher the concentration of hydrogen ions and the more acidic the client; the higher the pH, the lower the hydrogen ion concentration and the more alkaline the client.
- The normal ratio of bicarbonate to carbonic acid is 20:1, making body fluids slightly alkaline; the normal pH range is 7.35 to 7.45 (see Table 1, page 571).
- Normal acid-base status is maintained by the respiratory system, which eliminates or retains CO_2, and the kidneys, which eliminate or retain both hydrogen ions and HCO_3.
- Altered respiratory function can lead to hypoventilation, which causes retention of CO_2 and results in an increased concentration of hydrogen ions, producing respiratory acidosis.
- Alternatively, hyperventilation blows off excess CO_2 gas and reduces hydrogen, producing respiratory alkalosis.
- Only the kidneys can compensate for respiratory disturbances of pH.

- Metabolic acidosis and metabolic alkalosis can occur due to a variety of conditions that either increase or decrease acids or bases within the body.
- Both the respiratory and renal systems, if functioning optimally, can compensate for metabolic disturbances of pH.
- Acid-base status is usually monitored by way of serial ABG studies, which can identify not only whether a disturbance is present, but also whether the disorder is caused by respiratory or metabolic mechanisms and whether compensation has occurred.
- The components of the ABG used for assessment of acid-base status are pH, $Paco_2$, and HCO_3.

CAUSES

Acute Respiratory Acidosis (Uncompensated)

- Hypoventilation: acute respiratory failure, respiratory muscle damage/paralysis, asphyxia, chest wall/central nervous system (CNS) trauma, drug overdose, cardiopulmonary disease, inadequate mechanical ventilation

Chronic Respiratory Acidosis

Early (compensated)
Late (decompensated): failure to maintain compensation; ABGs deteriorating

- Chronic obstructive lung disease (COPD)
- Bronchiectasis
- Chronic bronchitis
- Emphysema

Respiratory Alkalosis

- Hyperventilation: psychogenic, fever, hypoxia, pulmonary edema, pulmonary embolism, pneumonia, early acute asthma, gram-negative sepsis, salicylate toxicity, CNS lesions/trauma, liver failure, excessive mechanical ventilation

Metabolic Acidosis

- Acid gain: lactic acidosis (shock, cardiac arrest), ketoacidosis (diabetes, starvation), renal failure
- Base loss: diarrhea

Metabolic Alkalosis

- Acid loss: vomiting, gastric lavage/nasogastric suction, diuretics, corticosteroids, aldosteroma
- Base gain: excessive HCO_3 ingestion/infusion, milk-alkali syndrome

Signs & Symptoms

Acute Respiratory Acidosis (Uncompensated)

- Slow and/or shallow breathing pattern
- Increased heart rate
- Diaphoresis
- Headache
- Restlessness, anxiety (early)
- Lethargy, coma (late)
- Cyanosis
- Dysrhythmias

Chronic Respiratory Acidosis

- Early (compensated): S/S of COPD
- Late (decompensated): S/S of respiratory failure

Respiratory Alkalosis

- Deep, rapid respirations
- Lightheadedness
- Dizziness
- Agitation
- Paresthesia
- Twitching
- Carpopedal spasms
- Muscle weakness
- Cardiac dysrhythmias (severe alkalosis)

Metabolic Acidosis

- Increased respiratory rate and depth (Kussmaul's respirations)
- Decreased blood pressure
- Cold, clammy skin
- Coma
- Arrhythmias

Metabolic Alkalosis

- Decreased respiratory rate
- Irritability
- Confusion

Acute Respiratory Distress Syndrome (ARDS)

OVERVIEW

- Acute respiratory distress syndrome (ARDS) is an acute form of noncardiac pulmonary edema that can proceed rapidly to acute pulmonary failure.
- The underlying pathology in ARDS is acute lung injury resulting from an unregulated systemic inflammatory response to acute injury or inflammation. Inflammatory cellular responses and biochemical mediators damage the alveolar-capillary membrane.
- Damage to type II pneumocytes reduces alveolar surfactants, producing profound alveolar collapse and stiff lungs.
- Ventilation is impaired, decreasing oxygenation of pulmonary capillary blood.
- While survival rates are improving, the mortality rate for ARDS exceeds 50%.

CAUSES

- Shock
- Aspiration/drowning
- Smoke inhalation
- Chemical inhalation (Cl_2, NO_2, NH_3)
- Chemical ingestion (hydrocarbon or Paraquat)
- Pneumonia: viral, bacterial, fungal, *Pneumocystis carinii*
- Sepsis, especially gram negative
- Trauma: chest/lung, head, long bone
- Embolism: disseminated intravascular coagulation (DIC), thrombus, fat, air, amniotic fluid
- Oxygen toxicity
- Blood transfusion
- Drug reactions/overdose
- Post cardiopulmonary bypass surgery
- Systemic disorders: pancreatitis, uremia, systemic lupus erythematosus (SLE), Goodpasture's syndrome

Signs & Symptoms

- Rapid, shallow breathing
- Tachycardia
- Hypoxemia, cyanosis
- Dyspnea, air hunger
- Intercostal/suprasternal retractions
- Rales and rhonchi
- Central nervous system (CNS) changes: anxiety/restlessness, mental dullness, motor deficits

Diagnostics

- Arterial blood gases (ABGs) initially reveal hypoxemia with a Po_2 of less than 50 mm Hg and respiratory alkalosis owing to the rapid respiratory rate. Large amounts of albumin may be present in the sputum late in the course of the disease.
- Pulmonary function testing shows decreased lung compliance with reduced vital capacity, minute volume, and functional vital capacity.
- Chest X-rays show a progression from:
  1. mild bilateral infiltrates, to
  2. ground glass appearance, to
  3. bilateral whiteouts.

MEDICAL INTERVENTIONS

- Surfactant therapy reduces surface tension, helping maintain open alveoli, decreasing the work of breathing, improving compliance and gas exchange, and preventing atelectasis.
- Inhaled nitric oxide reduces intrapulmonary shunting and improves oxygenation by dilating blood vessels in better-ventilated areas of the lungs.
- NSAIDs and other drugs to block the inflammatory response are under investigation; corticosteroids may be used late in the course of ARDS.
- The mainstay of ARDS management is endotracheal intubation and mechanical ventilation while the underlying problem is being identified and treated.

SELECTED NURSING DIAGNOSES
WITH INTERVENTIONS

Decreased Cardiac Output

- Monitor and record vital signs, including blood pressure and apical pulse, at least every 2 hours. Assess the client more frequently immediately after initiation of mechanical ventilation or the addition of positive end-expiratory pressure (PEEP). Correlate measurements with baseline vital signs.
- Measure and record urine output hourly.
- Assess the client's level of consciousness at least every 4 hours.
- Monitor pulmonary artery pressures, central venous pressure, and cardiac output readings frequently, every 1 to 4 hours.
- Assess heart and lung sounds frequently.
- Weigh the client daily, at the same time each day.
- Provide good skin care frequently, keeping the skin clean and dry and massaging pressure points.
- Maintain IV fluids as prescribed.
- Administer analgesics, sedatives, and neuromuscular blockers as needed.

Dysfunctional Ventilatory Weaning Response

- With ARDS, the pathologic processes of the disease and the severity of the impairment in gas exchange may be responsible for a prolonged or ineffective weaning process.
- Monitor and record vital signs every 15 to 60 minutes following changes in ventilator settings and during T-piece trials.
- Monitor ABG levels and pulse oximetry readings when the ventilator settings are changed.
- Prior to changing ventilator settings, auscultate lung sounds and hyperoxygenate and suction as needed.
- Place the client in Fowler's position.
- Fully explain all weaning procedures to the client, along with expected changes in the breathing sensation.
- Remain with the client during initial periods following changes of ventilator settings or T-piece trials.
- Limit procedures and activities during weaning periods.
- Provide diversion, such as television or radio.
- Start weaning procedures in the morning, when the

client is well rested and alert. Weaning may be discontinued overnight to allow adequate rest.

- When synchronous intermittent mandatory ventilation (SIMV) is used for weaning, decrease the SIMV rate by increments of two breaths per minute.
- Avoid administering drugs that may depress respirations during the weaning process (except as prescribed at night to facilitate rest while the client is on ventilator support).
- Once the client has been weaned, keep oxygen available at the bedside.
- If tolerated, place the client in prone position to improve oxygenation.
- Provide pulmonary hygiene with percussion, vibration, and postural drainage.
- Continue to assess the client's respiratory status, including lung sounds, vital signs, level of consciousness, or complaints of dyspnea.

CLIENT TEACHING

- Explain all procedures, tubes, equipment, and therapeutic interventions to the client and significant others as indicated. Reassure the client and significant others that endotracheal intubation and mechanical ventilation are temporary measures to support the client's lungs and respiratory function during the acute phase of the syndrome.
- Provide factual information about ARDS and its prognosis.
- If the client has been a smoker, stress the importance of avoiding smoking in the future to preserve lung function.

HOME CARE CONSIDERATIONS

- A referral to a home health nurse may be appropriate for the client recovering from ARDS.
- The client who survives ARDS may require psychologic support to assist in coping with the near-death experience.

For more information on Acute Respiratory Distress Syndrome, see Medical-Surgical Nursing *by LeMone and Burke, p. 168 and 1499.*

Adrenal Insufficiency (Hypofunction; Addison's Disease)

OVERVIEW

- A disorder that results in inadequate levels of glucocorticoids, mineralocorticoids, and androgens.
- Adrenal insufficiency is divided into two categories:
  1. *Primary:* due to lack of adrenal hormones. The most common form is Addison's disease, a condition resulting from failure of adrenal cortex function, with deficits of glucocorticoids, mineralocorticoids, and androgens.
  2. *Secondary:* due to lack of adrenocorticotropic hormone (ACTH).
- Addisonian crisis is a serious, life-threatening response to acute adrenal insufficiency. Primary problems are severe hypotension, circulatory collapse, shock, and coma.

CAUSES

Primary Insufficiency

- Addison's disease (autoimmune)
- Bilateral adrenalectomy
- Infections (tuberculosis, septicemia), neoplasms, trauma, or hemorrhage of the adrenal glands

Secondary Insufficiency

- Hypopituitarism (decreased ACTH)
- Surgical removal of ectopic ACTH-secreting tumors (e.g., oat-cell carcinoma of the lungs)
- Abrupt withdrawal of long-standing corticosteroid drugs

Signs & Symptoms

- Weakness, fatigability, fever
- Anorexia, nausea, vomiting, weight loss
- Myalgias, arthralgias
- Anxiety and irritability, emotional changes

- Hyperpigmentation of skin (especially areas such as knuckles, elbows, and palmar creases) and mucous membranes
- Hypoglycemia
- Hypotension, orthostatic hypotension
- Scant axillary and pubic hair in women

Diagnostics

- Plasma cortisol levels are decreased if disease is primary or secondary.
- Plasma aldosterone levels are decreased if disease is primary or secondary.
- Serum ACTH level is increased if primary, decreased if secondary.
- 24-hour urine is done to check for decreased cortisol excretion.
- ACTH stimulation testing shows decreased cortisol secretion in primary disease.
- Electrolytes show decreased sodium, increased potassium, and possibly increased calcium.
- Fasting blood glucose may be low.

MEDICAL INTERVENTIONS

- The primary treatment of Addison's disease is replacement of corticosteroids and mineralocorticoids, accompanied by increased dietary sodium.

SELECTED NURSING DIAGNOSES WITH INTERVENTIONS

Fluid Volume Deficit

- Monitor intake and output and assess for signs of dehydration.
- Monitor cardiovascular status: Take and record vital signs including orthostatic BPs, assess character of pulses, and monitor potassium levels.
- Weigh the client daily at the same time and in the same clothing.
- Encourage the client to maintain an oral fluid intake of 3000 mL per day and to increase salt intake.
- Teach the client to sit and stand slowly and provide assistance as necessary to avoid orthostatic hypotension.

- Encourage the client to verbalize concerns.
- Teach the client and significant others the effects of the illness and how to provide care. Family stability, an awareness of the serious nature of the disease, and the effectiveness of treatment all promote compliance.

CLIENT TEACHING

Include in the teaching plan:

- How to self-administer steroids.
- The importance of carrying at all times an emergency kit containing parenteral cortisone and a syringe and needle.
- The importance of wearing a MedicAlert bracelet or necklace.
- The need to increase oral fluid intake.
- The importance of maintaining a diet high in sodium and low in potassium.
- The importance of eating regular meals.
- The need to alter the medication dose when experiencing emotional or physical stressors.
- The importance of continuing health care.

DISCHARGE PLANNING/CONTINUING CARE

- Provide the client with referrals to community health services and support groups for information and follow-up health care.

For more information on Adrenal Insufficiency (Hypofunction; Addison's Disease), see Medical-Surgical Nursing *by LeMone and Burke, p. 708.*

Alzheimer's Disease

OVERVIEW

- Alzheimer's disease is a chronic, progressive, degenerative disorder of the cerebral cortex that results in severe cognitive dysfunction.
- It accounts for about half of all cases of dementia (presenile or senile onset).
- Histopathologic features include cortical neuronal cell loss, neurofibrillary tangles, and neuritic plaques.
- Gross pathologic features include extensive cortical, convolutional atrophy (especially frontal, parietal, and medial temporal regions), along with a concomitant enlargement of the ventricular system.
- Neuron loss produces deficits in neurotransmitters, primarily acetylcholine, but also norepinephrine, serotonin, somatostatin, and dopamine.
- Pathophysiologic features include histopathologic changes and decreased neurotransmitters, which reduce nerve conduction and result in profound impairment of memory and deterioration of intellect.
- The onset is insidious; disease progresses relentlessly to total disability.
- Death usually occurs within 3 to 15 (average, 8) years of diagnosis, due to secondary complications such as aspiration, malnutrition, trauma, or infection.

CAUSES

The exact cause is unknown but the following factors have been suggested:

- *Genetics:* familial clusters are known to exist and to follow an autosomal-dominant pattern linked to chromosome 21; very common in people with trisomy 21; genetic types manifest at an earlier age
- *Biochemistry:* deficiencies of neurotransmitters (above) are well documented
- *Environmental:* may include infection with a slow-growing virus, central nervous system (CNS) trauma, or toxicity
- *Immunologic:* may result from an autoimmune response

Signs & Symptoms

- Develop very insidiously

Early S/S

- Forgetfulness
- Memory loss (especially for recent events)
- Difficulty learning new information; decreased ability to concentrate
- Mental/behavioral changes including apathy, anxiety, depression, irritability, suspiciousness

Late S/S

- Progressive forgetfulness and memory loss
- Language disturbances: poor word choices, circumlocution, echolalia
- Motor manifestations: apraxia, myoclonus, Parkinsonism
- Incontinence
- Progressive mental/behavioral deterioration: delusions, hallucinations, wandering
- Progressive self-care deficit

Diagnostics

- Electroencephalogram (EEG) measures the brain's electrical activity; shows slowing of brain waves.
- Computed tomography (CT) scan shows cortical atrophy and ventricular enlargement.
- Magnetic resonance imaging (MRI) shows cortical atrophy and ventricular enlargement.
- Positron emission tomography (PET) shows reduced metabolic activity level of cerebral cortex; may be used to establish early diagnosis.

MEDICAL INTERVENTIONS

- Tacrine hydrochloride is the first medication specifically approved for the treatment of mild-to-moderate Alzheimer's disease. It improves memory in up to a third of clients.
- Antidepressant medications, mild sedatives such as benadryl, and low-dose haloperidol may be used to manage behavior problems.

SELECTED NURSING DIAGNOSES
WITH INTERVENTIONS

Altered Thought Processes

- Label rooms, drawers, and other items as appropriate.
- Keep environmental stimuli to a minimum. Decrease noise levels and speak in a calm, low voice. Take an unhurried approach.
- Limit questions to those that require a simple yes or no response.
- Orient the client to the environment, person, and time as able.
- Provide continuity in nursing staff.
- Repeat explanations simply and as needed to decrease anxiety.

Anxiety

- Assess for and note on care plan early behaviors of fatigue and agitation.
- Keep daily routine as consistent as possible.
- Schedule rest periods or quiet times throughout the day.

Hopelessness

- Assess the client's and significant others' responses to the diagnosis and understanding of Alzheimer's disease. Encourage expression of feelings.
- Provide realistic information about the disorder at the client's level of understanding. The client and family may need to have separate sessions.
- Avoid criticizing or judging expressed feelings.
- Support positive family bonds and enhance communciation among family members.
- Promote positive regard.
- Encourage the client to make as many decisions as possible.
- Encourage the client and significant others to seek spiritual guidance or other strategies that previously inspired hope.

Risk for Caregiver Role Strain

- Teach the caregivers self-care techniques, such as taking rest periods and avoiding fatigue.
- Have the caregivers list and partake regularly in activities they enjoy, such as walking.

- Refer the caregivers to local Alzheimer's disease support groups and to the national association. Suggest books on the topic.
- Refer the caregivers to Meals-on-Wheels, home health services, and other community services.

CLIENT TEACHING

- Explain to the client and caregivers the disorder and its consequences.
- Review medication regimen with both the client and the caregivers, and provide written instructions.
- If the client will be cared for at home, address safety considerations as well as the ability of caregivers to meet the client's needs, such as maintaining hygiene and other activities of daily living (ADLs).
- Suggest memory cues such as labeling drawers and rooms, and keeping the furniture and other items in each room in a consistent place.

HOME CARE CONSIDERATIONS

- Suggest obtaining a MedicAlert bracelet or necklace for the client in case he or she wanders and is unable to provide verbal identification.
- Refer the client and caregivers to the community services mentioned above, including long-term-care facilities.
- A home safety inspection may be appropriate.

For more information on Alzheimer's Disease, see Medical-Surgical Nursing *by LeMone and Burke, p. 1818.*

Amyotrophic Lateral Sclerosis (ALS)

OVERVIEW

- Amyotrophic lateral sclerosis (ALS) is a chronic, progressively disabling motor neuron disease that results in muscle atrophy and weakness.
- It is also known as Lou Gehrig's disease.
- ALS is the most common form of progressive motor neuron disease.
- Onset usually occurs between ages 40 to 70 years; incidence is slightly higher in males.
- ALS produces degeneration of both upper motor neurons (motor cortex and corticospinal tracts) and lower motor neurons (anterior horn cells of spinal cord and cranial nerves).
- Neuron degeneration causes muscle atrophy with progressive weakness that usually begins in the upper extremities and progresses to paralysis.
- Sensory, cognitive, and sphincter function remain intact throughout the disease.
- Death usually results within 3 to 5 (up to 15) years following diagnosis; usually from respiratory infection or paralysis.

CAUSES

- Approximately 5% to 10% of clients inherit ALS as an autosomal-dominant trait
- In most instances, the cause of ALS is unknown, although it is theorized that an autoimmune process or toxic accumulation of glutamine, a neurotransmitter, in neural synapses may lead to neuronal destruction.

Signs & Symptoms

- Muscle atrophy
- Muscle weakness/fatigue; usually begins in distal, upper extremities
- Fasciculations/spasticity
- Hyperreflexia
- Dysphagia

- Dysarthria (slurred speech), drooling
- Dyspnea, ineffective cough, shallow respirations
- Progression to flaccid quadriplegia and respiratory muscle paralysis with respiratory failure

Diagnostics

- No specific diagnostic tests are available.
- Electromyogram (EMG) shows abnormal electrical activity of involved skeletal muscles.
- Nerve conduction studies are usually normal.
- Cerebrospinal fluid (CSF) analysis shows increased protein content in some patients.
- Muscle biopsy shows atrophy of myofibrils; rules out primary muscle disease.

MEDICAL INTERVENTIONS

- Medical care for clients with ALS is mainly supportive. Riluzole, a drug that inhibits glutamate release, may slow the progression of ALS. As the disease progresses, nutritional and ventilatory support may be primary considerations.

SELECTED NURSING DIAGNOSES WITH INTERVENTIONS

Risk for Disuse Syndrome

- Assess current condition for baseline parameters, particularly skin over bony prominences, lung sounds, and vital signs.
- Lubricate and inspect skin. Obtain an alternating-pressure mattress.
- Institute active range-of-motion (ROM) exercises as the client is able. Perform passive ROM exercises every 2 hours when the client is turned.
- Maintain positive nitrogen balance and hydration status: monitor albumin levels, hemoglobin and hematocrit levels, and urine specific gravity.
- Monitor client for manifestations of infection. Specifically, assess urinalysis, especially if a urinary catheter is present.

Ineffective Breathing Pattern

- Monitor breathing pattern, air movement, and oxygen saturation.
- Turn the client at least every 2 hours.

- Elevate the head of the bed at least 30°, suction as indicated, and provide oxygen.
- Assess the client's temperature and lung sounds routinely. Obtain sputum culture as indicated.

CLIENT TEACHING

- Initial teaching centers on explaining the disease process, expected course, and prognosis.
- As the disease progresses, teach significant others how to suction the client and perform the Heimlich maneuver to treat aspiration.
- Teach methods to establish a bowel routine, considerations related to a urinary catheter, and symptoms of constipation or infection to report promptly.

HOME CARE CONSIDERATIONS

- Referral to a social worker to determine home care needs and financial assistance is helpful.
- Referral to a psychologic counselor to aid the client in facing the diagnosis may be appropriate. An ALS support group may also be helpful.

For more information on Amyotrophic Lateral Sclerosis, see Medical-Surgical Nursing *by LeMone and Burke, p. 1850.*

Anaphylaxis

OVERVIEW

- Anaphylaxis is an acute, life-threatening, systemic hypersensitivity reaction.
- It is mediated by IgE antibody on previously sensitized mast cells produced during previous exposure to the antigen.
- During the acute reaction, antigen and IgE binding release histamine and leukotrienes into the general circulation.

- Bronchospasm, massive vasodilation, and increased capillary permeability and leakage occur within seconds or minutes of exposure to the offending antigen.
- Anaphylaxis may progress rapidly to vascular collapse, shock, and possibly death.

CAUSES

- Most commonly caused by ingestion, infusion, and/or inhalation of significant amounts of antigen, the most common of which are:
  1. antibiotics (especially penicillin)
  2. sulfonamides
  3. local anesthetics
  4. salicylates
  5. iodine drugs used in diagnostic tests
  6. hormones/enzymes
  7. vaccines/serums
  8. foods, including seafood, eggs, berries, nuts, legumes, foods containing sulfites
  9. latex
  10. insect venom, including bees, hornets, wasps, yellow jackets, fire ants, spiders
  11. snake venom

Signs & Symptoms

- Onset of S/S usually within minutes of exposure to the offending antigen; may persist for 24 hours

General S/S

- Anxiety, sense of impending doom
- Weakness
- Urticaria
- Cutaneous wheals: well circumscribed, erythematous
- Angioedema
- Sweating

Cardiovascular S/S

- Hypotension
- Shock
- Cardiac dysrhythmia
- Possible cardiac arrest

Respiratory S/S

- Sneezing
- Nasal congestion, urticaria
- Watery rhinorrhea
- Hoarseness, stridor
- Wheezing, "tight chest"
- Hyperventilation
- Dyspnea, shortness of breath
- Respiratory failure

Gastrointestinal S/S

- Nausea
- Severe GI cramps
- Diarrhea

Neurologic S/S

- Dizziness
- Drowsiness
- Headache
- Seizures

Diagnostics

- Allergic skin testing may indicate antigenic substance; may also precipitate an acute anaphylactic response.
- Arterial blood gases (ABGs) obtained during acute phase can assess degree of respiratory failure; they usually indicate a decrease in pH, Pao_2, and total oxygen saturation, and an increase in $Paco_2$.
- Serum electrolytes: as shock progresses, glucose and sodium levels decrease and potassium levels increase.
- Differential white blood cell (WBC) count: eosinophils are increased during an anaphylactic response.

MEDICAL INTERVENTIONS

- IV fluid resuscitation with isotonic solution.
- Oxygen therapy, usually by mask or nasal cannula.
- Pharmacologic agents may include epinephrine to increase tissue perfusion and oxygenation, diphenhydramine to treat angioedema and urticaria, aminophylline drip for bronchospasm, and/or steroids for long-term care.

- Emergency tracheostomy may be necessary.

SELECTED NURSING DIAGNOSES

- Altered Tissue Perfusion
- Impaired Gas Exchange
- Ineffective Airway Clearance
- Anxiety

SELECTED NURSING INTERVENTIONS

- Ask all clients about allergies prior to administering any medications, using latex gloves, or hanging an IV.
- Assess for signs and symptoms of anaphylactic shock, including itching, edema, wheezing, dyspnea, cyanosis, anxiety, flushing, diaphoresis, hypotension, and bronchospasm.
- Assess airway. Prepare for possible emergency tracheostomy.
- Administer IV fluid resuscitation with isotonic solution.
- Decrease further absorption of antigen as appropriate by placing tourniquet between injection/sting site and heart, if possible. Apply ice pack to injection/sting site. If antigen was ingested, administer gastric lavage.
- Suction client as needed.
- Administer oxygen per physician prescription.
- Administer epinephrine per physician prescription: (1:1000) 0.3–0.5 mg/kg IM, SL, or inhaled, or (1:10,000) 0.5 mg in 10 mL IV slowly over 5 to 10 minutes.
- Administer diphenhydramine, 50–100 mg IM, per physician prescription.
- Administer an aminophylline drip per physician prescription.
- Administer steroids per physician prescription.
- Clearly mark all records with known allergies.

CLIENT TEACHING

- Teach the client to avoid the antigen/causative agent.
- Teach the use of the anaphylaxis kit (Epi pen) for emergencies.

HOME CARE CONSIDERATIONS

- Provide information on obtaining and wearing a MedicAlert bracelet to inform others of the client's susceptibility to a known antigen.
- Discuss where to obtain and keep an anaphylaxis kit.
- Stress the importance of having family members trained in CPR.

For more information on Anaphylaxis, see Medical-Surgical Nursing *by LeMone and Burke, p. 270.*

Anemia

Hypoproliferative (Nutritional, Marrow Damage)
Hemorrhagic (Acute, Chronic)
Hemolytic (Genetic, Acquired)

OVERVIEW

- Anemia is a reduction in hemoglobin concentration [Hgb] or red blood cell (RBC) count, each or both of which reduce hemoglobin (Hgb) volume and hematocrit (HCT).
- Reduced [Hgb] impairs ability to deliver oxygen to peripheral tissues.

CAUSES

- Three basic mechanisms can cause anemia (see Table 3, page 572):
  1. Hypoproliferation (insufficient RBC production): results from an inability of the bone marrow to make enough RBCs, either due to lack of a needed nutrient (B_{12}, folate, iron), reduced erythropoietin, or damage to the bone marrow (drugs, toxins, radiation)
  2. Hemorrhage (RBC loss due to bleeding): results from any acute or chronic bout of bleeding or RBC loss via the kidneys

3. Hemolysis (RBC destruction): results from either genetic disorders (sickle-cell anemia, glucose-6-phosphatase deficiency [G6PD]) or acquired conditions (drugs, toxins, infection, immune reactions, systemic disease)

Signs & Symptoms

- Severity of S/S depend on time-course, severity, and accompanying medical conditions such as cardiac, respiratory, or infectious disease; some clients are asymptomatic.
- Each type of anemia may have specific S/S. The general S/S of anemia are the result of a reduced oxygen-carrying capacity, and therefore tissue hypoxia. These include:
  1. pallor (skin, mucous membranes, nailbeds)
  2. shortness of breath (SOB)
  3. weakness, fatigue
  4. anorexia, weight loss
  5. tachycardia/tachypnea (compensatory)

Diagnostics

- Total Hgb measures the weight (g) of Hgb in a volume (dL) of blood; it is below normal in anemic conditions.
- Hematocrit is reduced in anemia.
- RBC count is reduced in some anemias.
- RBC indices are based on the total Hgb, HCT, and RBC count:
  1. Mean corpuscular volume (MCV) is the ratio of HCT to RBC count, giving a measure of RBC volume; it may be increased or decreased depending on type of anemia.
  2. Mean corpuscular hemoglobin (MCH) is the ratio of Hgb to RBC count, giving an estimate of the weight of Hgb in an average RBC; it is decreased in certain anemias.
  3. Mean corpuscular Hgb concentration (MCHC) is the ratio of Hgb weight to HCT, giving an estimate of the Hgb in an average RBC; it is decreased in certain anemias.
- RBC morphology is a microscopic evaluation of the size and shape of RBCs; many possible morpho-

logic changes are possible depending on the type of anemia.

MEDICAL INTERVENTIONS

- The pharmacologic treatment of anemia is determined by the cause.
- Dietary management is indicated for the client with a nutritional deficiency anemia.
- Blood transfusion may be indicated for clients with anemia resulting from a major blood loss. It may also be used to treat severe anemias.

SELECTED NURSING DIAGNOSES WITH INTERVENTIONS

Activity Intolerance

- Help the client and significant others identify ways to perform activities more slowly, in a different way, or with assistance.
- Help the client and significant others establish priorities in tasks to be done.
- Stress the importance of periods of rest throughout the day.
- Encourage the client to sleep 8 to 10 hours a night.
- Monitor the client's vital signs before and after activity. Discontinue activity if the client experiences chest pain, vertigo, breathlessness, palpitations, decreased heart rate, decreased respiratory rate, excessively increased respiratory rate, or decreased systolic blood pressure.
- Instruct the client to avoid smoking.

Risk for Decreased Cardiac Output

- Monitor vital signs, including breath sounds, respiratory rate and effectiveness, and pulse rate and rhythm.
- Assess for pallor, cyanosis, and dependent edema.
- Stop activity for signs of decreased cardiac output and report to physician.

CLIENT TEACHING

- Teach the client about the disorder, causative factors, if known, and manifestations that signal the need to seek medical help.

- Teach the client methods to conserve energy.
- Clients requiring iron supplementation should be instructed to take oral preparations after meals to reduce gastrointestinal (GI) irritability; to take liquid preparations through a straw to prevent staining of teeth; and to maintain a high-fiber diet and use stool softeners if required to reduce constipation.

HOME CARE CONSIDERATIONS

- Stress the importance of follow-up visits to the health care provider for blood count monitoring.
- A referral for counseling to facilitate decisions about pregnancy may be necessary for clients with inherited anemias.
- For clients with sickle cell anemia, discuss ways to reduce the risk of sickling and sickle cell crisis, such as avoiding excessive exercise, preventing hypothermia and dehydration, promptly treating infections, and notifying all care providers about their condition.

For more information, see the following pages in Medical-Surgical Nursing *by LeMone and Burke:*
Hypoproliferative anemia, p. 1267
Hemorrhagic anemia, p. 1267
Hemolytic anemia, p. 1271

Aneurysm

Aortic (Thoracic, Abdominal)
Peripheral (Femoral, Popliteal)
(For Cerebral, see
Cerebral Vascular Accident [CVA])

OVERVIEW

- An aneurysm is an abnormal dilation in a portion of an arterial wall.

- Aneurysms form from a weakness in the medial (muscle) layer of the vessel. The intima and adventitia then stretch.
- Dilation creates high arterial-wall tension in the area of aneurysm.
- Increased wall tension causes greater dilation. The vessel eventually bursts, resulting in massive hemorrhage.
- Types include:
  1. *Saccular*—a bubble in a portion of the arterial wall.
  2. *Fusiform*—dilation entirely encircles a portion of the arterial wall.
  3. *Dissecting*—blood separates layers of the arterial wall.
  4. *False*—rupture of an artery; blood collects next to vessel.
- Aortic aneurysms are the most common. Abdominal aortic aneurysms arise between the renal and iliac arteries. Thoracic aortic aneurysms arise between the subclavian and renal arteries, the most common site for dissecting aneurysms.
- Peripheral aneurysms include popliteal and femoral aneurysms. Both are extremely rare and result in compromised peripheral perfusion; similar to acute arterial occlusion.

CAUSES

- Atherosclerosis is the most common cause
- Connective-tissue disease and trauma are also causative
- Aneurysms may be idiopathic

Signs & Symptoms

- Most are asymptomatic unless dissecting or ruptured
- Ruptured aortic aneurysm causes massive hemorrhage, leading to:
  1. severe shock
  2. rapid loss of consciousness/seizures/coma
  3. probable death
- Dissecting aneurysms are excruciatingly painful

- Both ruptured and dissecting aneurysms are surgical emergencies requiring multiple blood transfusions

Diagnostics

- Cardiac enzyme levels may rule out a myocardial infarction.
- Imaging devices such as X-rays, transesophageal echocardiography, aortography, and abdominal ultrasonography may be used depending on the suspected location of the aneurysm.

MEDICAL INTERVENTIONS

- Pharmacologic agents include antihypertensive medications for aortic aneurysms, and/or beta-adrenergic blocking agents to lower blood pressure and control the rate and rhythm of the heartbeat. Following surgical correction of an aneurysm, anticoagulation and prophylactic antibiotic therapy may be prescribed.
- Immediate surgical intervention may be necessary to preserve life. The surgical repair of most aortic aneurysms involves excising the aneurysm and replacing it with a fabric graft, a procedure known as aneurysmectomy.

SELECTED NURSING DIAGNOSES

- Activity Intolerance
- Decreased Cardiac Output
- Fear
- Risk for Infection
- Self-Care Deficit
- Altered Thought Processes

SELECTED NURSING INTERVENTIONS

- Assess abdominal aorta for pulsating mass with lateral protrusion.
- Prepare client for surgery if needed.
- Provide emotional support for client and significant others.
- Insert large-gauge IV catheter if needed for blood administration.

- Monitor vital signs for indications of infection.
- Monitor neurologic and circulatory status for signs of occlusion.
- Report changes in color or sensation of extremities.
- Administer analgesics as prescribed, and monitor response.

CLIENT TEACHING

- Clients with small aneurysms need to be taught to control hypertension through making dietary changes, stopping smoking, limiting alcohol intake, and following the medication regimen.
- Teach postoperative clients how to prevent infection, care for wound, and recognize manifestations of complications; provide information on medications.
- Teach the client ways to prevent constipation and straining at stool. The client should also avoid prolonged sitting, lifting heavy objects, exercising strenuously, and having sexual intercourse for 6 to 12 weeks after surgery, as prescribed.

HOME CARE CONSIDERATIONS

- Referral to a home health nurse may be appropriate.

For more information on Aneurysm, see Medical-Surgical Nursing *by LeMone and Burke, p. 1230.*

Appendicitis

OVERVIEW

- Appendicitis is an inflammation of the vermiform appendix. It is the most common inflammatory disorder of the bowel.
- The vermiform appendix is a blind pouch attached to the cecum.
- Appendicitis begins with ulceration or obstruction of the proximal lumen of the appendix by a hard

mass of feces, parasites, a tumor, a calculus, or other agent. Following obstruction, the appendix becomes distended with fluid secreted by its mucosa. Pressure increases, leading to decreased blood flow, inflammation, edema, ulceration, infection, and necrosis, which can result in rupture. A ruptured appendix then causes local and/or disseminated peritonitis.

- Appendicitis is the most frequent disorder resulting in an abdominal surgical procedure.

CAUSES

- Impaction can result from a fecolith, stricture, neoplasm, barium swallow, or viral infection

Signs & Symptoms

Initial

- Abdominal pain: diffuse epigastric and/or periumbilical
- Over several hours pain increases in intensity and localizes to right lower quadrant (McBurney's point)
- Anorexia, nausea, vomiting (A/N/V)
- Rigid abdomen (muscle guarding)
- Rebound tenderness

Late

- Fever (99–102F or 37.2–38.9C)
- Tachycardia
- Rapid, shallow respirations
- Constipation, possible diarrhea
- Sudden disappearance of pain indicates perforation

Diagnostics

- White blood cell (WBC) count is increased.
- Immature WBCs (bands, stabs) are increased.
- Abdominal X-ray and/or ultrasound is performed to detect fecal mass or calculus.

MEDICAL INTERVENTIONS

- Pharmacologic agents include preoperative IV fluids to replenish or maintain vascular volume and antibiotics prior to, during, and after surgery.

- Appendectomy—surgical removal of the appendix—is the standard treatment for acute appendicitis.

SELECTED NURSING DIAGNOSES WITH INTERVENTIONS

Altered Tissue Perfusion: Gastrointestinal

- Monitor for perforation and peritonitis preoperatively. Notify the physician immediately if the client experiences a sudden relief of pain followed by increased generalized pain and abdominal distention.
- Monitor the client's vital signs.
- Maintain IV fluid replacement preoperatively and until the client is able to drink adequate amounts postoperatively.
- Postoperatively, assess the client's wound, abdominal girth, and pain status. Swelling of the wound, increased girth, or increased pain may indicate infection.

Pain

- Assess the client's pain, including its character, location, severity, and duration.
- Administer prescribed pain medications.
- Assess effectiveness of medication half an hour after administration. Notify the physician if the client has not experienced the desired level of pain relief.
- Provide alternative methods of pain relief, including distraction, therapeutic touch, massage, meditation, or visualization.

CLIENT TEACHING

- Preoperatively, provide instructions on turning, coughing, and deep breathing, as well as on postoperative pain management.
- Postoperative teaching includes wound or incision care, hand washing, and dressing change procedures. Tell the client and significant others to report immediately any swelling, redness, bleeding, warmth, or drainage.

HOME CARE CONSIDERATIONS

- A home health referral may be appropriate for wound care.
- Tell the client to avoid heavy lifting and strenuous activity for 4 to 6 weeks postoperatively.

For more information on Appendicitis, see Medical-Surgical Nursing *by LeMone and Burke, p. 796.*

Asthma

OVERVIEW

- Asthma is defined as a chronic inflammatory airway disorder characterized by recurrent episodes of bronchospasm, airway swelling, and increased thick mucus production.
- Bronchospasm results from a heightened responsiveness of bronchial smooth muscle to various stimuli.
- As airways close, air becomes trapped behind obstructed areas, causing hyperinflation of alveoli.
- It is usually a chronic disease that manifests as recurrent, acute attacks.
- Asthma is a common disorder that can occur at any age.

CAUSES

- Bronchospasm in asthmatics occurs as a response to a variety of stimuli.
- There are two major categories, which may coexist in some clients:
  1. *Extrinsic asthma:* most common in children and adolescents with personal or family history of allergy. Exposure to antigens results in release of chemical mediators in an IgE–mast cell interaction (type I hypersensitivity), which causes bronchospasm, increased secretions from goblet

cells, and mucosal swelling, all of which obstruct airflow and produce air trapping. Allergens include pollen, dust, mold, animal dander, feathers (pillows), sulfite food additives, and others.

2. *Intrinsic asthma:* frequently affects adults; personal or family history not as strongly positive as for extrinsic disorders. Stimuli include infection (especially viral), noxious fumes (cigarette smoke, solvents), fatigue, endocrine changes, changes in environmental temperature or humidity, exercise, aspirin (reduces bronchodilator prostaglandins); possible emotional component.

Signs & Symptoms

- Attacks occur in a paroxysmal pattern
- Severity may range from mild to life-threatening *status asthmaticus*
- Extrinsic attacks are usually preceded by contact with a known allergen
- Intrinsic attacks most often accompany lower respiratory tract infection
- S/S may begin suddenly or insidiously and include:
  1. dyspnea/shortness of breath
  2. wheezing (auscultated, may be audible), rhonchi
  3. hyperresonant lung fields (trapped gas)
  4. coughing (dry; later tenacious)
  5. tightness in chest
  6. nasal flaring, pursed-lip breathing
  7. accessory muscle use
  8. tachypnea/tachycardia
  9. diaphoresis
  10. anxiety
  11. decreased vocalization (must pause due to dyspnea)
- *S/S of status asthmaticus,* the acute respiratory failure due to asthma, are:
  1. cyanosis
  2. reduced breath sounds, reduced wheezing, ineffective cough
  3. pulsus paradoxus
  4. lethargy, confusion

Diagnostics

- Pulmonary function tests performed during an attack show reduced flow rates and decreased forced expiratory volume at 1 second (FEV_1). Vital capacity is decreased but residual capacity and total lung volume are increased.
- Arterial blood gases (ABGs) initially show hypoxemia with a low PaO_2 and mild respiratory alkalosis with an elevated pH and low $PaCO_2$ due to the client's tachypnea. When airflow and ventilation are severely compromised, significant hypoxemia and respiratory acidosis occur.
- Chest X-ray performed during an attack shows possible hyperinflation with areas of atelectasis (absorption type, due to mucus plugging).
- Complete blood count (CBC) with white blood cell (WBC) differential may show increased eosinophils ($250–400/\mu l$); often correlates well with severity of clinical symptoms.
- Skin testing for specific antigens may reveal sensitivity.
- Inhalation challenge test checks significance of allergens identified by skin testing.

MEDICAL INTERVENTIONS

- Drugs used for *long-term control* of asthma include anti-inflammatory agents such as cromolyn sodium, long-acting bronchodilators such as methylxanthines, and leukotriene modifiers.
- *Quick-relief* medications often are administered by inhalation to provide prompt relief of bronchoconstriction and airflow obstruction. Short-acting beta-adrenergic agonists (rapid-acting bronchodilators), anticholinergic drugs, and systemic corticosteroids fall into this category.

SELECTED NURSING DIAGNOSES WITH INTERVENTIONS

Ineffective Airway Clearance
- Assess the adequacy of respirations every 1 to 2 hours. Assess respiratory rate and depth, chest movement or excursion, and breath sounds.

- Assess the client's cough effort.
- Assess sputum for color, consistency, and amount.
- Assess the client's skin color, temperature, and level of consciousness every 1 to 2 hours or as indicated.
- Assess ABG results and pulse oximetry readings. Notify the physician of abnormal values or changes in status.
- Position the client in Fowler's, high-Fowler's, or orthopnea position to facilitate breathing and lung expansion.
- Administer oxygen as prescribed.
- Administer nebulizer treatments and provide humidification as prescribed.
- Initiate or assist with chest physiotherapy, including percussion and postural drainage.
- Increase the client's fluid intake.
- Provide endotracheal suctioning as needed.

Ineffective Breathing Pattern

- Assess respiratory rate, pattern, and breath sounds every 1 to 2 hours or as indicated. Look for manifestations of ineffective breathing, including rapid rate, shallow respirations, nasal flaring, use of accessory muscles, intercostal retractions, and diminished or absent breath sounds.
- Monitor vital signs and laboratory results.
- Assist the client with activities of daily living (ADLs) as needed.
- Provide rest periods between schdeuled activities and treatments.
- Assist the client to use techniques to control breathing pattern, including pursed-lip breathing, abdominal breathing, and relaxation techniques.
- Administer medications, including bronchodilators and anti-inflammatory drugs, as prescribed. Monitor for effects and side effects.

Anxiety

- Assess the client's level of anxiety.
- Assist the client to identify usual coping skills that have been successful in the past.
- Provide physical and emotional support for the client. Remain with the client during acute episodes of severe anxiety. Schedule time every 1 to

2 hours to be with the client who is mildly or moderately anxious, and reassure the client that the call light will be answered promptly.

- Listen actively to the client's concerns. Do not deny or negate the fear of dying or of being unable to breathe.
- Provide clear, concise directions and explanations about procedures. Avoid presenting more information than the client is able to assimilate.
- Include the client in care planning and decision making as appropriate, without making excessive demands on the client.
- Reduce excessive environmental stimuli and maintain a calm demeanor.
- Allow supportive significant others to remain with the client.
- Assist the client to use relaxation techniques such as guided imagery, muscle relaxation, and meditation.

CLIENT TEACHING

- In the acute-care setting, the teaching needs of the client are related primarily to diagnostic and treatment procedures. Include teaching about the specific medications prescribed and their effects and side effects. Instruct about procedures such as pulmonary function testing, nebulizer treatments, and so on.
- Help the client find ways to avoid any suspected triggers for the asthma attacks. Also discuss the availability of flu shots and immunizations against pneumococcal pneumonia.
- Assist clients to identify stress management techniques they can incorporate into their lifestyles.
- Teach the client to take prophylactic medication as prescribed; effectiveness depends on adequate blood levels. Stress the importance of not exceeding the recommended dose of inhalers; fatal respiratory failure has occurred due to reduced sensitivity to overused drug therapy. Also warn clients against discontinuing glucocorticoids abruptly, as this may precipitate an Addisonian-like crisis.

HOME CARE CONSIDERATIONS

- Instruct the client and significant others regarding correct prophylactic and emergency medication use.
- Teach client how to effectively use metered-dose inhalers (MDI). Stress the importance of using prompt-relief medications as prescribed and avoiding their overuse. Instruct client to contact primary care provider if asthma attacks are increasing in frequency or severity.
- Discuss measures to prevent acute asthma attacks, such as avoiding strenuous exercise in cold air and secondhand smoke.
- Discuss the importance of preventing exposure to cigarette smoke with parents of an asthmatic child. Refer to smoking-cessation clinics or help groups as appropriate.
- Have the client's living partners prepare the home environment by removing offending agents as much as possible with special attention to the client's sleeping area. Air-conditioning often improves air quality.
- Provide referral to a local or regional agency for further teaching and support as needed.

For more information on Asthma, see Medical-Surgical Nursing *by LeMone and Burke, p. 1425.*

Bell's Palsy

OVERVIEW

- Bell's palsy is an idiopathic palsy (paralysis) of the face.
- It is the result of reduced conduction in the facial nerve (cranial nerve [CN] VII), a major motor nerve of the face.
- It produces (usually) an acute unilateral paralysis of the muscles of facial expression.
- The palsy usually resolves spontaneously in a few weeks or months.
- It is seen at all ages, but is most common in people aged 20 to 40 years.
- It is the most common type of facial palsy.

CAUSES

- Idiopathic
- Viral infection (herpes simplex virus [HSV], mumps) suspected
- Other causes of facial palsy are hemorrhage, local trauma, meningitis, neoplasm, stroke, infection

Signs & Symptoms

- Onset of S/S is rapid; peak paralysis is reached in 2 to 5 days
- Aching pain, behind the ear or in the jaw, may precede facial paralysis for several days
- Taste sense may be lost ipsilaterally
- Unilateral:
  1. facial weakness, flaccidity
  2. mask-like face, smooth forehead
  3. drooping of mouth, with drooling
  4. loss or distortion of taste sensation
  5. excessive tearing
  6. inability to puff out cheeks, raise eyebrows, smile or frown, show teeth, whistle
  7. incomplete eyelid closure resulting in wide palpebral fissure and upward and outward rotation of eyeball when closure is attempted (Bell's phenomenon)

- Electromyography (EMG) may distinguish between acute and chronic nerve changes.

MEDICAL INTERVENTIONS

- Treatment is unnecessary in most cases; 60% recover completely without treatment.
- A 5- to 7-day course of corticosteroids (e.g., prednisone) followed by gradual tapering of the dose over 5 days may shorten the recovery period.
- Eye protection with lubricating drops and/or ointment and an eye patch, if closure is not possible, is helpful.

SELECTED NURSING DIAGNOSES

- Risk for Altered Nutrition: Less than Body Requirements
- Risk for Injury
- Body Image Disturbance

SELECTED NURSING INTERVENTIONS

- Assess the degree of involvement and the resulting deficits.
- Nursing interventions are aimed primarily at teaching the client and family about the disease and how to prevent injury and maintain nutrition (see below).

CLIENT TEACHING

- The loss of the corneal reflex and the inability to close the eyelid increase the risk of corneal dryness and abrasion. Teach the client to use artificial tears four times a day and to wear an eye patch at night and sunglasses or goggles when outdoors or when exposed to dust or sprays.
- The facial paralysis makes it difficult for the client to chew and swallow. Drooling is common. Teach the client to chew slowly on the unaffected side and to avoid hot foods. A diet of frequent small soft meals is also helpful. Teach the client to inspect and clean the mouth carefully after meals.

- Teach the client to massage the affected side of the face and manually close the eyelid several times a day to maintain muscle tone. Encourage the client, as function returns, to wrinkle the forehead, open and close the eyes, whistle, and so on, several times daily.

HOME CARE CONSIDERATIONS

- Encourage the client to obtain medical follow-up care if the condition does not resolve spontaneously within a few months.

For more information on Bell's Palsy, see Medical-Surgical Nursing *by LeMone and Burke, p. 1867.*

Benign Prostatic Hyperplasia (BPH)

OVERVIEW

- Benign prostatic hyperplasia (BPH) is a hyperplasia of prostate glandular, stromal, and smooth muscle tissues.
- It almost universally affects males older than 45 years.
- The mean age for development of signs and symptoms is 60 to 65 years of age with symptomatic BPH developing earlier in African American males than in European Americans.
- It occurs in all male populations, but is less common in Asian countries.
- BPH begins in the periurethral area and progresses to involve the rest of the gland, and results mainly in S/S of urinary obstruction.
- Obstruction and retention result in a higher incidence of urinary tract infection.
- Only about 10% of clients require surgical intervention such as transurethral resection of the prostate (TURP) or incisional prostatectomy.
- BPH is not a risk factor for cancer of the prostate.

CAUSES

- Possibly due to a change in the estradiol-to-dihydrotestosterone ratio in older males

Signs & Symptoms

- Urinary frequency, nocturia
- Urinary hesitancy, difficulty starting urine stream
- Incomplete bladder emptying
- Postvoiding dribble
- Enlarged bladder
- Possible hematuria
- Urinary incontinence
- Enlarged prostate gland on rectal examination
- Complete obstruction: anuria, bladder pain, renal insufficiency

Diagnostics

- Prostate-specific antigen (PSA) is measured to help differentiate BPH from prostate cancer.
- Urodynamic evaluation, uroflowmetry in particular, is useful to determine the peak urinary flow rate. In general, a flow rate of less than 10 mL/second is considered indicative of obstruction.
- Ultrasonography may be used to estimate the size of the gland and assess bladder or upper urinary tract changes associated with BPH.
- Intravenous urography is normal in most men with BPH and is reserved for those with hematuria or evidence of upper urinary tract disease.
- Urethrocystoscopy may be performed in clients with hematuria.

MEDICAL INTERVENTIONS

- Excessive smooth muscle contraction in BPH may be blocked with the adrenergic-antagonist terazosin.
- Since the hyperplastic tissue is androgen dependent, treatment with finasteride, which inhibits conversion of testosterone to dihydrotestosterone (DHT) in androgen-sensitive tissue, is helpful in some men.

- Surgery for BPH includes transurethral incision of the prostate (TUIP), TURP, and simple prostatectomy.
- Minimally invasive procedures such as balloon urethroplasty, laser or microwave hyperthermia, and intraurethral stents to maintain patency of the urethra can be done as outpatient procedures, although their long-range effectiveness is yet to be determined.

SELECTED NURSING DIAGNOSES WITH INTERVENTIONS

Ineffective Management of Therapeutic Regimen
- Assess the client's severity of symptoms.
- Teach the client methods to minimize symptoms and prevent infection.
- Advise the client to restrict alcohol intake, especially at night, to minimize problems with nocturia.

Fluid Volume Excess
- Assess the client for manifestations of fluid volume excess and dilutional hyponatremia.
- Monitor fluid balance. Weigh the client daily at the same time each day.
- Restrict fluids and administer diuretics as prescribed.
- Administer replacement therapy as prescribed.

CLIENT TEACHING

- Provide the client with information about the disease process and treatment options.
- Tell the client to maintain a fluid intake of 2 to 3 L per day of nonalcoholic beverages, unless contraindicated.
- Teach the client Kegel exercises to decrease potential for urinary incontinence.
- Explain to the client that he may pass clots for up to 2 weeks postoperatively. Increasing fluid intake should clear the urine in one or two voidings. Tell the client to notify the physician if blood in the urine continues.
- Tell the client to avoid strenuous activity, heavy labor, and heavy lifting for 6 weeks postoperatively.

HOME CARE CONSIDERATIONS

- If the client is discharged with a catheter following outpatient surgery, provide catheter care instructions.
- Address the client's concerns about sexuality following prostate surgery, providing referral to counseling or support services as indicated.

For more information on Benign Prostatic Hyperplasia, see Medical-Surgical Nursing *by LeMone and Burke, p. 1972.*

Bladder Cancer

OVERVIEW

- Bladder cancer is a malignant neoplasm of the urinary bladder.
- It is the most common malignancy of the urinary system.
- In the male, it accounts for 7% of all new cases, and is the fourth most common type of cancer.
- In the female, it accounts for 2% of all new cases, and is the ninth most common type of cancer.
- Most (90%) are carcinomas of the transitional tissue of the bladder mucosa.
- Bladder cancer is usually a squamous cell or deeper adenocarcinoma; sarcomas occur less frequently, but are more virulent.
- The 5-year survival rate is 90% (early); 45% (with regional metastasis); and 9% (with distant metastasis).
- It is usually seen in people 60 to 70 years of age; it occurs 3 to 4 times more commonly in males than in females.

CAUSES

The precise cause of bladder cancer is unknown. However, risk factors include:

- Smoking (smokers have twice the risk of nonsmokers)

- Male gender
- European American race (European Americans have twice the risk of African Americans)
- Chronic or recurrent urolithiasis or urinary tract infection (UTI)
- Environmental exposure to carcinogens: 2-napthylamine, benzidine, aniline dye
- Occupations: hairdressers; spray painters; weavers; rubber, cable, leather, or petroleum workers
- Drug exposure: cyclophosphamide, phenacetin
- Geographic locations with high rates of infection with *Schistosoma haematobium*

Signs & Symptoms

- Gross/microscopic hematuria
- Dysuria
- Frequency, nocturia
- Urgency
- Late S/S: obstruction, pain, evidence of secondary lesions

Diagnostics

- Urinary cytology from voided, catheter, or cystoscopic specimens for detection of tumor or pre-tumor cells.
- Cystoscopic visual examination and biopsy.
- Intravenous pyelography (IVP) may show obstruction, deformity of the bladder wall, or bladder filling or emptying defects.
- Abdominal/pelvic computed tomography (CT) scan may show bladder lesion.
- Routine physical examination, blood studies, chest x-ray.

MEDICAL INTERVENTIONS

- Surgery ranges from simple resection of noninvasive tumors to removal of the bladder and surrounding structures, including hysterectomy in women. A urinary diversion is also created to provide for urine collection and drainage.
- Radiation is an adjunctive therapy used in the treatment of bladder cancer. It may reduce the tumor size prior to surgery, or it may be used palliatively in clients with inoperable tumors.

- Chemotherapy is an adjunctive therapy. Systemic agents include cyclophosphamide, doxorubicin, or a combination regimen of cisplatin, methotrexate, and vinblastine.

SELECTED NURSING DIAGNOSES WITH INTERVENTIONS

Altered Patterns of Urinary Elimination

- Monitor urinary output from all catheters, stents, and tubes for amount, color, and clarity—hourly for the first 24 hours postoperatively, then every 4 to 8 hours.
- Label all catheters, stents, and their drainage containers. Maintain separate closed gravity drainage systems for each.
- Secure ureteral catheters and stents with tape, to prevent kinking or occlusion by the client. Maintain gravity flow by keeping drainage bag below the level of the kidneys.
- Encourage the intake of 3000 mL of fluid per day.
- Monitor urine output closely for the first 24 hours after the removal of any stents or ureteral catheters.
- Encourage client to engage in activity as tolerated.

Risk for Impaired Skin Integrity

- Postoperatively, assess the skin surrounding the stoma for redness, excoriation, or signs of breakdown. Assess for leakage of urine from any catheters, stents, or drains.
- Ensure gravity drainage of urine-collection device or empty bag every 2 hours.
- Change urine-collection appliance as needed, removing any mucus from stoma.

Risk for Infection

- Maintain separate closed drainage systems, keeping drainage bags lower than the kidney, and prevent loops or kinks in drainage tubing, which impede urine flow.
- Monitor for signs of infection.
- Teach the client and significant others the signs and symptoms of infection and self-care measures to prevent UTI.

CLIENT TEACHING

- Teach the client and significant others care of the urinary stoma: skin and stoma care, prevention of urine reflux and infection, pouch emptying, pouch change, and use of night drainage.
- Encourage the client to maintain a fluid intake of at least 2 L per day.
- Teach the client to be alert for signs of tumor recurrence, and to maintain a regular schedule of urologist visits for follow-up care.

HOME CARE CONSIDERATIONS

- Provide a home health referral for continued teaching and monitoring related to management of the urinary stoma.
- Explain the need for a urine culture every 3 to 6 months and an IVP every year.
- Provide a list of local companies where the client may purchase necessary equipment or supplies.
- Provide information about national and local support groups, such as the United Ostomy Association and the American Cancer Society.

For more information on Bladder Cancer, see Medical-Surgical Nursing *by LeMone and Burke, p. 918.*

Bone Tumor, Primary

OVERVIEW

- Bone tumors are benign or malignant neoplasms arising from bone or bony structures.
- They are most common in the pelvis, proximal long bones, ribs, and vertebrae.
- They may arise from cartilage (chondroma or chondro sarcoma), bone (osteoma or osteosarcoma), collagen (fibrosarcoma), or bone marrow (giant cell tumor).

- Primary malignant tumors are rare, accounting for about 1% of all adult cancers and about 15% of pediatric cancers.
- Tumors arising in bone and cartilage are more common in males.
- Tumors arising in collagen and bone marrow are more common in females.
- Adolescents have the highest risk for developing osteosarcoma; its incidence peaks again in people in their 50s to 60s.
- Most types display rapid bone destruction and metastasis (to lung or other bones).
- The course and prognosis depend on the specific type of cancer.

CAUSES

- Unknown
- Suggested: heredity, trauma, radiation

Signs & Symptoms

- Bone pain (most common): dull, more common at night
- Weakness or limp
- Visible mass
- Tenderness, redness, swelling over tumor site
- Pathologic fracture
- Late: fever, cachexia, immobility

Diagnostics

- X-ray, computed tomography (CT) scan, or MRI may show tumor location, size, and invasion of adjacent tissues.
- Biopsy (needle or percutaneous needle) determines the type of tumor present.
- Serum alkaline phosphatase (a bone enzyme) is usually elevated.

MEDICAL INTERVENTIONS

- Chemotherapeutic agents are administered to shrink the tumor before surgery, to control recurrence of tumor growth after surgery, or to treat metastasis of the tumor.

- Radiation therapy may be used in combination with chemotherapy.
- The goal of surgery is to eliminate the bone tumor completely.

SELECTED NURSING DIAGNOSES WITH INTERVENTIONS

Risk for Injury

- Instruct clients in ways to avoid falls or injury to the tumor site.

Pain

- Develop strategies for controlling both acute pain (from surgery, fracture, or inflammation) and chronic pain (from progression of the disease).
- Provide assistive devices (e.g., canes, walkers, crutches) when the client ambulates.

Impaired Physical Mobility

- Begin muscle-strengthening and active and passive range-of-motion (ROM) exercises immediately after surgery. A continuous passive motion machine may be used after surgical procedures to either upper or lower extremities.
- For the client who has had an amputation, encourage active ROM exercises for all uninvolved joints.
- Encourage exercises that help strengthen the triceps muscles to assist in use of crutches or other devices.
- For the client who has undergone amputation of a lower extremity, encourage quadriceps and gluteal setting exercises and leg raises.

CLIENT TEACHING

- Review pain medication regimen, including dosage, effects, side effects, and timing of medication administration.
- Discuss activity and weight-bearing restrictions. Teach clients how to use assistive devices such as crutches, walkers, trapeze, and so on, correctly. Also teach prescribed exercises for optimum range of mobility.
- Teach wound care as appropriate. Provide a list of local resources for supplies.

HOME CARE CONSIDERATIONS

- Refer to physical therapy for ambulation training and appropriate muscle group strengthening exercises.
- Ensure referral to a prosthetic specialist for the client with an amputation.
- Tell the client to notify the physician immediately if the client notices increased swelling, discoloration, or changes in sensation. Stress to the client the importance of lifelong monitoring and follow-up care with the oncologist.
- Discuss hospice services and support groups for clients with metastatic disease.

For more information on Bone Tumor, Primary, see Medical-Surgical Nursing *by LeMone and Burke, p. 1564.*

Brain Tumor, Benign and Malignant

OVERVIEW

- Brain tumors may be primary tumors of CNS tissue (neurons, neuroglia), primary tumors arising from nonneural tissues (meninges, pituitary gland, pineal gland), or metastatic tissues.
- Both benign and malignant neoplasms can result in significant neurologic deficits and death.
- Tumors of neuroglia include astrocytoma (glioblastoma, glioma), oligodendroglioma, and ependymona; neural cell tumors include neuroblastoma and ganglion cell tumors; nonneural tissue tumors include meningiomas, pineal and pituitary tumors.
- Primary neoplasms can occur at any age, most often between 40 and 60 years of age.

CAUSES

- Unknown
- There may be a hereditary factor: 16% of clients with primary brain tumors have a family history of cancer
- Cranial irradiation and exposure to some chemicals may increase the risk of astrocytomas and meningiomas

Signs & Symptoms

- Onset is usually insidious; seizure is the first sign in about 15% of clients

General S/S

- Headache, especially in morning
- Vomiting, with or without nausea
- Lethargy
- Confusion, disorientation, forgetfulness
- Personality changes
- Seizures
- S/S of increased intracranial pressure

Focal S/S

- Frontal lobe: impaired memory, cognition/judgment; personality/mood changes, apathy, lethargy, ataxia, apraxia, aphasia, incontinence
- Temporal lobes: abrupt changes in personality (affective/psychotic), mood, appetite, libido; hallucinations (auditory); partial-complex seizures; contralateral visual-field cuts; dilated pupils; contralateral hemiparesis
- Parietal lobes: receptive aphasia with contralateral hemianopia (left); spatial disorientation, constructional apraxia, and contralateral hemianopsia (right)
- Occipital lobe: seizures, visual agnosia, visual-field cuts
- Cerebellum: tremors, nystagmus, incoordination, ataxia, nuchal headache
- Cranial nerves: ptosis, diplopia, changes in sense of smell and ocular movement, ipsilateral drooping of face, loss of cough/swallow/gag reflex, tongue protrusion; unilateral hearing loss, tinnitus, ataxia (cranial nerve [CN] VIII); decreased

facial sensation, facial weakness/paralysis (CN VII); schwannoma of CN VIII can compress CN VII and cause facial features

Diagnostics

- Biopsy can distinguish between normal, benign, or malignant tissue.
- Brain scan may show increased radioisotope uptake, indicative of tumors; especially useful for meningiomas.
- Cerebral angiography may show abnormal cerebral perfusion patterns suggestive of tumor location.
- Computed tomography (CT) may show tumor location and size and the presence of hydrocephalus or tissue shifts
- Electroencephalogram (EEG) may show localized abnormal brain wave function indicative of neoplastic growth.
- Lumbar puncture with cerebrospinal fluid (CSF) analysis may rule out infection; show increased pressure, neoplastic cells, or chemical changes.
- Magnetic resonance imaging (MRI) may show tumor location and size and the presence of hydrocephalus or tissue shifts.
- Positron emission tomography (PET) may show altered normal brain tissue metabolism versus abnormal brain neoplasm metabolism.
- X-ray of cranium may show tumor calcification or erosion of bony skull.

MEDICAL INTERVENTIONS

- Various chemotherapeutic agents are used in the treatment of brain tumors.
- Radiation therapy may be administered alone or as an adjunct to surgery.
- Neurosurgery is used to remove tumors, to reduce the size of a tumor, or for symptom relief.

SELECTED NURSING DIAGNOSES WITH INTERVENTIONS

Anxiety

- Assist the client through routine medical procedures, including blood work and radiologic studies.

- Reinforce, clarify, and repeat information that has been provided.
- Encourage client and significant others to verbalize feelings, questions, and fears; provide realistic information appropriate to their level of understanding.
- Review strengths and effective coping skills.
- Arrange for a member of the clergy to visit if the client so desires.
- Assess the client's and significant others' knowledge and response to hospitalization and impending surgery.
- Provide preoperative teaching. If possible, show the client and significant others the CCU or ICU and introduce them to personnel who will care for the client after surgery. Discuss the anticipated postoperative changes in both the client's appearance and behavior.
- Allow time for the client and significant others to be together.

Risk for Infection

The client who has had intracranial surgery is at risk for infection from multiple invasive lines, the scalp wound, and the introduction of bacteria into the operative area.

- Assess and report leakage of CSF and provide interventions to prevent contamination of the area leaking CSF.
- Implement interventions to prevent infection: use strict aseptic technique, keep the client's hands away from dressings, and administer prescribed antibiotics.
- Assess and report manifestations of infection, including increased temperature, redness, swelling, drainage, pain, fever, chills, increasing headache, neck stiffness, photophobia, or positive Kernig's or Brudzinski's sign.

Altered Protection

- Monitor for manifestations of increased intracranial pressure, including restlessness, decreasing level of consciousness, headache, vomiting, seizures, decreasing sensory and motor function, changes in pupil size and reaction, changes in vital signs, and abnormal posturing.

- Implement interventions to decrease the risk of increased intracranial pressure:
  1. Elevate the head of the bed 15° to 30° unless contraindicated.
  2. Avoid neck flexion or rotation.
  3. Do not take rectal temperatures.
  4. Avoid clustering activities that increase intracranial presssure, such as suctioning, turning, bathing.
  5. Administer prescribed medications to prevent vomiting.
  6. Do not suction for more than 15 seconds at one time.
  7. Tell the client to avoid—if possible—coughing, sneezing, and straining to have a bowel movement.
  8. Maintain prescribed fluid restrictions and administer prescribed diuretics.
  9. Maintain patency of drains or shunts.
- Maintain a quiet, calm, softly lighted environment.
- Implement interventions to prevent seizures or, if they occur, to prevent injury:
  1. Pad side rails of bed.
  2. Place bed in lowest position and keep side rails up.
  3. Have oral airway and suction equipment immediately available.
  4. Administer prescribed anticonvulsants.
  5. If seizure occurs maintain a patent airway, do not restrain client, do not force anything into the client's mouth, and provide physical and emotional support.
- Carefully monitor hydration status.

CLIENT TEACHING

- Teach the client and significant others about the disease process, treatment, and prognosis.
- Teach safety measures for motor deficits, sensory deficits, lack of coordination, seizures, and cognitive deficits as appropriate.
- Review medication information, including dosage, effects, and side effects.
- Discuss nonpharmacologic comfort measures for nausea, vomiting, and pain.

- Suggest different methods of communication if aphasia is present, and measures to improve vision if visual deficits are present.

HOME CARE CONSIDERATIONS

- Tell the client to report to the physician any manifestation such as a stiff neck, increasing headache, elevated temperature, new motor or sensory deficits, vision changes, or seizures.
- Provide information on how to purchase wigs and hairpieces if desired.
- Provide referrals to support groups and community resources such as the local chapter of the American Cancer Society.
- A referral to a rehabilitation service or home health nursing service may be appropriate.

For more information on Brain Tumor, Benign and Malignant, see Medical-Surgical Nursing *by LeMone and Burke, p. 1750.*

Breast Cancer

OVERVIEW

- Breast cancers are malignant neoplasms of breast tissues.
- They are the most common malignant neoplasm in women and the second most common malignancy causing death in women.
- Malignancy in women less than 35 years of age is most often familial and more serious.
- One in every eight women will be diagnosed with breast cancer.
- Incidence rose 4% per year in 1980s, but now has leveled off.
- Incidence is lower in African American women than in European American women; however, mortality rate is higher as it often is detected at a later stage and survival rates are lower at all stages.

- Breast cancer is hormone dependent and does not develop in the absence of estrogen.
- It may remain noninvasive or invasive without metastasis for long periods of time.
- Overall 5-year survival rate is 92% (if detected early); 76% (with regional metastasis); 21% (with distant metastasis).
- Breast cancer rarely occurs in men (1000 cases per year).

CAUSES

Causes remain elusive; however, several risk factors are known:

Genetics
- Family history of malignant neoplasia
- Point mutation in p53 tumor-suppressor gene
- Mutation of BRCA1 gene on chromosome 17
- BRCA-2, a gene on chromosome 11, increases risk of breast cancer in both men and women
- Family history of breast malignancy in first degree family member (mother, sister)

Hormones
- Early menarche (<11 years)/late menopause (>52 years)
- Nulliparity
- Late first pregnancy
- Estrogen replacement therapy or oral contraceptive use

Environment
- Radiation; especially if exposure occurs between 10 and 14 years of age
- High fat diet, moderate to high alcohol intake

Other
- Age: rises continuously with age
- History of cancer in contralateral breast
- History of endometrial/ovarian cancer
- History of stress
- European American race
- Middle/upper socioeconomic groups
- Obesity

Signs & Symptoms

- Breast lump palpable if larger than 1 cm. Characteristically, the lump is:
  1. hard or stony
  2. painless (most common)
  3. irregular in shape
  4. "fixed" or immovable
  5. often found in upper, outer quadrant
- Advanced disease may show:
  1. nipple discharge
  2. nipple retraction
  3. breast dimpling, contour changes
  4. inflammation (redness, heat, edema)
  5. *peau d'orange* appearance
  6. palpable axillary lymph nodes
  7. ulceration of breast

Diagnostics

- Diagnostic mammography is used to help decide whether an identified lesion needs further diagnostic studies or may be reexamined at a later time.
- Ultrasonography can differentiate cystic lesions from solid ones.
- Biopsy (fine needle, core needle, or surgical) is used to differentiate benign lesions from malignant ones.
- Chest x-ray can identify chest metastasis.
- Scans of bone, brain, and liver can identify distant metastasis.

MEDICAL INTERVENTIONS

- Surgery is the treatment of choice for breast cancer. Surgical excisions range from removal of the lump itself, called a lumpectomy, to removal of the entire breast, the underlying chest muscles, and the lymph nodes under the arms, called a radical mastectomy.
- Radiation therapy is typically used following breast cancer surgery.
- Adjuvant chemotherapy has become the standard of care for the majority of breast cancer cases with

axillary lymph node involvement. Hormonal therapy may be used to shrink the tumor or to delay postsurgical recurrence.

- Tamoxifen, a drug that interferes with estrogen activity, is used to prevent breast cancer in women at high risk and as adjunctive therapy for stages II, III, and IV breast cancer; its use is under investigation for carcinoma in situ.

SELECTED NURSING DIAGNOSES WITH INTERVENTIONS

Anxiety

- Provide opportunities for the client to express her thoughts and feelings.
- Discuss with the client her knowledge of breast cancer.
- Have the client discuss her immediate concerns about resuming her life at home and the changes she must make.
- Explain the surgical procedure. Tell the client what to expect regarding preoperative medications, anesthesia, and recovery.
- Explain that it is normal to have decreased sensation in the surgical area.

Decisional Conflict

- Provide an opportunity for the client to ask questions; answer questions as simply and directly as possible. Make eye contact with the client and pay attention to body language.
- Focus on immediate concerns and provide up-to-date written material for the client to review.
- Listen to the client in a nonjudgmental manner during her decision-making process.
- If the client wishes, provide opportunities for her to meet other women who have had breast cancer surgery.
- Facilitate a team approach with the surgeon, anesthesiologist, oncologist, plastic surgeon, and other health professionals.

Anticipatory Grieving

- Listen attentively to client's expression of grief and watch for nonverbal cues (failure to make eye contact, crying, silence).

- Allow time to interact with the client; do not rush interaction.
- Explain that it is normal to have periods of depression, anger, and denial after breast surgery.
- If the client wishes, involve the partner in helping the client cope with her grief. Remember that the partner may also be grieving.

Risk for Infection

- Assess the surgical dressings for bleeding, drainage, color, and odor every 4 hours for 24 hours and document findings.
- Observe the incision and IV sites for pain, redness, swelling, and drainage. Assess the drainage system for patency and adequate suction. Note the color and amount of drainage.
- Change dressings and IV tubing using aseptic technique, and document.
- Encourage the client to eat a protein-rich diet. Discuss the client's nutritional status with the dietitian and request a consultation with the client.
- Teach the client how to care for the drainage system.
- At discharge, teach the client to watch for signs and symptoms of infection: fever, redness, or hardness at the surgical site, or purulent drainage. Any of these signs should be reported to the physician.
- Explain to the client that she may experience scaling, flaking, dryness, itching, rash, or dry desquamation of the involved skin, particularly after radiation therapy.
- Tell the client to avoid deodorants and talcum powder on the affected side until the incision is completely healed.

Risk for Body Image Disturbance

- Encourage the client to verbalize her thoughts and feelings.
- Assess how the client views her body.
- Explain that redness and swelling will fade with time.
- Include significant others if possible when discussing the plan of care and activities of daily living (ADLs). Request consultation with a psychologist or other professional if the client is interested.

- Offer pamphlets and suggest books and videos that might increase the client's understanding of what lies ahead. Document her response.
- Offer referral to support groups with women experiencing similar problems. Some women may prefer one-on-one counseling.
- Encourage the client to look at her incision when she feels ready. Often the reality is not as frightening as the client had imagined. Explain that it is normal to be afraid to look.
- Make it clear that it is up to the client to decide whether and how she will involve others in her care.
- Let the client know that there is no rush in deciding about a prosthesis or reconstruction. She may choose neither.
- If the client is interested in breast reconstruction, provide written material and encourage her to talk with a plastic surgeon and with women who have had reconstruction.

CLIENT TEACHING

In addition to the above teaching:

- Teach the client the continued need to perform breast self-examination.
- Teach the client postoperative exercises. An exercise program should be developed in consultation with the physician and physical therapist.
- Review with the client the signs of metastasis to the lungs, liver, and bones and stress the importance of promptly reporting these signs to the physician.
- Encourage a wholesome, balanced diet. Tell the client that vitamin supplements can help in promoting healing and recovery.

HOME CARE CONSIDERATIONS

- Review the client's medication regimen and her schedule of follow-up visits for radiation, chemotherapy, wound care, and so on.
- Refer the client to breast cancer support groups to share her thoughts, feelings, experiences, and information about treatments, side effects, insurance, and other practical aspects of living with breast cancer.

- Discuss the client's options for reconstructive surgery and the option of using a prosthesis. Provide information on how to pursue these options, such as how soon she can consider reconstructive surgery and where to purchase a prosthesis.

For more information on Breast Cancer, see Medical-Surgical Nursing *by LeMone and Burke, p. 2054.*

Bronchiectasis

OVERVIEW

- Bronchiectasis is an abnormal and permanent dilation of bronchi and destruction of their walls.
- It is usually seen in medium-sized (segmental, subsegmental) airways.
- It may be focal, with limited airways affected, or diffuse, with a widespread pattern.
- Bronchial dilation is associated with inflammatory and fibrous changes.
- Affected airways contain pools of purulent material; chronic, recurrent infections are common.
- The most distal airways may be occluded by secretions or closed completely owing to the overgrowth of fibrous tissues.
- There are three types:
  1. *Cylindrical (fusiform)* is a uniform dilation of a portion of the wall; ends abruptly where joining smaller obliterated airway.
  2. *Varicose* is an irregular or beaded pattern of dilation resembling varicose veins.
  3. *Saccular (cystic)* is a ballooning at the periphery; no recognizable airways are beyond.
- Bronchiectasis results in a chronic, obstructive type of respiratory disease.

CAUSES

Infectious

- Inflammatory mediators released by neutrophils in response to infection damage respiratory epithelium and impair mucociliary clearance.
- Epithelial damage, in turn, increases susceptibility to infection, leading to a cycle of inflammation and airway damage, impaired clearance of microorganisms, and further infection.
- A number of organisms have been implicated:
  1. Viruses include measles, adenovirus, and influenza virus
  2. Bacteria include *Staphylococcus aureus, Klebsiella* species, and anaerobes
  3. Tuberculosis or other mycobacteria

Noninfectious

- Severe inflammatory response to exposure to a toxic substance (inhalation of a toxic gas such as ammonia, or aspiration of gastric contents)
- Hypersensitivity response to inhaled substances, e.g., allergic bronchopulmonary aspergillosis, an immune response to *Aspergillus* organisms
- Rarely in autoimmune disorders such as ulcerative colitis, rheumatoid arthritis, and Sjogren's syndrome.
- Genetic and/or congenital disorders associated with bronchiectasis include cystic fibrosis, Williams-Campbell syndrome, tracheomegaly, Young's syndrome, alpha$_1$-antitrypsin deficiency, yellow-nail syndrome.

Signs & Symptoms

- Initially may be asymptomatic
- Usually a history of chronic cough, producing copious mucopurulent secretions
- Hemoptysis: small amounts to massive hemorrhage
- Rales, rhonchi, or wheezes on auscultation
- Chronic disease results in hypoxemia, clubbing of fingernails, S/S of cor pulmonale

Diagnostics

- A chest x-ray may show peribronchial inflammation, thickened walls, cystic air spaces, obliterated lumens, "tram track" or "ring shadow" patterns.
- Computed tomography (CT) scans are sensitive diagnostic tests that can show high-resolution outlines of airways in cross section.
- Bronchoscopy can show the source of secretions and/or bleeding.
- Pulmonary function tests reveal decreased vital capacity and expiratory flow.
- Arterial blood gases (ABGs) may show hypoxemia.
- Complete blood count (CBC) may show a normocytic, normochromic anemia and leukocytosis.

MEDICAL INTERVENTIONS

- Antibiotics are prescribed at the first indication of an infection, and may be used prophylactically as well. Inhaled bronchodilators also may be ordered. Oxygen may be prescribed if the client is hypoxemic.
- Chest physiotherapy is a vital component of client care.
- Bronchoscopy may be necessary to remove retained secretions or obstruction.
- If lung destruction is localized and unresponsive to conservative management, surgical lung resection may be performed.

SELECTED NURSING DIAGNOSES

- Ineffective Airway Clearance
- Ineffective Breathing Pattern
- Impaired Gas Exchange
- Altered Nutrition: Less than Body Requirements
- Self-Care Deficit

SELECTED NURSING INTERVENTIONS

- Assess respiratory rate and pattern, ABGs, and signs of hypoxia and hypercapnea.
- Administer low-flow oxygen therapy.
- Maintain client in high-Fowler's position.
- Administer medications as prescribed, and monitor effects and side effects.

- Provide adequate hydration, 2 to 3 L per day unless contraindicated.
- Perform chest physiotherapy, assessing breath sounds before and after treatment.
- Maintain quiet, calm environment.
- Assist client with energy conservation, and plan frequent rest periods.

CLIENT TEACHING

- Teach the client how to use pursed lip breathing and diaphragmatic breathing techniques.
- Teach the client the proper use of all medications, including inhalers, nebulizers, and so on.
- Review stress management techniques, such as relaxation and meditation.
- Tell the client to avoid irritants such as smoke, dust, and powders.
- Teach the client the signs and symptoms of hypoxia and hypercapnea.

HOME CARE CONSIDERATIONS

- A referral to a smoking cessation program may be appropriate.
- Encourage the client to obtain pneumonia vaccine and annual influenza immunizations.

For more information on Bronchiectasis, see Medical-Surgical Nursing *by LeMone and Burke, p. 1447.*

Bronchitis, Acute

OVERVIEW

- Acute bronchitis or inflammation of the bronchi usually follows an upper respiratory infection
- Inflammation leads to vasodilation and edema of the mucosal lining of the bronchi, increasing mucus production

- Acute bronchitis occurs most commonly in people with impaired physiologic defenses and cigarette smokers

CAUSES

- Infectious bronchitis may be caused by bacteria or viruses; common bacteria include *Streptococcus pneumoniae* and *Haemophilus influenzae*
- Inhalation of toxic gases or chemicals can lead to inflammatory tracheobronchitis

Signs & Symptoms

- Fever
- Cough, initially nonproductive, later becoming productive; often occurs in paroxysms
- Tachypnea, possible dyspnea
- Chest pain, substernal or chest wall pain
- General malaise
- Bronchovesicular breath sounds on auscultation

Diagnostics

- A chest x-ray can differentiate between bronchitis (no consolidation) and pneumonia (consolidation).

MEDICAL INTERVENTIONS

- Pharmacologic agents include aspirin or acetaminophen to relieve fever and malaise. A broad-spectrum antibiotic may be prescribed, since approximately 50% of cases of acute bronchitis are bacterial in origin.
- An expectorant cough medication is recommended for use during the day, and a cough suppressant at night to facilitate rest.

SELECTED NURSING DIAGNOSES

- Ineffective Airway Clearance
- Knowledge Deficit
- Sleep Pattern Disturbance
- Impaired Home Maintenance Management

SELECTED NURSING INTERVENTIONS

- Clients with acute bronchitis are rarely hospitalized, and most nursing interventions are directed toward teaching.

CLIENT TEACHING

- If the client is a smoker, stress the importance of smoking cessation.
- Tell the client to increase fluid intake to 2 to 3 L per day unless contraindicated.
- Review the use and effects of prescribed medications. Instruct the client to use sedatives, narcotics, and tranquilizers cautiously.

HOME CARE CONSIDERATIONS

- A referral to a smoking cessation program may be appropriate.

For more information on Bronchitis, Acute, see Medical-Surgical Nursing *by LeMone and Burke, p. 1391.*

Bronchitis, Chronic

OVERVIEW

- Chronic bronchitis is a form of chronic obstructive pulmonary disease (COPD).
- It usually coexists with some degree of emphysema.
- It consists of a chronic, progressive inflammation of large bronchi with loss of cilia, airway swelling, and hyperplasia and hypertrophy of mucus-secreting glands in airway walls.
- Small airways (bronchioles) show increased inflammatory cells, goblet-cell hyperplasia, peribronchiolar fibrosis, mucus plugs, and hypertrophied smooth muscle.

- Chronic bronchitis is associated with excess mucopurulent secretions, cough, and expectoration lasting for 3 or more months each year for more than 2 consecutive years.
- It is a leading cause of morbidity, disability, and mortality in the United States.
- Hypoxemia and hypercarbia appear earlier and are more severe than in the predominantly emphysematous patient.

CAUSES

- Smoking (including passive smoke), is the most common correlate
- Air pollution, especially sulfur dioxide, nitrous dioxide, particulate matter; much higher incidence in urban, industrial areas
- Occupational exposure to organic or inorganic noxious gases or dusts
- Familial/genetic factors may be operative but have not been proved

Signs & Symptoms

- Chronic and productive cough; precedes dyspnea; exacerbated by inhalation of irritant and cold damp air (winter)
- Expectorations are copious, thick, and white, gray, or yellow in color
- Frequent pulmonary infection
- Dyspnea, first on exertion; later at rest
- Shortness of breath
- Bronchospasm with wheezing, rhonchi
- Respiratory rate normal to slightly increased
- Cyanosis
- Coarse rhonchi and wheezes on auscultation
- S/S of right heart failure (cor pulmonale): peripheral edema, puffy appearance, distended neck veins, weight gain
- Appearance referred to as "blue bloater"

Diagnostics

- Pulmonary function tests show slightly increased minute volume, increased residual volume; decreased vital capacity; decreased FEV_1.

- Arterial blood gases (ABGs) show severe hypoxemia and hypercapnia.
- Chest x-ray may show an increase in bronchovesicular markings.
- Complete blood count (CBC) shows severe polycythemia (compensatory to low PaO_2).

MEDICAL INTERVENTIONS

- Pharmacologic agents may include antibiotics, bronchodilators, and corticosteroids.
- Smoking cessation is vital.
- Pulmonary hygiene measures include hydration, effective cough, percussion, and postural drainage.
- Clients with an acute exacerbation may require oxygenation and inspiratory positive-pressure assistance with a face mask or intubation and mechanical ventilation.

SELECTED NURSING DIAGNOSES

- Impaired Gas Exchange
- Ineffective Airway Clearance
- Risk for Infection
- Activity Intolerance
- Anxiety
- Sleep Pattern Disturbance

SELECTED NURSING INTERVENTIONS

- Assess respiratory rate and pattern, ABGs, and signs of hypoxia and hypercapnea.
- Administer low-flow oxygen therapy as prescribed.
- Maintain client in high-Fowler's position.
- Administer medications such as bronchodilators and corticosteroids as prescribed, and monitor for effects and side effects.
- Perform chest physiotherapy, assessing breath sounds before and after treatment.
- Maintain a quiet, calm environment; plan frequent rest periods; and assist the client with energy conservation.

CLIENT TEACHING

- Teach the client breathing, coughing, and relaxation techniques.

- Review the medication regimen, including the use of inhalers and nebulizers.
- Encourage the client to quit smoking.
- Teach the client the signs and symptoms of hypoxia and hypercapnea.

HOME CARE CONSIDERATIONS

- A referral to a smoking cessation program may be appropriate.
- Encourage pneumonia vaccine and annual immunizations against influenza, and suggest the client avoid persons with influenza or upper respiratory tract infections.

For more information on Bronchitis, Chronic, see Medical-Surgical Nursing *by LeMone and Burke,* *p. 1434.*

Calcium Imbalance

Hypercalcemia
Hypocalcemia

OVERVIEW

- Calcium is one of the body's most plentiful minerals.
- Most (98%) calcium is combined with phosphate and hydroxide to form hydroxyapatite crystals, which impart structural rigidity to the bones and teeth.
- Only 1% to 2% of the total body calcium is contained in the extracellular fluid (ECF); however, a normal concentration of calcium ions [Ca^{++}] in ECF is critical to the normal function of excitable tissue throughout the body (nerve and all types of muscle), and for proper enzyme function and blood clotting.
- Regulation of calcium is achieved via the hormones parathyroid hormone (PTH) and calcitonin, and vitamin D.
- PTH is secreted by the parathyroid glands in response to low serum calcium, and raises calcium by:
  1. increasing bone resorption, liberating calcium from bone.
  2. conserving calcium at the renal tubules.
  3. improving calcium absorption from the GI tract.
- Calcitonin is secreted by C cells in the thyroid gland in response to elevated calcium and lowers calcium by inhibiting bone resorption.
- Vitamin D is formed in the skin, activated in the kidney, and increases the intestinal absorption of calcium; excess vitamin D can cause increased bone resorption.
- Serum calcium concentration measures the total calcium in the blood; normal serum calcium is 8.8 to 10.4 mg/dL.
- Calcium is present in three forms in the blood:
  1. about 50% is ionized;

2. almost 50% is bound to plasma proteins, mainly albumin; and
3. a trace amount is combined with nonprotein anions such as phosphate, citrate, and carbonate.

- Ionized calcium is freely diffusible and important physiologically, influencing neuromuscular irritability, nerve impulse transmission, muscle contraction, and blood coagulation.
- The ratio of ionized calcium to other forms depends on:
  1. serum albumin content: decreased albumin leads to decreased bound calcium, which leads to decreased total calcium content; ionized calcium concentration should remain unchanged.
  2. phosphorus concentration: decreased phosphorus leads to increased ionized calcium; increased phosphorus leads to decreased ionized calcium; calcium and phosphorus can combine when phosphorus is elevated.
  3. plasma pH: increased pH (alkalosis) leads to decreased ionized calcium; decreased pH (acidosis) leads to increased ionized calcium.
- Calcium imbalance, either hypercalcemia or hypocalcemia, can be a medical emergency.
- Hypercalcemia may represent increased total serum calcium levels or an increased ratio of ionized to total calcium.
- Hypocalcemia may represent reduced total serum calcium levels or a decreased ratio of ionized to total calcium.
- Hypercalcemia can cause cardiac arrhythmias and/or arrest.
- Hypocalcemia can cause tetany and/or convulsions.

CAUSES

Hypercalcemia

- Primary hyperparathyroidism: increased bone resorption, intestinal absorption, and renal reabsorption of calcium
- Malignancy: breast and lung cancers, multiple myeloma
- Hyperthyroidism
- Immobilization

- Drugs: thiazide diuretics, lithium, alkaline antacids such as calcium carbonate
- Vitamin D or vitamin A intoxication
- Renal transplant

Hypocalcemia

- Hypoparathyroidism, primary or surgical
- Acute pancreatitis: calcium ions combine with fatty acids released by lypolysis
- Hypomagnesemia: malnourished alcoholics, cisplatin therapy
- Hyperphosphatemia
- Alkalosis: promotes increased calcium:albumin binding
- Lack of vitamin D or insufficient sun exposure
- Malabsorption: partial gastrectomy with gastrojejunostomy, ileal bypass, Crohn's disease, pancreatic insufficiency, hepatobiliary disease
- Rapid or massive blood transfusion with citrated blood: citrate added to banked blood to prevent clotting and extend the life of the blood binds calcium, reducing ionized calcium concentrations
- Drugs: loop diuretics, anticonvulsants (phenytoin, phenobarbital), phosphates, mithramycin, calcitonin
- Alcoholism
- Sepsis
- Other: thyroid carcinoma, AIDS

Signs & Symptoms

Hypercalcemia

- Neuromuscular: muscle weakness, fatigue, depressed deep tendon reflexes (DTRs)
- Gastrointestinal: constipation, anorexia, nausea, vomiting
- Behavior: confusion, impaired memory, personality changes
- Renal: polyuria, polydipsia; renal colic
- Cardiovascular: bradycardia, heart block (AV or bundle branch block); hypertension

Hypocalcemia

- Neuromuscular:

  1. Tetany: circumoral and distal peripheral paresthesias (tingling around the mouth, of the hands and feet); extremity and facial muscle spasms; laryngeal spasm
  2. Trousseau's sign: blood pressure cuff on upper arm inflated to above systolic pressure for 3 minutes produces carpal spasm (palmar flexion with finger spasms)
  3. Chvostek's sign: tapping over facial nerve just in front of ear produces ipsilateral facial muscle contraction

- Cardiovascular: decreased cardiac output, hypotension; bradycardia, ventricular tachycardia, asystole
- CNS manifestations: convulsions; anxiety, depression, confusion, psychoses

Diagnostics

Hypercalcemia

- Total serum calcium: >10.5 mg/dL.
- Ionized serum calcium: >5.5 mg/dL.
- PTH levels increased in primary or secondary hyperparathyroidism.
- EKG shows shortened ST segment and Q-T interval, and sometimes a prolonged P-R interval.

Hypocalcemia

- Total serum calcium <8.7 mg/dL (if serum albumin increases, serum calcium should also rise proportionately).
- Ionized serum calcium <4.0 mg/dL.
- PTH levels are decreased in hypoparathyroidism; may be elevated with some secondary types of hypocalcemia.
- Magnesium and phosphorus: increased levels may identify cause of hypocalcemia.
- EKG shows prolonged Q-T interval secondary to prolonged ST segment; also shows ventricular tachycardia (torsades de pointes).

MEDICAL INTERVENTIONS

Hypercalcemia

- Pharmacologic therapy includes administration of IV saline solution to dilute the serum, and diuretics to increase urinary excretion of calcium and saline.
- When rapid reversal of hypercalcemia is required, IV sodium phosphate or potassium phosphate may be administered.

Hypocalcemia

- IV calcium is given to prevent or treat tetany and convulsions.
- Clients with chronic hypocalcemia may receive oral calcium supplements and oral vitamin D to restore normal serum calcium levels.

SELECTED NURSING DIAGNOSES

Hypercalcemia

- Decreased Cardiac Output
- Risk for Constipation
- Risk for Injury
- Risk for Altered Nutrition: Less than Body Requirements
- Impaired Physical Mobility

Hypocalcemia

- Decreased Cardiac Output
- Risk for Impaired Gas Exchange
- Risk for Injury
- Risk for Altered Nutrition: Less than Body Requirements

SELECTED NURSING INTERVENTIONS

Hypercalcemia

- Force fluids to prevent renal damage and dehydration.
- Administer loop diuretics per physician prescription (avoid thiazide diuretics).

- Provide acid-ash foods (meats, fish, poultry, eggs, cranberries, plums, prunes).
- Encourage mobility or bed exercise.
- Provide safe environment.
- Orient client to surroundings.
- Assess client's level of consciousness.
- Monitor intake and output.
- Strain urine for calcium stones.
- Monitor vital signs, EKG, serum electrolytes, and digitalis levels.
- Assess renal function to identify signs of nephropathy.

Hypocalcemia

- Administer IV calcium gluconate in D5W slowly (less than 1 g/hr) per physician prescription. (Calcium gluconate can cause tissue to slough if it infiltrates.)
- Administer oral calcium supplements per physician prescription after meals.
- Follow seizure precautions.
- Provide quiet environment.
- Keep emergency tracheostomy tray at bedside for respiratory emergency secondary to laryngeal spasm.
- Monitor serum calcium levels.
- Perform frequent respiratory assessments for signs of respiratory distress.
- Monitor EKG for changes indicative of heart block or ventricular dysrhythmias.
- Check for Trousseau's and Chvostek's signs, and report their presence to the physician.
- Since calcium supplements may precipitate digitalis toxicity, monitor digitalis levels carefully, when indicated.

CLIENT TEACHING

Hypercalcemia

- Provide the client with a list of foods high in calcium and teach the client to limit intake of these foods.
- Encourage the client to follow a low-calcium, acid-ash diet.

- Instruct the client to maintain a fluid intake of 3 L per day.
- Review the client's use of over-the-counter drugs for presence of calcium, and instruct client to avoid these drugs.

Hypocalcemia

- Teach the client the purpose of calcium and vitamin D in the body and the importance of maintaining adequate levels of calcium and vitamin D in the diet.
- Give the client a list of foods and dietary supplements rich in calcium and vitamin D.
- Instruct the client to take oral calcium 1 to 1.5 hours after eating.

HOME CARE CONSIDERATIONS

Hypercalcemia

- Instruct client to discontinue use of calcium and vitamin D supplements.
- Teach the client about the use of diuretics if prescribed.
- Instruct the client to maintain a fluid intake of 2.5 to 3 quarts per day.

Hypocalcemia

- Instruct the client to increase calcium through diet (dairy products, broccoli, collard greens, tofu); supplements (calcium carbonate); and through vitamin D intake (sunlight, milk, liver, eggs).
- Teach the client the S/S of decreased calcium: tetany and carpopedal spasm.

For more information, see the following pages in Medical-Surgical Nursing *by LeMone and Burke:*
Hypercalcemia, p. 141
Hypocalcemia, p. 138

Cancer

OVERVIEW

- Cancer is a group of cellular diseases characterized by mutations in DNA; abnormal, uncontrolled cell growth; and loss of cell differentiation (specialized structure and function).
- Clones of abnormal cells form nests of malignant neoplasms (tumors).
- Malignant cells invade surrounding tissues, and may break away from the primary tumor to metastasize to distant sites in the body.
- Cancers tend to grow rapidly; crowd, invade, and destroy normal tissue; recur, if removed; and metastasize to distant tissues via the blood or lymph.
- *Primary* malignant neoplasms are those that grow in the tissue of origin.
- *Secondary (metastatic)* neoplasms grow in tissues distant from the tissue of origin.
- Types of cancer include:
  1. Carcinomas (nonglandular epithelial tissue)
  2. Adenocarcinomas (glandular epithelial tissue)
  3. Sarcomas (connective tissue, muscle, bone)
  4. Leukemias (blood cells [usually white blood cells])
  5. Lymphomas/myelomas (lymphatic cells, tissues, organs)
  6. Seminomas (embryonic structures)
  7. Melanoma (melanocytes)
  8. Meningioma (meninges)
- Cancer (all types, combined) is the second leading cause of death in the United States.
- Untreated cancer is usually fatal.

CAUSES

- Genetics: mutations can be passed from parent to child; some cancers display a high degree of incidence within families
- Viruses: can carry mutations into cells and insert abnormal genes in the human genome; several cancers are known to occur by this mechanism

- Environment: many pollutants, chemicals, gases, toxins, and exposure to radiation are known to initiate or promote cell transformation
- Lifestyle: stress, diet, occupation, infections such as Epstein-Barr and certain STDs, and use of substances such as tobacco, alcohol, and recreational drugs contribute to the risk for cancer

Signs & Symptoms

- Depend on specific disease
- Generally asymptomatic in early stages
- Late, systemic S/S include pain, anorexia, weakness, weight loss/cachexia, frequent infection

Diagnostics

Grading

- Measures the degree of cell disorganization (de-differentiation).
- Grading uses a scale (usually I to IV) with higher numbers indicating the least differentiation and thus most disorganized malignant cells.

Staging

- Categorizes the extent of the disease.
- An internationally recognized staging system is the TNM system. Each specific metastatic disease will have different criteria regarding these categories:
  1. T—tumor size (primary site)
  2. N—node involvement (regional)
  3. M—metastasis, absence or presence (at distant site)
- Cytologic examination is carried out on specimens from biopsied tissues, tumors, body secretions, or body fluids.
- *Tumor markers* are molecules detectable in serum or other body fluids that are used as a biochemical indicator of the presence of a malignancy. High levels of tumor markers mandate follow-up diagnostic studies.
- Oncologic imaging includes X-ray imaging, computed tomography (CT), magnetic resonance imaging (MRI), ultrasonography, radioisotope

scans, angiography, use of tagged antibodies, and use of direct visualization (e.g., sigmoidoscopy, endoscopy, etc.).

- Laboratory tests may be used to rule out nutritional disorders and other noncancerous conditions that may be causing the client's symptoms. However, some laboratory tests are useful in screening for specific cancerous conditions. See the specific condition for more information.

MEDICAL INTERVENTIONS

- Chemotherapy involves the use of cytotoxic chemicals to decrease tumor size, to prevent or treat suspected metastases, and, in some cancers, to effect a cure. Chemotherapy is used to disrupt the cell cycle in various phases by interrupting cell metabolism and replication. It also works by interfering with the ability of the malignant cell to synthesize needed enzymes and chemicals. Phase-specific drugs work during specific phases of the cell cycle; non–phase-specific drugs work through the entire cell cycle.
- Surgery is used for diagnosis and staging of more than 90% of all cancers and for primary treatment of more than 60%. Ideally, the entire tumor is removed.
- Radiation therapy may be used to kill the tumor, to reduce its size, to decrease pain, or to relieve obstruction. Lethal injury to DNA is believed to be the primary mechanism by which radiation kills cells.
- Immunotherapy (or biotherapy) is used to modify the biologic processes that support tumor growth, often by enhancing immune responses. Immunotherapy is still considered experimental and may be used to prevent tumor development in certain high-risk people or treat advanced and metastatic disease.
- Bone marrow transplantation is used to stimulate nonfunctioning marrow or replace diseased bone marrow. It is used to treat leukemias and may be used in treating some solid tumors such as breast cancer.

- Pharmacologic management of pain includes opioid and nonopioid analgesics as well as adjuvant medications to enhance the effect of the analgesic.

SELECTED NURSING DIAGNOSES WITH INTERVENTIONS

Anxiety

- Assess the client's level of anxiety.
- Establish a therapeutic relationship.
- Encourage the client to acknowledge and express feelings.
- Review the coping strategies the client has used in the past and build on past successful behaviors.
- Identify resources in the community that can help the client manage anxiety-producing situations.
- Provide specific information for the client about the disease, its treatment, and what may be expected.
- Provide a safe, calm, and quiet environment for the client in panic. Administer antianxiety medications per physician prescription.

Body Image Disturbance

- Assist the client and significant others to cope with the loss or change in appearance by providing a supportive environment, encouraging the client and significant others to express feelings, giving matter-of-fact responses to questions, identifying new coping strategies, and enlisting family and friends in reaffirming the client's worth.
- Teach the client and/or significant others to participate in the care of the afflicted body area.
- Teach the client specific strategies for minimizing physical changes, such as dressing to enhance appearance, using an ice cap or tight headband during chemotherapy treatments to decrease the amount of drug that reaches the hair follicles, and referring the client to support programs.

Anticipatory Grieving

- Use therapeutic communication skills to provide an open environment for the client and significant others to express their feelings and discuss their concerns.

- Answer questions about illness and prognosis honestly, while encouraging hope.
- Encourage the client to continue working and participating in activities he or she enjoys for as long as possible.
- Encourage the dying client to update his or her will and make funeral and burial plans to help the client maintain a sense of control.

Risk for Infection
- Monitor the client's vital signs.
- Monitor WBC counts frequently, especially for the client receiving chemotherapy that is known to cause bone marrow suppression.
- Teach the client and significant others to avoid crowds, small children, and people with infections when the WBC count is low and to practice scrupulous personal hygiene.
- Teach the client and significant others to protect the skin and mucous membranes from injury.
- Encourage the client to consume a diet rich in protein, minerals, and vitamins, especially vitamin C.

Altered Nutrition: Less than Body Requirements
- Assess the client's current eating patterns and identify factors that impair food intake.
- Evaluate the degree of malnutrition by checking laboratory values for total serum protein, albumin, and so on.
- Calculate nitrogen balance and creatinine-height index. Calculate skeletal muscle mass and compare findings with normal ranges.
- Take anthropometric measurements and compare them with standards.
- Teach the client the principles of maintaining good nutrition; adapt the client's diet to medical restrictions and current preferences.
- Encourage small, frequent meals. Cold and highly seasoned foods may appeal to clients with reduced sense of taste. Manage nausea and vomiting by administering antiemetic drugs and encouraging the client to eat small, frequent, low-fat meals, to avoid liquids with meals, and to sit upright for an hour after meals.
- Teach the client to supplement meals with nutritional supplements such as Ensure Plus or Isocal.

- Teach the client and significant others to keep a food diary to document the client's intake.
- Teach the client and significant others to administer parenteral nutrition via a central line or other vascular access device (VAD). Teach safety measures and care of the VAD. Provide an emergency phone number for help.

Other nursing diagnoses may be appropriate. See listings for each specific type of cancer.

CLIENT TEACHING

- Teach the client about the specific type of cancer and the treatment options available.
- Teach the client relaxation techniques, stress management, meditation, and so on.
- Provide the client with information about prescribed medications, effects, and side effects.
- Teach the client and significant others how to use any equipment placed in the home.
- Teach the client when to see the doctor for follow-up care.

HOME CARE CONSIDERATIONS

- Assist in making arrangements for transportation for follow-up appointments for medical care, chemotherapy, and/or radiation.
- Encourage the client to contact the American Cancer Society and other local cancer support groups.
- Make sure the client has the equipment and supplies needed for home care, and provide information on where to obtain further supplies. For the client needing complex care, a referral to a home health nurse is appropriate.
- Stress the importance of long-term medical follow-up care.
- Because people do not learn well under stress, provide the client and significant others a phone number to call for concerns and questions. Phone calls to the client for several days after the client arrives home are also appropriate.
- For the client with terminal disease, hospice care may be appropriate and should be discussed with the client and significant others.

Cross Reference: *Bladder Cancer; Bone Cancer; Brain Neoplasm, Benign and Malignant; Breast Cancer; Cervical Cancer; Colorectal Cancer; Endometrial Cancer; Hodgkin's Disease; Kaposi's Sarcoma; Leukemia; Lymphoma; Melanoma; Multiple Myeloma; Ovarian Cancer; Pancreatic Cancer; Prostate Cancer; Skin Cancer; Testicular Cancer. For more information on Cancer, see* Medical-Surgical Nursing *by LeMone and Burke, p. 311.*

Candidiasis (Moniliasis, Yeast Infection, Thrush)

OVERVIEW

- Candidiasis is an infection of the mucous membranes, nails, skin, or blood by fungi of the *Candida* genus.
- Mucous membranes of the vagina, oropharynx (thrush), esophagus, and GI tract are most frequently infected.
- *Candida* organisms are part of the normal vaginal environment, causing problems only when they multiply rapidly in response to antibiotic therapy, increased estrogen levels, fecal contamination, or other factors.
- Occasionally, the organisms may develop into a candidemia (hematologic infection), and infect various organ systems (brain, kidney, lung).
- Candidemia is most common in immunocompromised patients, such as those with HIV/AIDS, malignancy, diabetes, sepsis, trauma/burn injury, and history of IV drug use.
- The prognosis depends on the site and extent of infection as well as the state of the patient's resistance.

CAUSES

- Many *Candida* species are normal floral organisms that overgrow if the environment changes, as during antibiotic therapy and hyperglycemia, or if the host enters a period of immunosuppression

- *Candida albicans* is the most common species, but several others (*glabrata, guilliermondi, krusei, parapsilosis, tropicalis*) can cause deep infection and death in immunocompromised patients

Signs & Symptoms

- Depend on area of infection
- Oral lesions appear as discrete or confluent patches in the mouth and throat and on the tongue
- Vulvovaginal candidiasis causes intense pruritis; a creamy white, curdy discharge; and dysuria and dyspareunia
- Skin infection appears as red, macerated areas and/or pustules, usually around nailbeds (paronychia), glans penis (balanitis), or anus; drier areas may be red, papular, and scaly
- Nails are red, swollen, or crumbling
- Esophageal infection usually causes dysphagia
- Systemic infection may produce general signs and symptoms of fever, chills, rash, and prostration, or S/S specific to one organ system, such as meningitis, pneumonia, renal insufficiency, endocarditis, arthritis, osteomyelitis, myositis, or brain abscess

Diagnostics

- Wet smear (of mucous membrane, skin, nail scrapings) may show psuedohyphae; should be confirmed with culture (not diagnostic alone for superficial lesions).
- Biopsy for deeper lesions
- Culture of blood, cerebrospinal fluid (CSF), joint fluid

MEDICAL INTERVENTIONS

- Over-the-counter antifungal creams and suppositories are available for vaginal yeast infections.
- Oral antifungal agents, such as fluconazole, ketoconazole, clotrimazole troches, and nystatin troches, are used to treat thrush.

SELECTED NURSING DIAGNOSES

- Impaired Skin Integrity
- Risk for Sexual Dysfunction
- Altered Nutrition: Less than Body Requirements
- Pain
- Knowledge Deficit

SELECTED NURSING INTERVENTIONS

- Explain to the client the disease process and its transmission, prevention, and treatments.
- The client with a vaginal yeast infection should be told about the importance of having her partner evaluated and treated for infection.
- Administer prescribed antifungal agents as appropriate to site. Cover antifungal products in moist areas with a moisture barrier cream.
- Assess for signs of systemic infection.
- Provide the client with thrush small frequent feedings. Provide good oral hygiene and lidocaine-based mouthwash prior to eating.
- Suggest the use of cool compresses, vinegar douches, and sitz baths to alleviate the discomfort of vaginal yeast infections.

CLIENT TEACHING

- Discuss the disease process, prevention, and treatment, including administration of antifungals and side effects.
- Encourage the client with a vaginal yeast infection to consume daily 8 ounces of yogurt containing live active cultures to help restore normal vaginal flora.

HOME CARE CONSIDERATIONS

- Stress the importance of treating the client's sexual partner as appropriate.
- Tell the client that follow-up care is required for recurrence of symptoms.

For more information on Candidiasis, see Medical-Surgical Nursing *by LeMone and Burke, p. 580.*

Cardiomyopathy

OVERVIEW

- Cardiomyopathy is a primary or secondary disease of the myocardium (heart muscle) that affects its structure and/or function, leading to heart failure.
- Three types, based on pathophysiologic features, are recognized.

Dilated (Congestive)

- Damage to myofibrils, producing contractile dysfunction and dilation of all heart chambers, especially the ventricles; produces a very large heart that can be seen on x-ray; can begin as right or left but results in biventricular failure, dysrhythmias, and emboli; the most common type.

Hypertrophic

- Decreased compliance and significant hypertrophy of left ventricular muscle, especially the septal portion; cavity space does not increase, restricting filling; obstruction to outflow from ventricle, which lowers stroke volume and increases end systolic volume and workload; pulmonary congestion occurs.

Restrictive

- Fibrosis and scarring of myocardium and endocardium produce a stiff heart that restricts filling, lowering stroke volume.

CAUSES

Dilated

- No known positive cause, but associated with toxins (alcohol, drugs, radiation), metabolic disorders, or infectious (especially viral) agents as well as accompanying pregnancy/puerperium and systemic disease (neuromuscular, connective tissue, storage)

Hypertrophic

- Genetic, congenital idiopathic

Restrictive

- Infiltrative disease (amyloidosis, sarcoidosis, hematochromocytosis, neoplasms); storage diseases (glycogen, mucopolysaccharidoses); endomyocardial fibrosis; eosinophilic endomyocardial disease

Signs & Symptoms

Dilated

- S/S of left, then right, congestive heart failure, dysrhythmias, emboli formation, S_3, S_4 gallop

Hypertrophic

- May be asymptomatic until sudden death, or may present with dyspnea, angina, fatigue, syncope, cardiac dysrhythmias

Restrictive

- S/S of right heart failure, S_3, S_4 gallop

Diagnostics

- EKG shows dysrhythmias associated with each type.
- Echocardiography can show chamber size, wall enlargement/thinning, abnormal wall motions.
- Chest x-ray may show cardiomegaly, pulmonary congestion, or pleural effusion.
- Angiography may reveal dilated, hypokinetic ventricles.
- Biopsy can distinguish specific types.
- Hemodynamic studies can distinguish specific types.

MEDICAL INTERVENTIONS

- Pharmacologic agents include vasodilators, diuretics, angiotensin converting enzyme (ACE) inhibitors, and cardiac glycosides. Beta-blockers are the drugs of choice to reduce anginal symptoms and syncopal episodes for clients with hypertrophic cardiomyopathy.

- Cardiac transplant is the definitive treatment for dilated cardiomyopathy.

SELECTED NURSING DIAGNOSES

- Decreased Cardiac Output
- Fatigue
- Ineffective Breathing Pattern
- Anxiety
- Fear
- Altered Role Performance
- Anticipatory Grieving

SELECTED NURSING INTERVENTIONS

- Administer prescribed medications and monitor the client for effects and side effects.
- Assess heart and lung sounds and peripheral pulses, monitor blood pressure, and assess for symptoms of heart failure.
- Assess the client's level of comfort and ability to tolerate activity. Provide frequent rest periods and assistance with activities of daily living (ADLs) as needed.
- Discuss all treatment options with the client and significant others, including the need for cardiac transplant, if indicated. Encourage the client and significant others to discuss their questions, concerns, and fears. Assist the client to verbalize fears of potential loss.
- Assess past experiences of the client and significant others with loss, their existing support systems, and current grief work. Discuss phases of the greiving process with the client and family.

CLIENT TEACHING

- Teach the client and significant others about the disease process, its ultimate outcome, and treatment options.
- Teach self-care measures such as activity restrictions, dietary changes, and pharmacologic measures to reduce symptoms or prevent complications.
- Clients who are undergoing invasive procedures for diagnosis and treatment of cardiomyopathy require preoperative and postoperative teaching.

HOME CARE CONSIDERATIONS

- Discuss treatment options such as an implanted automatic internal defibrillator for clients who experience potentially lethal dysrhythmias and cardiac transplantation.
- Encourage significant others to maintain current skills in administering CPR because of the risk of sudden death associated with some cardiomyopathies.
- For clients who have undergone cardiac transplant, emphasize the need for lifetime immunosuppression to prevent rejection of the transplanted organ. Stress the risks of infection postoperatively related to immunosuppression. Teach the client and significant others to recognize manifestations of organ rejection and to report them promptly to the physician.
- Referral to home health care may be appropriate.
- Referral to a psychologic counselor or support group may help the client and/or significant others cope with the diagnosis and prognosis.

For more information on Cardiomyopathy, see Medical-Surgical Nursing *by LeMone and Burke, p. 1152.*

Carpal Tunnel Syndrome

OVERVIEW

- Carpal tunnel syndrome is a disorder in which the medial nerve is entrapped within the carpal tunnel of the wrist.
- It is the most common nerve entrapment syndrome.
- It is most commonly seen in women 30 to 60 years of age.

CAUSES

- Occupational risk factors include computer workers, assembly line workers, switchboard operators (e.g., any job requiring repetitive hand movements)
- Any condition that causes swelling or obstruction of the wrist, such as rheumatoid arthritis, tendinitis, pregnancy, renal failure, menopause, diabetes mellitus, hypothyroidism/myxedema, amyloidosis, or trauma

Signs & Symptoms

- Pain in thumb, forefinger, middle finger, and half of fourth finger; more severe at night and in morning; pain may radiate to shoulder
- Paresthesia, numbness, tingling, burning
- Weakness, clumsiness, decreased ability to clench fist
- Atrophic nails, dry and shiny skin
- Thenar muscle atrophy
- Decreased response to pinpricks
- Positive compression test—application of inflated blood pressure cuff elicits S/S
- Positive Phalen's test—flexion of both wrists to 90 degrees while pressing dorsal aspects of hands together elicits pain or paresthesia
- Positive Tinel's test—light percussion over median nerve elicits tingling

Diagnostics

- Electromyogram (EMG) shows median nerve conduction velocity delayed >5 milliseconds.

MEDICAL INTERVENTIONS

- Pharmacologic agents usually include nonsteroidal anti-inflammatory drugs (NSAIDs). The physician may opt to inject corticosteroids into the joint.
- Surgery entails resection of the carpal ligament to enlarge the tunnel.

SELECTED NURSING DIAGNOSES WITH INTERVENTIONS

Pain

- Ask the client to rate the pain on a scale of 0 to 10 before and after interventions.
- Encourage the use of immobilizers.
- Apply ice.
- Apply heat.
- Administer NSAIDs per physician's prescription.

Impaired Physical Mobility

- Provide care to alleviate pain.
- Consult the physical therapist for exercises per physician's prescription.
- Suggest occupational rehabilitation to the client and physician.

CLIENT TEACHING

- Teach the client about the injury, its causes, and treatment, including medication regimen.
- Help the client explore ways of avoiding further injury.
- Caution the client to avoid hot temperatures to the affected hand.

HOME CARE CONSIDERATIONS

- Discuss measures to prevent carpal tunnel syndrome in clients with high-risk occupations, including use of wrist supports with computer keyboard and mouse, and appropriate keyboard height.
- A hand and forearm splint may help relieve pain, particularly when worn at night.
- Tell the client who has undergone surgery to avoid heavy lifting with the affected hand for at least 4 to 6 weeks.

For more information on Carpal Tunnel Syndrome, see Medical-Surgical Nursing *by LeMone and Burke, p. 1614.*

Cataract

OVERVIEW

- A cataract is an opacity of the lens or lens capsule of the eye.
- As the lens ages, its fibers and proteins change and degenerate, losing clarity. The process usually begins at the periphery of the lens, gradually spreading to the central portion. Opacity reduces the amount of light reaching the retina.
- It is a very common cause of vision loss.
- Cataracts are most common in people older than 70 years of age.

CAUSES

- Genetic: primary or accompanying many other genetic disorders (Alport's, Conradi's, cri du chat, and Down syndromes; Crouzon's disease)
- Congenital: most often secondary to intrauterine exposure to rubella, but also to herpes simplex virus (HSV), varicella zoster virus (VZV), cytomegalovirus (CMV), and syphilis
- Senile: occurs due to age-related changes in water and protein content
- Traumatic: may be unilateral; blunt, penetrating blows; burns
- Toxic: heavy smoking, chemicals (naphthalene), drugs (corticosteroids, ergot, phenothiazines)
- Radiation: long-term UVB exposure (sunlight), ionizing, infrared
- Accompanying other eye disorders: detached retina, glaucoma, retinitis, uveitis
- Secondary to metabolic disorders: diabetes mellitus, Fabry's disease, Wilson's disease, Lowe's syndrome, galactosemia, myxedema, chronic hypercalcemia

Signs & Symptoms

- Painless, gradual loss of visual acuity (clouding, blurring)
- Milky white lens
- Reports of headlight glare at night; better vision in dim light

Diagnostics

- Indirect ophthalmoscopy shows a dark area in red reflex.
- Slit-lamp examination shows opacity.
- Visual acuity tests correlate amount of lens involved to function.

MEDICAL INTERVENTIONS

- Surgical removal is the only treatment for cataracts at this time. No medical therapies are available to prevent or treat them.

SELECTED NURSING DIAGNOSES

- Sensory/Perceptual Alteration: Visual
- Risk for Injury
- Anxiety
- Fear

SELECTED NURSING INTERVENTIONS

- Explain the nonemergent nature of the condition, and help the client to determine the extent to which the cataract is affecting daily life. Provide information and support to help the client decide when to proceed with surgery.
- Many clients may fear blindness. Maintain a caring, understanding attitude when teaching and listening to the client to help the client cope with this fear prior to surgery.
- Ensure that the pre- and postoperative environment is safe for the client and free of obstructions.
- Provide preoperative teaching regarding the surgery and expected outcomes and limitations.

- Administer pre- and postoperative medications per physician's prescription.
- Maintain the client in semi-Fowler's position or turn the client to the side that did not have surgery.
- Report to the physician any signs of drainage, severe pain, nausea, vomiting, or changes in vision in the eye that did not have surgery.

CLIENT TEACHING

- Advise the client to use eyeglasses, sunglasses, or an eyeshield for protection both day and night.
- Teach the client to use an eye shield at night to avoid inadvertent damage to eye sutures while sleeping.
- Tell the client to avoid coughing, sneezing, heavy lifting, bending at waist, and sleeping on operative side as per the physician's instructions.
- Review the administration of eye drops and ointments with the client and significant others.
- Tell the client to avoid washing the hair until several days after the surgery, and to keep the head tilted back. The client also should avoid getting water into the eyes during showering.
- Remind the client that changes in activities in daily living (ADLs) may be required owing to vision changes after the surgery or with use of prescribed contact lenses or eyeglasses.

HOME CARE CONSIDERATIONS

- A home safety assessment is appropriate for this client to prevent accidents.
- Remind the client of the importance of follow-up visits with the ophthalmologist.
- Tell the client to abstain from driving, operating machinery, or participating in sports activities until the physician has approved resuming these activities.

For more information on Cataract, see Medical-Surgical Nursing *by LeMone and Burke, p. 1907.*

Cerebral Vascular Accident (CVA, Stroke, Brain Attack)

OVERVIEW

- A cerebral vascular accident (CVA) is a sudden reduction in cerebral perfusion secondary to a thrombus, embolus, or hemorrhage.
- Reduction in blood flow reduces available oxygen and can result in temporary deficits or permanent brain damage.
- CVA is the third leading cause of death in the United States; 500,000 cases per year resulting in about 200,000 deaths and significant neurologic damage.

CAUSES

- *Thrombosis* is the most common cause in middle-aged and older persons; it results from occlusion of a (usually extracerebral) vessel, (e.g., carotids) with atheromatous plaques; may be preceded by transient ischemic attack (TIA); risk factors include smoking, sedentary lifestyle, and atherosclerosis
- *Embolus* is the second most common cause; it can occur at any age, and is associated with pre-existing peripheral thrombophlebitis, atherosclerosis, rheumatic heart disease, endocarditis, valve disease, or cardiac dysrhythmias or following open heart surgery; usually involves the middle cerebral artery; risk factors include smoking; oral contraceptive use; sedentary lifestyle
- *Hemorrhage* is the least common cause; it can occur at any age; a vessel ruptures secondary to aneurysm, hypertension, or trauma; also results from blood dyscrasias

Signs & Symptoms

- Vary with location and extent of each type of lesion
- General S/S include weakness; dizziness; contralateral hemiparesis or hemiplegia; changes in cognition or levels of consciousness; seizures;

communication difficulties (agnosia, aphasia, apraxia); coma
- Onset and prognosis vary according to type:
  1. Thrombotic—gradual development of S/S, onset over minutes, hours, days; prognosis good
  2. Embolic—sudden onset of S/S, not related to activity; usually immediate maximum deficits; prognosis fair to good
  3. Hemorrhagic—sudden onset, with continued development or worsening of S/S; onset associated with activity; headache and nuchal rigidity (stiff neck due to meningeal irritation of blood); may be rapid development of deepening coma; poor prognosis

Diagnostics

- Lumbar puncture may be bloody, if hemorrhagic type.
- Computed tomography (CT) scan shows edema, lesions, structural details with high accuracy.
- Positron emission tomography (PET) scan gives blood flow and metabolic activity data; especially useful for thrombotic or embolic CVA.
- Magnetic resonance imaging (MRI) delineates size and location of lesion only.
- Ophthalmoscopy shows signs of hypertension or atheromatous blood vessel changes.
- Angiography shows arterial vessel shadow and can identify narrowing, blockage, or rupture.
- EEG can assess localized damage.

MEDICAL INTERVENTIONS

- Antiplatelet agents are often used to treat clients with TIAs or who have had a previous CVA.
- Thrombolytic and anticoagulant drug therapy is often prescribed for thrombotic CVA during the stroke-in-evolution phase, but is contraindicated in complete stroke because it may increase the risk of cerebral hemorrhage.
- Antithrombotic drugs, which inhibit the platelet phase of clot formation, have been used as a preventive measure for clients at risk for embolic and thrombotic CVA.

- Calcium channel blockers are under investigation and have been used in clinical trials to reduce cerebral vasospasm.
- Surgery may be performed to prevent the occurrence of a CVA or to restore blood flow when a CVA has already occurred.

SELECTED NURSING DIAGNOSES WITH INTERVENTIONS

Altered Tissue Perfusion: Cerebral

- Monitor respiratory status and airway patency. Suction as necessary, position client in side-lying position, and administer oxygen as prescribed.
- Monitor neurologic status by assessing mental status and level of consciousness, strength, reflexes, pain, posturing, and so on.
- Continuously monitor cardiac status, observing for dysrhythmias.
- Monitor body temperature.
- Maintain accurate intake and output records. Measure urinary excretion via a Foley catheter.
- Monitor the client for seizures. Pad the side rails, and administer prescribed anticonvulsants.

Impaired Physical Mobility

- Encourage active range-of-motion (ROM) exercises for unaffected extremities and perform passive ROM exercises for affected extremities every 4 hours during the day and evening shifts and once during the night shift. Support the joint during passive ROM exercises.
- Turn the client every 2 hours around the clock. Maintain body alignment, and support extremities in proper position with pillows.
- Monitor the lower extremities each shift for symptoms of thrombophlebitis. Assess for Homan's sign (pain on passive dorsiflexion of the foot). Assess for increased warmth and redness in calves. Measure the circumference of the calves and thighs.
- Do not use a footboard. Use hand splints only as directed by the physician and physical therapist to prevent flexion contractures of the fingers and wrists.
- Collaborate with the physical therapist as the client gains mobility, using consistent techniques to

move the client from the bed to the wheelchair or to help the client ambulate.

Self-Care Deficit

- Encourage the client to use the unaffected arm to bathe, brush teeth, comb hair, dress, and eat.
- Teach the client and significant others to put on clothing by first dressing the affected extremities and then dressing the unaffected extremities.
- Collaborate with the occupational therapist in scheduling times for training for upper-extremity functioning necessary for activities of daily living (ADLs). Encourage the use of assistive devices if required for eating, physical hygiene, and dressing.

Impaired Verbal Communication

- Approach and treat the client as an adult. Do not assume that the client who does not respond verbally cannot hear. Allow adequate time for the client to respond. Face the client and speak slowly. When you do not understand what the client has said, be honest and say so. Use short, simple statements and questions.
- Accept the client's frustration and anger as a normal reaction to the loss of function.
- Try alternate methods of communication, including writing tablets, flash cards, and computerized talking boards.

CLIENT TEACHING

- Teach the client about CVA, its causes, treatment, and prevention.
- Discuss the client's strategies for self-care, mobility, and coping skills. Provide teaching as appropriate.
- Review medications, including dosage, effects, and side effects.

HOME CARE CONSIDERATIONS

- Review home and equipment modifications and use as appropriate, including, for example, a wheelchair, walker, raised toilet seat, grab bars in the bathroom, bath chair, vise lid opener, long-handled shoe horn, and so on.
- Referral to a home health nurse, physical and occupational therapy may be appropriate.

- Initiate communications with a long-term-care facility about the established plan of care if the client is going to such a setting for rehabilitation or care.
- Refer the client to Meals-on-Wheels, eldercare groups, social services, the National Stroke Association, stroke clubs, support groups, and respite care, as appropriate.

For more information on Cerebral Vascular Accident, see Medical-Surgical Nursing *by LeMone and Burke, p. 1764.*

Cervical Cancer

OVERVIEW

- Cervical cancer is classified as *preinvasive or invasive.*
- *Preinvasive* cervical changes are confined to the superficial layers of the cervix and represent a long (10 years) latent period of cervical intraepithelial neoplasia, beginning as mild dysplasia (premalignant) and ending in carcinoma in situ (malignant).
- *Invasive carcinoma* represents the extension of the above through the basement membrane, separating superficial cells from deeper tissues below; metastasis is via lymphatics.
- Invasive cervical cancer is the third highest reproductive-tract cancer in women, with approximately 15,700 new cases diagnosed annually, causing about 4900 deaths per year.
- It is usually (80%) squamous-cell carcinoma; others are adenocarcinoma.
- Distant metastasis is to liver, lungs, and bone.
- Death rates have dropped dramatically over the past 40 years owing to the widespread use of the Pap smear as a screening tool.
- Five-year survival rates are 68% (all stages combined); 91% (early invasive); 100% (preinvasive, carcinoma in situ).

CAUSES

Considered by most experts to be a sexually transmitted disease caused chiefly by human papilloma virus (HPV). Risk factors include:

- Sexual intercourse prior to age 16
- Multiple sexual partners, history of prostitution
- Multiparity, early first pregnancy
- Low socioeconomic class
- History of sexually transmitted diseases, especially HPV
- History of chronic cervicitis, untreated
- Smoking
- Age greater than 50 years (invasive)

Signs & Symptoms

- Preinvasive and early invasive carcinoma are asymptomatic.
- Abnormal bleeding or spotting after intercourse are common early signs; this may increase to intermenstrual or heavy menstrual bleeding.
- Yellowish vaginal discharge, lumbosacral back pain, and urinary symptoms also may develop.
- S/S of advanced carcinoma include bowel/bladder dysfunction or fistula formation; severe pelvic pain; bone pain; anorexia/weight loss/cachexia; fatigue

Diagnostics

- Pap smear, recommended yearly, shows abnormal desquamated cervical cells which can be categorized into classes (I to V) of increasing severity.
- Colposcopy magnifies cervix, and application of iodine dye (Schiller's test) isolates areas of abnormal-appearing tissue for biopsy.
- Biopsy determines degree of cellular neoplasia and depth of lesion.
- Various scans (bladder, bone, lung), and lymphangiogram are used to locate distant metastasis.

MEDICAL INTERVENTIONS

- Surgical interventions include conization, vaginal hysterectomy, and radical hysterectomy. Pelvic

exenteration, used for recurring cancers, involves removal of some or all of the pelvic organs, and may require urinary diversion and colostomy.
- Radiation therapy is used to treat the late stages of cervical cancer.

SELECTED NURSING DIAGNOSES

- Anxiety
- Fear
- Risk for Sexual Dysfunction
- Risk for Infection
- Risk for Injury
- Risk for Body Image Disturbance

SELECTED NURSING INTERVENTIONS

- Assess the client's level of anxiety, concerns about sexual functioning, and adjustment to altered body image.
- Provide routine pre- and postoperative care as appropriate for pelvic surgeries. Explain what the client should expect after surgery, including transfer to a critical care unit, invasive tubes, IV lines, and so on.
- After surgery, assess for potential complications such as wound infection, hemorrhage, pneumonia.
- Implement a sanitary pad count for vaginal procedures.
- Assess the client's level of pain, and administer prescribed pain medications. Provide perineal irrigations or sitz baths as prescribed.

CLIENT TEACHING

- Teach the client about the disease process, its causes, treatment, and prognosis. Discuss medications—their dosage, effects, and side effects.
- Teach self-care appropriate to the client's treatment. For instance, the client with a total exenteration will require teaching for colostomy care and possible referral to an enterostomal specialist.
- Discuss the importance of long-term monitoring of the amount, type, and duration of vaginal discharge.

HOME CARE CONSIDERATIONS

- Teach all women, particularly young women, about the importance of regular pelvic examinations and PAP smears. Include teaching about risk factors for cervical cancer and measures to reduce the risk.
- Provide the client with information about complications, including signs of infection, that should be reported immediately to the physician.
- Counsel the client about the need for long-term follow-up care.
- Schedule a consultation with a dietitian to provide the client with an individualized dietary plan.
- A referral to a sex therapist may be appropriate to assist the client in coping with the psychologic and physical changes associated with cervical cancer and its treatment.

For more information on Cervical Cancer, see Medical-Surgical Nursing *by LeMone and Burke,* p. 2029.

Cervicitis

OVERVIEW

- Cervicitis is an inflammation of endocervical tissues, most frequently due to infection.
- Both acute and chronic forms may occur.
- Untreated cervicitis can lead to endometriosis or salpingitis.

CAUSES

- Usually due to infection, particularly sexually transmitted diseases such as chlamydia, gonorrhea, trichomonas, or ureaplasma
- Can also be due to *Staphylococcus, Streptococcus* or *Escherichia coli,* or viruses (HSV, HPV)

Signs & Symptoms

- Discharge from endocervix; type depends on causative organism
- Pelvic pain, dyspareunia or postcoital
- Intermenstrual spotting
- Visually inflamed cervix

Diagnostics

- Pelvic examination reveals inflamed cervix.
- Pap smear reveals inflammatory or dysplastic cells.
- Culture and sensitivity identifies causative organism and preferred antibiotic.

MEDICAL INTERVENTIONS

- Pharmacologic agents include antibiotics and antiviral drugs such as acyclovir, depending on the causative organism.
- Surgical interventions include cryosurgery, electrocoagulation, and laser treatment. These are reserved for clients with persistent symptoms.

SELECTED NURSING DIAGNOSES

- Pain
- Risk for Sexual Dysfunction
- Impaired Tissue Integrity

SELECTED NURSING INTERVENTIONS

- Administer prescribed antibiotic or antiviral medications and monitor effects and side effects.
- Assess for signs and symptoms of systemic infection, especially elevated temperature.
- Assess the client's pain on a scale of 0 to 10 before and after treatment.
- Administer prescribed pain medications and assess effectiveness.

CLIENT TEACHING

- Teach the client how to practice safe sex (e.g., use of latex condoms, increased risk with multiple partners, etc.).

- Stress the importance of having the client's sexual partner(s) evaluated and treated to prevent reinfection.
- Explain the importance of completing all of the prescribed medication regimen.

HOME CARE CONSIDERATIONS

- Encourage follow-up visits for gynecologic care as per physician's instructions.

Chlamydial Infection

OVERVIEW

- Chlamydia is the most common sexually transmitted disease in the United States; it affects an estimated 4 million people each year.
- The causative organism, *Chlamydia trachomatis,* is an obligate intracellular bacterial parasite.
- In women, *C. trachomatis* causes cervicitis, urethritis, and proctitis, and is the most common cause of pelvic inflammatory disease (PID).
- Chlamydial infection during pregnancy has been associated in some studies with premature delivery and/or postpartum endometritis.
- Newborns delivered vaginally to infected mothers may acquire chlamydial infection, with 25% to 50% developing conjunctivitis and 10% to 20% developing chlamydial pneumonitis.
- The major cause of nongonococcal urethritis in males, *C. trachomatis* also causes epididymitis, prostatitis, and proctitis.
- Reiter's syndrome is a potential complication of the infection that consists of conjunctivitis, urethritis in men, cervicitis in women, arthritis, and mucocutaneous lesions.
- Lymphogranuloma venereum is a regional pelvic infection by certain strains (L2 most common) that cause inguinal or pelvic lymphadenopathy and inguinal ulceration and adhesion formation.
- In immunocompromised clients, chlamydia can cause pneumonia.

CAUSES

- Multiple strains of *Chlamydia trachomatis*
- Almost always transmitted sexually, orally, or congenitally from mother to newborn

Signs & Symptoms

- May be asymptomatic
- Cervicitis: yellow mucopurulent discharge, cervical edema, fragility, and eventually erosion
- PID: tenderness or pain of abdomen and pelvic region, fever, chills, bleeding/discharge, lymphadenopathy, S/S of urethritis, infertility
- Urethritis: erythema, dysuria, frequency, pruritis, purulent discharge
- Epididymitis: scrotal edema and pain
- Prostatitis: low back pain, painful ejaculation, S/S of urethritis
- Proctitis: rectal ulceration, rectal pain, mucus discharge, bleeding, tenesmus
- Lymphogranuloma venereum: painless skin lesion (vesicle or ulcer), regional lymphadenopathy, fever, chills, myalgia, headache, backache, weight loss

Diagnostics

- Identification of polymorphonuclear leukocytes (PMNs) on Gram stain of urethral (males) or cervical discharge provides presumptive evidence of infection.
- Tests for antibodies to chlamydia, such as direct fluorescent antibody test (DFA) and an enzyme-linked immunosorbent assay (ELISA), are less specific than tissue cultures but more rapid and readily available.
- Polymerase chain reaction (PCR) or ligase chain reaction (LCR) tests are highly sensitive, specific tests that can be performed on urine and vaginal swab specimens.

MEDICAL INTERVENTIONS

- The drugs of choice for chlamydial infection in men and nonpregnant women are oral doxycycline or tetracycline. For pregnant women, erythromycin is the alternative therapy.

SELECTED NURSING DIAGNOSES

- Pain
- Sexual Dysfunction
- Anxiety

SELECTED NURSING INTERVENTIONS

- Assess the client's level of pain. Teach the client about the medication regimen as well as nonpharmacologic measures to reduce pain.
- Provide a supportive, nonjudgmental environment for the client to discuss feelings and ask questions. Allow time and privacy to address the client's concerns.
- Encourage open communication between the client and his or her sexual partner(s).
- Help the client to focus on the present situation as a means of identifying coping mechanisms needed to reduce anxiety.

CLIENT TEACHING

- Teach the client the need to comply with the treatment regimen, to refer partner(s) for examination and treatment, and to use condoms to avoid reinfection.
- Review with the client the complications of untreated chlamydial infection.

HOME CARE CONSIDERATIONS

- Tell the client to avoid sexual activity until the chlamydia has been eradicated.
- Provide the client with a pamphlet or other literature on sexually transmitted diseases and their prevention and treatment.
- Discuss safer sex practices to reduce future risk of STDs.

For more information on Chlamydial Infection, see Medical-Surgical Nursing *by LeMone and Burke, p. 2090.*

Cholecystitis

OVERVIEW

- Cholecystitis is an acute or chronic inflammation of the gallbladder.
- Acute inflammation is due to abrupt obstruction of bile duct with cholelithiasis (gallstones); blood and lymph drainage is reduced, producing stasis; bacteria infiltrate and proliferate; and the inflammatory reaction causes tissue edema (cholangitis), resulting in ischemia and necrosis.
- Chronic inflammation is almost always due to the presence of stones, which result in persistent mechanical irritation.

CAUSES

The exact cause of cholelithiasis and thus cholecystitis is unknown. Risk factors include:

- Age greater than 40 years
- Female sex
- Increased estrogen secondary to pregnancy, multiparity, oral contraceptive use, or estrogen replacement therapy
- High-fat, high-cholesterol diet
- Antilipemic medication
- Very low calorie diet for rapid weight loss
- Systemic disease, such as diabetes mellitus, ileal disorders, hemolytic anemias, liver disease, or pancreatitis

Signs & Symptoms

- Pain:
    1. severe epigastric right-upper-quadrant (RUQ) pain
    2. sudden onset, increasing intensity
    3. radiates to back or referred to right scapula
    4. precipitated by a fatty meal (fat intolerance)
- Indigestion
- Flatulence
- Nausea, vomiting

- Low-grade fever, chills, diaphoresis
- Possible jaundice with clay-colored stools
- Increased white blood cell (WBC) count

Diagnostics

- Ultrasound of gallbladder is extremely accurate in locating stones.
- Oral cholecystogram identifies stones.
- Percutaneous transhepatic cholangiography will distinguish between gallbladder disease and pancreatic carcinoma.
- Positive Murphy's sign (client inspires while examiner holds fingers under liver border; inspiration causes pain due to gallbladder inflammation).

MEDICAL INTERVENTIONS

- Laparoscopic cholecystectomy, or removal of the gallbladder and its stones, is the treatment of choice for clients with recurrent gallbladder disease. Simple or open cholecystectomy may be necessary for clients with acute cholecystitis.
- Gallbladder stones may be fragmented using extracorporeal shock wave lithotripsy. This procedure uses ultrasound to align the stones with the source of shock waves. Because of a significant risk of recurring stone formation after the procedure, gallstone dissolution agents (medical litholytic therapy) generally are prescribed for an indefinite period following lithotripsy.
- Gallstone dissolution is an alternative to surgical intervention for clients who refuse surgery or are not candidates for it. UDCA and CDCA alter the processes by which gallstones are formed and can completely dissolve existing stones within 2 years. The recurrence of stone formation following litholytic therapy is high, however.

SELECTED NURSING DIAGNOSES WITH INTERVENTIONS

Pain

- Teach clients to avoid fat in their diets, and why.
- If dietary therapy is not effective, administer prescribed medications.

- If severe pain is unrelieved by other methods, administer prescribed narcotic analgesia.
- Monitor temperature every 4 hours; elevations may indicate presence of an infection or inflammation.
- Assist the client to a Fowler's position to decrease diaphragmatic pressure on the inflamed area.

Risk for Impaired Gas Exchange

Following a cholecystectomy, clients may have difficulty with effective breathing because of the high abdominal incision.

- Institute a regimen of turning, deep breathing, and coughing at least every 2 hours and use of an incentive spirometer every hour while awake, and begin early ambulation at least four times daily.
- Provide proper analgesia for the postoperative client.

Risk for Infection

Infection following a cholecystectomy with T-tube insertion may arise from varying sources.

- Assess for signs of systemic and localized infection during the immediate postoperative period by monitoring temperature every 4 hours.
- Assess the wound at least every 4 hours.
- Perform abdominal assessment at least every 4 hours.

CLIENT TEACHING

- Explain the role of bile and the function of the gallbladder in terms that the client and significant others can understand.
- Discuss treatment alternatives with the client as appropriate.
- Preoperatively, prepare the client for what to expect regarding type of surgery, pain, possible nausea, and nursing assessments, as well as self-care to prevent problems such as pneumonia.
- Postoperatively, teach the client and significant others about pain control, T-tube care, and monitoring for and preventing infection.
- Teach the client the importance of maintaining a low-fat diet, and provide the client with a list of foods high in fat and some low-fat alternatives.

HOME CARE CONSIDERATIONS

- A home care referral for wound and T-tube care may be appropriate.
- Ensure that the client has a scheduled follow-up visit with the surgeon for T-tube removal.

For more information on Cholecystitis, see Medical-Surgical Nursing *by LeMone and Burke, p. 512.*

Chronic Obstructive Pulmonary Disease (COPD)

OVERVIEW

- COPD is defined as chronic airway obstruction secondary to a number of diseases that produce airway collapse or inflammation that result in airway bronchospasm/swelling, and excess mucus.
- Usually more than one primary disease contributes to the overall obstructive process.
- These conditions result in airflow resistance and limitation during expiration, with distal gas trapping, and irreversible distal lung distention.
- COPD eventually leads to pulmonary insufficiency, pulmonary hypertension, cor pulmonale (right-heart failure due to lung disease), and respiratory failure.
- It is the most common cause of lung disease, affecting more than 18 million people in the United States.
- COPD is the second leading cause of disability in the United States.

CAUSES

- Asthma
- Bronchiectasis
- Chronic bronchitis
- Cystic fibrosis (genetic)
- Emphysema (genetic/nongenetic)

- Any combination of above
- Risk factors include cigarette smoking, air pollution, recurrent pulmonary infection, and allergies

Signs & Symptoms

- Usually appear in middle age, except with cystic fibrosis, which is present at birth
- Dyspnea on exertion is usually first symptom; early, exertional, progresses to rest
- Shortness of breath
- Cough
- Breath sounds: diminished or adventitious (rales, rhonchi, wheeze); depend on type, stage
- S/S specific to type. See Asthma; Bronchiectasis; Chronic Bronchitis; Emphysema

Diagnostics

- Chest x-ray shows increased AP chest diameter, diaphragm position, lung markings, hyperinflation, and cardiac silhouette.
- Arterial blood gases (ABGs) assess status of ventilation-perfusion and identify respiratory insufficiency or failure.
- Pulmonary function tests can show reduced vital capacity, increased residual volume, increased total lung capacity, decreased FEV_1 (one minute forced expiratory flow volume).
- Sputum culture and sensitivity identifies infectious bacteria and effective antibiotic.
- Complete blood count (CBC) can show increased red blood cells (RBCs), if hypoxemia (compensatory); increased white blood cells (WBCs), if infection.
- EKG may show right-heart strain, atrial/ventricular dysrhythmias.

MEDICAL INTERVENTIONS

- Immunization against pneumococcal pneumonia and yearly influenza vaccine are recommended. A broad-spectrum antibiotic is prescribed if infection is suspected.
- A therapeutic trial of bronchodilator therapy is initiated for all clients with symptomatic COPD.

- Corticosteroid therapy is used primarily for clients who have asthmatic bronchitis as a component of their COPD or who do not respond to bronchodilators. Alpha$_1$-antitrypsin replacement therapy is available for clients with emphysema due to a genetic deficiency of the enzyme.
- Home oxygen therapy may be required.
- Smoking cessation is vital to slow the progression of COPD.

SELECTED NURSING DIAGNOSES WITH INTERVENTIONS

Ineffective Airway Clearance

- Perform respiratory assessment every 1 to 2 hours or as indicated. Assess rate and pattern; cough and secretions; and breath sounds.
- Assess skin color and mental status frequently.
- Monitor arterial blood gas (ABG) results.
- Maintain pulse oximetry and monitor values.
- Assess hydration status by weighing the client, measuring intake and output, and monitoring status of mucous membranes and skin turgor.
- Encourage a fluid intake of at least 2000 to 2500 mL per day unless contraindicated.
- Position the client to facilitate maximal lung ventilation. Encourage movement and activity to tolerance.
- Assist the client to cough at least every 2 hours while awake.
- Provide tissues and a paper bag for disposal of expectorated sputum.
- Refer the client to a respiratory therapist and assist with or perform percussion and postural drainage as needed.
- Provide endotracheal, oral, or nasopharyngeal suctioning as needed.
- Provide for rest periods between treatments and procedures.
- Administer prescribed expectorant and bronchodilator medications. Correlate timing with respiratory treatments.
- Provide humidified oxygen therapy as prescribed.
- Prepare for intubation and mechanical ventilation if the client's condition deteriorates.

- Assess the client's knowledge and understanding of the choices involved and possible consequences for each.
- Acknowledge the client's concerns, values, and beliefs, and listen nonjudgmentally.
- Spend time with the client, allowing the client to express feelings.
- Help the client to plan a course of action for quitting smoking and adapt it as necessary.
- Demonstrate respect for the client's decisions and right to choose.
- Provide referral to a counselor or other professional as needed.

CLIENT TEACHING

- Teach effective breathing techniques, such as pursed-lip breathing and diaphragmatic or abdominal breathing; and effective coughing techniques, such as controlled coughing and huff coughing.
- Teach the client to maintain adequate fluid intake, at least 2 to 2.5 quarts of fluid daily.
- Stress the importance of avoiding respiratory irritants, including cigarette smoke and cold, dry air, and of avoiding exposure to infection.
- Discuss with the client the importance of maintaining adequate food intake, eating small, frequent meals, and using nutritional supplements to provide adequate kilocalories.
- Provide instruction on the proper use of medications, including their effects and side effects.

HOME CARE CONSIDERATIONS

- Tell the client to report promptly to the physician any of the following signs or symptoms: fever, increase in sputum production, purulent (green or yellow) sputum, upper respiratory tract infection, increased shortness of breath, decreased activity tolerance or appetite, and increased need for oxygen.
- Review the use of home oxygen, nebulizers, and any special home equipment.
- Advise clients to obtain and wear an identification band and carry a list of their medications at all times.

- A referral to a smoking cessation program may be appropriate.
- A home care referral for oxygen therapy may be appropriate.

For more information on Chronic Obstructive Pulmonary Disease, see Medical-Surgical Nursing *by LeMone and Burke, p. 1433.*

Cirrhosis

OVERVIEW

- Cirrhosis is diffuse fibrosis with nodular regeneration of the liver resulting from irreversible chronic injury to liver parenchyma. Fibrous tissue replaces normal functioning liver tissue and forms constrictive bands disrupting vascular and biliary flow within the liver.
- It is the final common pathway for a number of liver diseases.
- Cirrhosis is twice as common in men as in women.
- Several types of cirrhosis exist:
  1. *Alcoholic (Laennec's):* the most common type, shows diffuse, micronodular, fatty liver
  2. *Postnecrotic (postviral):* usually associated with hepatitis B or hepatitis C infection; displays a macronodular lesion, widespread loss of hepatocytes, hepatic bands, and nests of regenerating liver cells of varying size
  3. *Biliary:* results from injury to or prolonged obstruction of the biliary system; can be primary or secondary; *primary* type has infiltration by immune cells, destroys bile duct system, fibrosis is micronodular or macronodular; *secondary* type has ruptured bile ducts and formation of "bile lakes" and cholesterol deposits in cells
  4. *Cardiac:* displays a patchy pattern with red areas (congestion) and pallid areas (fibrosis) resulting from prolonged right heart failure with chronic liver congestion and hypoperfusion.

5. *Other:* inherited and metabolic disorders, drugs and toxins, graft-versus-host disease, and jejunoileal bypass also may cause cirrhosis.

- Cirrhosis ultimately results in liver failure and portal hypertension.

Liver Failure

- Results from a progressive decrease in the number of functioning liver cells (hepatocytes) and the replacement of normal liver tissue with shrunken, fibrotic, and nodular tissue with altered structure of both the functional (parenchymal) and the supporting (stromal) tissues. Less portal blood can enter the liver, reducing the amount of intestinal blood processed by the liver and creating a "portal to systemic shunt." This "unfiltered" blood enters the general circulation; fluid and electrolyte disturbances and toxicity result.

Portal Hypertension

- Occurs because the changed liver structure disrupts the normal physics of blood flow within the liver. This causes a rise in pressure within the portal venous system and also a shunting of blood, mainly backward to the gastrointestinal organs, raising pressure in those areas that results in varices formation, with possible hemorrhage; congestion of abdominal organs; and ascites.

CAUSES

- *Alcoholic:* chronic alcohol ingestion, especially if accompanied by malnutrition
- *Postnecrotic:* follows various infections or parasitic infestations, but mostly (75%) after hepatitis B virus (HBV) or hepatitis C virus (HCV)
- *Biliary:* primary—accompanies intrahepatic obstruction due to inflammation, may be autoimmune; secondary—results from partial or complete blockage of extrahepatic ducts
- *Cardiac:* produced when right-sided heart failure induces venous congestion
- *Metabolic:* inherited defect in a metabolic pathway

Signs & Symptoms

Liver Failure

- Skin: dry, pigmented, itchy; spider angiomas; purpura/ecchymoses; possible jaundice (retention of toxins and/or bleeding disorders due to liver failure)
- Peripheral edema (decreased plasma proteins, altered hemodynamics)
- Hematologic: anemia, bleeding tendency (decreased clotting factors)
- Gastrointestinal: anorexia, nausea, vomiting; constipation or diarrhea; hepatomegaly; abdominal ache; hematemesis/melena (increased portal pressure)
- Respiratory: pleural effusion, dyspnea, hypoxemia (heart failure)
- Endocrine: testicular atrophy, gynecomastia, menstrual irregularities, reduced body hair (altered hormone metabolism)
- Central nervous system: encephalopathy, lethargy, motor and cognitive deficits; asterixis, a hand-flapping tremor (due to lack of ammonia and other waste product detoxification)
- Hepatorenal syndrome: azotemia, oliguria, hyponatremia, and hypotension (altered renal perfusion)

Portal Hypertension

- Varices (esophageal, gastric, rectal); may hemorrhage (due to increased portal venous pressure)
- Splenomegaly due to congestion from increased portal pressure
- Ascites due to increased hydrostatic pressure in abdominal vessels and lack of plasma proteins

Diagnostics

- Liver biopsy shows specific pattern of liver destruction.
- Serum chemistry shows increased liver enzymes, AST, ALT, alkaline phosphatase, and LDH; decreased plasma proteins, increased bilirubin.
- Bleeding studies show increased prothrombin time.
- Complete blood count (CBC) shows anemia.

MEDICAL INTERVENTIONS

- Pharmacologic agents include diuretics and medications such as lactulose and neomycin to reduce the nitrogenous load. Vitamin supplements and antacids may also be indicated. Medications that are metabolized by the liver are avoided.
- Surgery may be indicated for the client with biliary cirrhosis to restore patency of the ducts and relieve obstruction. The client with esophageal varices may have sclerotherapy. Clients with severe ascites may require paracentesis, the aspiration of ascitic fluid from the abdominoperitoneal cavity. When the client develops a portal hypertension with bleeding varices, a surgical shunt may be indicated. Liver transplantation is another option for clients with cirrhosis.
- Dietary support is essential for the client with cirrhosis. Sodium intake is restricted to less than 2 g per day, and fluids may be limited to 1500 mL per day. If hepatic encephalopathy is present, protein is restricted. Vitamin and mineral supplements are prescribed based on laboratory values.

SELECTED NURSING DIAGNOSES WITH INTERVENTIONS

Fluid Volume Excess

- Monitor weight daily using a consistent technique. Monitor for fluid shifts. Monitor intake and output strictly.
- Assess client's urine specific gravity.
- Provide a diet low in salt and with restricted fluids.

Altered Thought Processes

- Avoid factors that may precipitate hepatic encephalopathy. Cautious and judicious use of medications and appropriate monitoring can eliminate iatrogenic causes.
- Assess neurologic signs, and monitor for signs of early encephalopathy: changes in handwriting, speech, and development of asterixis.
- Provide a low-protein diet as prescribed, and teach the client and significant others the importance of dietary restrictions.
- Administer medications or enemas as prescribed.

- Orient the client as possible to surroundings, person, and place. Provide simple explanations for nursing interventions.

Risk for Injury: Bleeding

- Monitor vital signs for early signs of bleeding.
- Institute bleeding precautions (e.g., avoid injections, avoid rectal temperatures and enemas, use only soft toothbrush, assess oral cavity for bleeding gums, assess ecchymotic areas and areas of purpura, etc.).
- Monitor coagulation studies and platelet count.

Risk for Impaired Gas Exchange

- Position client in high-Fowler's position with feet elevated. Avoid the supine position when possible.
- Monitor respirations as needed. Obtain oxygen saturation level if indicated. Monitor arterial blood gases (ABGs).
- Administer oxygen as indicated and prescribed.

Impaired Skin Integrity

- Inspect the skin for injury at least every shift.
- Use warm rather than hot water when bathing.
- Initiate measures to prevent dry skin.
- Turn the client at least every 2 hours, use an alternate pressure mattress, and assess for skin breakdown.
- If indicated, protect the skin from injury by applying mittens to client's hands. Clients with encephalopathy may not understand the need to refrain from scratching.

CLIENT TEACHING

- Teach the client and significant others the importance of proper nutrition (high-calorie, low-sodium, low-protein if encephalopic) and vitamin and mineral supplementation.
- If alcohol is the etiologic factor, reinforce with the client and significant others the importance of avoiding alcohol ingestion.
- Discuss the medication regimen, effects, and side effects.
- Stress the importance of avoiding over-the-counter medications unless approved by the physician.

HOME CARE CONSIDERATIONS

- Include significant others when caring for the client with cirrhosis, especially when the etiologic agent is alcohol abuse. Coordinate appropriate referrals for home care, including follow-up visits to community health agencies and, if needed, Alcoholics Anonymous or similar rehabilitation and support groups.
- Stress the importance of long-term medical follow-up, and what signs and symptoms to report immediately to the physician. For example, the client with a shunt should immediately report increasing abdominal girth and feelings of fullness.
- Referral to a nutritionist, social worker, and/or psychologist may be indicated, especially for the client with alcoholic cirrhosis.

For more information on Cirrhosis, see Medical-Surgical Nursing *by LeMone and Burke, p. 526.*

Colorectal Cancer

OVERVIEW

- Colorectal cancers are malignant neoplasms (usually adenocarcinomas) of the colon and/or rectum.
- Of all cancers, colorectal cancer is the third most common, in incidence and mortality, in the United States.
- It tends to grow slowly and remain localized for long periods.
- Neoplasms spread via the lymphatic and circulatory systems.
- Five-year survival rates depend on stage at diagnosis: early/local—91% for colon, 83% for rectum; regional spread, 60%; distant metastasis, 7%.

CAUSES

The specific cause of colorectal cancer is unknown. Risk factors include:

- Age greater than 40 years
- Genetics: higher incidence in those with preexisting familial polyposis or ulcerative colitis
- Diet: high in fat, especially animal fat; high calorie; low fiber

Signs & Symptoms

- Occult, or frank, chronic, or intermittent bleeding
- S/S of iron deficiency anemia
- Anorexia, nausea, vomiting
- Weight loss
- Alternating diarrhea and constipation
- Narrow or ribbon-like stools
- Black, tarry stools
- Change in bowel habits
- Palpable abdominal mass
- S/S of obstruction, intermittent
- Cramping or vague lower abdominal pain

Diagnostics

- Digital rectal exam detects 15% to 20% of tumors.
- Hemoccult test detects presence of blood in stool.
- Endoscopy (colonoscopy preferred) allows visualization of entire colon wall to the ileocecal valve to detect tumors; also allows for tissue collection for biopsy.
- Tissue biopsy is conducted with endoscopy to confirm that tissue is cancerous.
- Complete blood count (CBC) may show iron-deficiency anemia.

MEDICAL INTERVENTIONS

- Surgical resection of the tumor, adjacent colon, and regional lymph nodes is the standard treatment for colorectal cancer. Surgical resection of the bowel may be followed by a colostomy for diversion of fecal contents.
- Radiation therapy may be used in addition to surgery or to slow the progression of inoperable tumors.

- Chemotherapeutic agents such as oral levamisole and IV fluorouracil are used postoperatively as adjunctive therapy.

SELECTED NURSING DIAGNOSES WITH INTERVENTIONS

Pain

- Assess the client frequently for adequate pain relief. Ask the client to rate pain on a scale of 0 to 10, and document the level of pain.
- Assess the effectiveness of pain medications one half hour after administration. Monitor for effects and adverse effects.
- Assess the incision postoperatively for signs of inflammation or swelling. Assess drainage catheters and tubes for patency.
- Assess the abdomen for distention, tenderness, and bowel sounds.
- Administer pain medication prior to an activity or procedure.
- Provide nonpharmacologic relief measures, such as positioning, diversional activities, management of environmental stimuli, and relaxation.
- Splint the incision with a pillow, and teach the client how to self-splint the incision when coughing and deep breathing.

Altered Nutrition: Less than Body Requirements

- Assess the client's readiness for enteral feedings after surgery or diagnostic procedures using data such as statements of hunger, presence of bowel sounds, passage of flatus, and minimal abdominal distention.
- Monitor and document food and fluid intake.
- Weigh the client daily.
- Maintain total parenteral nutrition and central IV lines as prescribed.
- When oral intake is resumed, develop a meal plan with the client.

Anticipatory Grieving

- Work to develop a trusting relationship with the client and significant others.
- Listen actively to the client and significant others, encouraging them to express their fears and concerns regarding the loss.

- Provide a referral to cancer support groups, social services, or counseling as appropriate.

Risk for Sexual Dysfunction

The client undergoing ostomy surgery is at risk for sexual dysfunction.

- Provide opportunities for the client and significant other to express their feelings about the ostomy.
- Provide consistent colostomy care with an accepting attitude.
- Encourage expression of sexual concerns.
- Reassure the client and significant other that physical illness and prescribed interventions usually have a temporary effect on sexuality.
- Refer the client and significant other to social services or a counselor for further intervention.
- Arrange for a visit from a member of the United Ostomy Association.

CLIENT TEACHING

- Teach the client home management and care of the colostomy pouch and stoma. Provide suggestions for incorporating care into routine activities of daily living (ADLs).
- Teach the client the signs and symptoms of postoperative complications, such as wound infection and intestinal obstruction.

HOME CARE CONSIDERATIONS

- A variety of referrals may be appropriate, including referrals to an enterostomal therapy nurse, a dietitian, a home health nurse, and a psychologist.
- The client should be referred to local chapters of the United Ostomy Association and the American Cancer Society, and be informed of the locations of local suppliers of ostomy appliances.
- The client with an inoperable tumor needs information about hospice and home care.

For more information on Colorectal Cancer, see
Medical-Surgical Nursing *by LeMone and Burke,*
p. 844.

Condyloma Acuminata (Genital Warts)

OVERVIEW

- Condyloma acuminata are genital warts caused by one of the 70 types of human papilloma virus (HPV).
- The incubation period ranges from 3 weeks to 18 months.
- It is the most common sexually transmitted disease in the United States.
- It is a risk factor for cervical cancer, and is associated with cancer of the penis, anus, vagina, and vulva.

CAUSES

- Infection of skin and/or mucous membrane with various strains of HPV (6, 11, 30, 42–45, 51, 54)
- Transmitted by sexual contact; facilitated by trauma at inoculation site
- Increased susceptibility in immunocompromised patients

Signs & Symptoms

- Characteristic leafy-looking warts
- Warts located on external genitalia, perineum, anus, and/or vagina or cervix
- Itching
- Bleeding
- Secondary infection
- May be asymptomatic, and growths may not be noticed by the client

Diagnostics

- Visual inspection can identify most lesions.
- Pap smear may show atypical cells of the cervix.
- Colposcopy magnifies skin or mucous membranes for closer inspection.
- Biopsy may be used to assess for transformation to neoplasia.

MEDICAL INTERVENTIONS

- Topical pharmacologic agents used to treat genital warts include podofilox and podophyllin.
- Warts may be removed by cryotherapy, electrocautery, or surgical excision. Carbon dioxide laser surgery is common for removal of extensive warts.

SELECTED NURSING DIAGNOSES WITH INTERVENTIONS

Impaired Tissue Integrity

- Discuss the need for prompt treatment and for sexual abstinence until lesions have healed.
- Discuss the need for the client's sexual partner to be examined and treated.
- Stress to the female client the increased risk of cervical cancer and the importance of an annual Pap smear.

Fear

- Allow the client to express specific fears and feelings about the procedure chosen to remove the warts. Explain the procedure, approximate recovery time, possible complications and ways to avoid them, and ways to cope with complications that might occur.
- Explain that the procedure is performed using only local anesthesia.
- Encourage verbalization of fears related to changes in and limitations of sexual activity.

CLIENT TEACHING

- Teach the client about the disease process, prevention, treatment, and necessary follow-up care.
- Stress the importance of abstaining from sexual activity until all warts have been removed from both the client and the sex partner.

HOME CARE CONSIDERATIONS

- Tell the client to schedule a follow-up visit with the physician 3 months after treatment.
- Encourage the female client with cervical dysplasia related to condyloma to follow the physician's

instruction to obtain a Pap smear within 6 months following treatment.
- Discuss safer sex practices to reduce the risk of contracting STDs.

For more information on Condyloma Acuminata, see Medical-Surgical Nursing *by LeMone and Burke, p. 2091.*

Coronary Artery Disease (CAD)

OVERVIEW

- Coronary artery disease (CAD) is defined as impaired coronary vessel flow, most often secondary to plaque formation.
- Most cases are due to atherosclerosis.
- Atheromas (or plaques) form over many years and progressively narrow the arterial lumen.
- Impaired coronary perfusion results in ischemia of the myocardium.
- CAD is the most common form of heart disease and the major cause of death in the United States.
- It can result in angina, acute myocardial infarction (MI), dysrhythmias, or heart failure.

CAUSES

- Atherosclerosis causes most cases; it produces plaques and may cause vessels to spasm
- Platelet aggregation/thrombosis
- Congenital vessel anomalies/arteritis
- Syphilis
- Risk factors include:
  1. genetics: familial history of heart disease, hyperlipidemia, CAD
  2. male gender, post-menopausal females
  3. diet: high in fat, carbohydrate, cholesterol
  4. lifestyle: sedentary; high stress/Type A personality

5. obesity
6. diabetes mellitus
7. hypertension
8. smoking

Signs & Symptoms

- Angina (pain due to myocardial ischemia):
  1. a burning, squeezing, chest pain
  2. originates in the precordial or substernal region
  3. may radiate to the left arm, neck, jaw, or shoulder
  4. usually occurs during or follows strenuous activity/sexual intercourse
  5. may be precipitated by cold exposure, excitement, or a large meal
  6. typically relieved with rest
- Weakness, dizziness
- Nausea, vomiting, indigestion
- Diaphoresis, cool skin
- Palpitations
- Shortness of breath

Diagnostics

- EKG may show ischemia or dysrhythmias, especially during angina attacks.
- Treadmill or bicycle stress test may precipitate angina and/or dysrhythmias.
- Coronary angiography can identify coronary narrowing and collateral vessels.
- Myocardial perfusion imaging detects areas of decreased blood flow.
- Serum lipids show elevated LDL/VLDL, decreased HDL, increased triglycerides, and increased cholesterol.

MEDICAL INTERVENTIONS

- Conservative management includes following a low-fat, low-cholesterol diet, smoking cessation, control of contributing conditions, stress reduction, and moderate exercise.

- Pharmacologic agents include prophylactic low-dose aspirin therapy, oral estrogen replacement for postmenopausal women, and drugs to lower LDL levels, including niacin or nicotinic acid, bile acid–binding resins, and cholesterol-synthesis inhibitors.

SELECTED NURSING DIAGNOSES

- Altered Nutrition: More than Body Requirements
- Altered Tissue Perfusion: Cardiac
- Activity Intolerance
- Pain

SELECTED NURSING INTERVENTIONS

- Teach and provide support for risk-factor modification to slow the progress of the disease. See the Client Teaching section below.
- Assess the location, severity, and quality of the client's pain. Ask the client to rate the pain on a scale of 0 to 10. Discuss prescribed pain medication management.
- Encourage the client to space activities to allow rest periods.

CLIENT TEACHING

- Strongly encourage the client to stop all forms of tobacco use. Discuss the effects of smoking and provide information on smoking cessation programs.
- Discuss American Heart Association dietary recommendations with the client, emphasizing the role of diet in heart disease.
- Encourage regular moderate physical activity and exercise as approved by the physician. Provide information about manifestations of exercise intolerance and what to do if these are noted.
- Provide tips for stress management, including relaxation techniques, stress reduction classes, and so on. Provide referrals as necessary.

HOME CARE CONSIDERATIONS

- Provide the client with referrals to cardiac rehabilitation programs, classes, support groups, and information resources for risk-factor modification techniques as appropriate.

- Discuss the importance of maintaining a regular schedule of aerobic exercise to promote cardiovascular health. The client should check with his or her physician before engaging in weight training or isometric exercises.
- Discuss the role of hormone replacement therapy in reducing the risk of CAD in postmenopausal women.
- Emphasize the need for continued lifelong follow-up care.

For more information on Coronary Artery Disease, see Medical-Surgical Nursing *by LeMone and Burke,* p. 1065.

Cor Pulmonale

OVERVIEW

- Cor pulmonale is right ventricular hypertrophy (RVH) secondary to diseases of the lung, thorax, or pulmonary circulation.
- It is preceded by pulmonary hypertension, which increases the workload of the right ventricle.
- Obvious right-heart failure may or may not be present.
- Cor pulmonale accounts for approximately 20% of hospital admissions for heart failure.

CAUSES

- Pulmonary embolism
- Adult respiratory distress syndrome (ARDS)
- Chronic obstructive pulmonary disease (COPD)
- Lung fibrosis
- Lung resection
- Various other causes: obesity, myxedema, thoracic muscle conditions, kyphoscoliosis, high altitude

Signs & Symptoms

- Cough
- Dyspnea on exertion, breathlessness
- Tachypnea, hypocapnia
- Weakness/fatigue
- S/S of right-heart failure: peripheral or visceral edema

Diagnostics

- Chest x-ray shows enlargement of pulmonary vessels.
- Echocardiogram measures increased right ventricular wall thickness and an enlarged right ventricle.
- Magnetic resonance imaging (MRI) measures wall thickness, chamber volume, and ejection fraction.
- Cardiac catheterization measures intracardiac pressures accurately.
- Pulmonary capillary wedge pressure (PCWP) will be >30/15 mm Hg.
- Arterial blood gases (ABGs) usually show reduced Pao_2, reduced $Paco_2$, and elevated pH (hyperventilation).
- Hematocrit (HCT) may be >50% if cor pulmonale is chronic.

MEDICAL INTERVENTIONS

- Treat specific underlying cause.
- General treatment of RVH includes oxygen therapy, sodium and fluid restriction, and diuretics.

SELECTED NURSING DIAGNOSES WITH INTERVENTIONS

Fluid Volume Excess

- Assess the client's respiratory status, including respiratory rate, effort, any shortness of breath, dyspnea, cough, orthopnea, or paroxysmal nocturnal dyspnea (PND). Auscultate lung sounds at least every 4 hours.
- Notify the physician immediately if the client develops air hunger, an overwhelming sense of

impending doom or panic, tachypnea, the need to sit straight up in bed, or a cough productive of large amounts of pink, frothy sputum.

- Monitor and record intake and output. Notify the physician if urine output drops to less than 30 mL per hour.
- Weigh the client daily.
- Maintain bed rest, with the head of the bed elevated to 45°.
- Assess for other manifestations of fluid volume excess, including jugular venous distention, peripheral edema, and cardiac rhythm changes.
- Monitor and record hemodynamic parameters. Note changes in pulmonary artery pressures and systemic vascular resistance and decreases in cardiac output and blood pressure.
- Administer diuretics and other medications as prescribed.
- Restrict fluids as instructed. Encourage the client to choose the time and type of fluid consumed, scheduling the majority of the intake in the morning and afternoon. Offer ice chips and frequent mouth care.

Activity Intolerance

- Assess vital signs and cardiac rhythm before and after the client engages in activity.
- Monitor for signs of activity intolerance such as tachycardia, changes in blood pressure, diaphoresis, chest pain, excessive fatigue, palpitations, and so on.
- Organize nursing care to allow for rest periods.
- Assist the client as needed with self-care activities. Encourage the client to perform activities of daily living (ADLs) independently within prescribed limits.
- Plan and implement a progressive activity plan. Employ passive and active range-of-motion (ROM) exercises as appropriate. Consult with a physical therapist on the activity plan.
- Provide written and verbal information about activity after discharge.

CLIENT TEACHING

- Teach the client the importance of a low-sodium diet. Provide the client with a list of foods high in sodium to be avoided. Emphasize the need for high-potassium foods to clients taking diuretics.

- Caution the client to avoid sedatives and nonprescription medications that depress ventilatory drive.
- Additional teaching may be appropriate for the client experiencing other manifestations of heart failure.

HOME CARE CONSIDERATIONS

- Encourage the client to keep regular appointments with the cardiologist to monitor the disease and the effects of therapy.
- Refer the client to a smoking cessation program as appropriate. A cardiac support group or rehabilitation program may also be beneficial.
- The client may require a referral for home health care, especially if elderly or in need of suction or oxygen therapy at home.
- Stress the importance of pneumococcal and annual influenza vaccinations.

For more information on Cor Pulmonale, see Medical-Surgical Nursing *by LeMone and Burke,* *p. 1457.*

Crohn's Disease

OVERVIEW

- Crohn's disease is a chronic inflammatory disease of the gastrointestinal (GI) tract, most often affecting the distal ileum or colon.
- Bowel mucosa is inflamed in an intermittent pattern, producing a "cobblestone" appearance; inflamed areas are surrounded by normal-appearing tissue.
- Inflammation penetrates all bowel layers, producing deep ulcerations with possible fissures; adjacent mesentery and lymphatics may also be inflamed.
- Complications can include abscess or fistula formation, perforation, or obstruction.

- The incidence of bowel cancer may be increased with Crohn's disease.
- Systemic manifestations are often present and can include arthritis (migratory); inflammation of eye, mucous membranes, or skin; renal calculi formation; amyloidosis.
- The course can be rapidly fulminating, but most often presents with a series of exacerbations and remissions.
- The disease is seen with increased frequency in Jewish and Eastern European people, and within families; it affects both sexes equally.
- There is a bimodal age distribution, with the first age peak seen in the late teen years; the second peak is in the 55- to 60-year-old age group.

CAUSES

- The precise cause of Crohn's disease is unknown; possible mechanisms include genetic, autoimmune, infectious (bacteria, viruses), and psychogenic factors

Signs & Symptoms

- Diarrhea (may or may not be bloody)
- Steatorrhea (fatty stools) are possible
- Right-lower-quadrant pain, may be steady and constant, or colicky in nature
- Weight loss and/or deficiency states
- Fever
- Fatigue

Diagnostics

- Sigmoidoscopy/colonoscopy will show ulcerative lesions.
- Bowel biopsy will show extent of bowel wall involvement.
- Barium enema can show mucosal changes.
- Complete blood count (CBC) may show anemia from chronic inflammation, blood loss, and malnutrition. It may also show leukocytosis owing to inflammation.

MEDICAL INTERVENTIONS

- Pharmacologic agents include anti-inflammatory drugs such as sulfasalazine and corticosteroids, as well as antidiarrheal preparations. Broad-spectrum antibiotics may be used to prevent or treat infections. Antispasmodics may be used to reduce abdominal cramping.
- Dietary management is indicated, and may include the use of elemental enteral feedings such as Ensure. Milk and milk products may be eliminated. Clients with symptoms of obstruction or narrowing may need a low-roughage diet.
- Surgical intervention in Crohn's disease is limited to clients with complications such as bowel obstruction.

SELECTED NURSING DIAGNOSES WITH INTERVENTIONS

Altered Nutrition: Less than Body Requirements

- Weigh daily and maintain accurate intake, output, and dietary records.
- Monitor the results of laboratory studies that indicate the client's nutritional status.
- Provide the prescribed diet: high kilocalorie, high protein, low fat, with restricted dairy intake if lactose intolerance is suspected.
- Provide parenteral nutrition as necessary.
- Arrange for dietary consultation. Provide for the client's food preferences as allowed.
- Administer prescribed nutritional supplements.
- Include significant others in teaching and dietary discussions.

Diarrhea

- Monitor and record the frequency and characteristics of bowel movements.
- Measure abdominal girth and auscultate bowel sounds every shift as indicated.
- Administer antidiarrheal medications as prescribed.
- Limit the client's food intake if the diarrhea is acute, to allow the bowel to rest.

CLIENT TEACHING

- Teach the client and significant others about the disease, prescribed medications, and dietary management. Instruct them in manifestations of complications and their appropriate management.
- Present information on stress management and teach the importance of adequate rest.
- Teach the client to avoid GI stimulants such as nicotine, caffeine, pepper, and alcohol.
- If the client is to be discharged with a central catheter and home parenteral nutrition, provide written and verbal instructions on catheter care and trouble-shooting as well as administration of total parenteral nutrition (TPN).

HOME CARE CONSIDERATIONS

- Referral to a home health nurse is often appropriate for the client with TPN.
- Refer the client to the local chapter of the Crohn's and Colitis Foundation for support services.

For more information on Crohn's Disease, see Medical-Surgical Nursing *by LeMone and Burke, p. 832.*

Cushing's Syndrome

OVERVIEW

- Cushing's syndrome is a complex syndrome of excess glucocorticoid activity; it results in widespread metabolic, cardiovascular, neurologic, and immunologic changes.
- It can be primary or secondary, and is usually iatrogenic.
  1. *Primary:* results from excess steroid secretion from the adrenal gland itself; most common in women 20 to 40 years of age.

2. *Secondary:* is due to increased secretion of adrenocorticotropic hormone (ACTH) from the pituitary gland (*Cushing's disease*), or an ectopic focus.
3. *Iatrongenic:* glucocorticoid therapy is commonly given for hypersensitivity reactions, autoimmune disease, or for severe inflammatory conditions; it produces exactly the same S/S as disease forms.

CAUSES

- *Primary:* benign adrenal adenoma (85%); adrenal carcinoma
- *Secondary:* benign pituitary adenomas; hypothalamic-pituitary dysfunction; ectopic secretion of ACTH as in oat-cell carcinoma, pancreatic carcinoma; carcinoid of thymus
- *Iatrogenic:* long-term glucocorticoid therapy (prednisone, prednisolone, Solu-Medrol)

Signs & Symptoms

- Protein catabolism: muscle atrophy/weakness, capillary fragility (ecchymosis), osteoporosis (decreased bone matrix), striae, poor wound healing
- Fat metabolism: central obesity: moon face, buffalo hump, rotund trunk, thin extremities
- Carbohydrate metabolism: glucose intolerance, secondary diabetes mellitus (DM)
- Fluid and electrolytes: sodium retention/potassium wasting, fluid retention, edema, weight gain
- Cardiovascular: hypertension, arteriosclerosis, decreased stress response
- Immunologic: reduced inflammatory/immunologic response, increased infection rate
- Neurologic: memory loss, poor concentration, mood swings, frank psychosis
- Reproductive: oligo/amenorrhea, virilism, hirsutism, and acne in women; impotence in men

Diagnostics

- Plasma cortisol level is elevated in both primary and secondary types.

- 24-hour urine for cortisol is elevated in both primary and secondary types.
- Low-dose dexamethasone suppression test identifies Cushing's syndrome, but not type.
- High-dose dexamethasone suppression test is positive if pituitary-hypothalamic dysfunction is present, negative if disease is secondary to an ACTH-secreting adenoma.
- Plasma ACTH level is increased with ACTH-secreting neoplasms (pituitary or ectopic), reduced if primary.
- Visualization studies (ultrasound, angiography, CT scan) may reveal adrenal, pituitary, or ectopic neoplasms.

MEDICAL INTERVENTIONS

- Pharmacologic treatment may be used as an adjunct to surgery or radiation or for clients with inoperable malignancies. Mitotane suppresses the activity of the adrenal cortex and decreases peripheral metabolism of corticosteroids. Metyrapone inhibits cortisol synthesis by the adrenal cortex.
- Radiation therapy may be indicated to destroy the pituitary gland. Lifelong replacement of pituitary hormones is then necessary.
- Surgical removal of the pituitary gland is indicated when Cushing's syndrome is the result of a pituitary disorder. Lifelong replacement of pituitary hormones is then necessary. When Cushing's is caused by an adrenal cortex tumor, an adrenalectomy may be performed.

SELECTED NURSING DIAGNOSES WITH INTERVENTIONS

Fluid Volume Excess
- Weigh the client at the same time each day and in the same clothes.
- Record accurate intake and output each shift.
- Monitor blood pressure, rate and rhythm of pulse, respiratory rate, and breath sounds.
- Assess for peripheral edema and jugular vein distention.

- Teach the client and significant others the reasons for restricting fluids and the importance of limiting fluids if instructed.

Risk for Injury

- Maintain a safe environment in the health care facility: reduce clutter, maintain adequate lighting, and so on.
- Teach the client home safety measures.
- Monitor the client for signs of fatigue.
- Encourage the client to use assistive devices for ambulation or to ask for help if needed. Non-skid slippers or shoes are also appropriate.

Risk for Infection

- Place the client in a private room and limit visitors.
- Monitor the client's vital signs every 4 hours.
- Use principles of medical asepsis and sterile asepsis when caring for the client.
- If wounds are present, assess the color, odor, and consistency of wound drainage. Also assess for increased pain in and around the wound.
- Teach the client to increase intake of protein and vitamins A and C.

Body Image Disturbance

- Encourage the client to express feelings and to ask questions about the disorder and its treatment.
- Ask the client to discuss strengths and previous coping strategies. Enlist the support of significant others in reaffirming the client's worth.
- Discuss signs of progress in controlling symptoms (e.g., decreased facial edema).

CLIENT TEACHING

- Teach the client the importance of home safety and provide tips for ensuring a safe home environment (e.g., non-skid rugs, shower rails).
- Stress the importance of maintaining the prescribed dietary supplements and fluid restrictions as instructed.
- Since clients often require medications for the rest of their lives, and dosage changes are likely, teach the client the importance of taking medications as indicated, and of having regular health assessments to maximize wellness.

HOME CARE CONSIDERATIONS

- For clients with iatrogenic Cushing's, emphasize the importance of gradually discontinuing corticosteroid therapy to avoid the risk of acute adrenal insufficiency with severe hypotension, circulatory collapse, shock, and coma.
- Provide clients with information on obtaining a MedicAlert bracelet or necklace and stress the importance of wearing it.
- A referral to social services or a community health service may be appropriate because of the complexity of the treatment and care required.

For more information on Cushing's Syndrome, see Medical-Surgical Nursing *by LeMone and Burke,* *p. 702.*

Decubitus Ulcers (Pressure Ulcers, Bedsores)

OVERVIEW

- Decubitus ulcers are defined as cellular necrosis of skin, subcutaneous, and/or deep tissues.
- They are usually localized over bony prominences.
- Pressure ulcers develop from external pressure that compresses blood vessels, and from friction and shearing forces that tear and injure vessels.
- The older adult is at increased risk for development of pressure ulcers because the dermis is thinner, with decreased vascularity, decreased sebaceous gland activity, and decreased strength and elasticity.

CAUSES

Risk factors include:

- Reduced mobility (common in bed- or wheelchair-bound clients)
- Altered level of consciousness (LOC)
- Inadequate nutrition
- Susceptible skin/subcutaneous tissue due to edema, infection, fever, incontinence, cachexia, or obesity

Signs & Symptoms

- Stage I: skin redness (not blanchable)
- Stage II: cracked or peeling skin (partial-thickness loss)
- Stage III: broken skin with subcutaneous damage and exudate (full-thickness loss)
- Stage IV: deep ulcer, through fascia to muscle and bone

Diagnostics

- Culture and sensitivity (C&S) will identify pathogens and the appropriate antibiotic.

MEDICAL INTERVENTIONS

- Pharmacologic agents include antibiotics to eradicate any infection present, and a variety of topical products to aid healing.
- Surgical debridement may be necessary if the ulcer is deep, if subcutaneous tissues are involved, or if an eschar (scab or dry crust) has formed over the ulcer. Large wounds may require skin grafting.

SELECTED NURSING DIAGNOSES WITH INTERVENTIONS

The nursing diagnoses appropriate for the client with a decubitus ulcer are *Risk for Impaired Skin Integrity* and *Impaired Skin Integrity*. The interventions below are used to identify adults at risk and treat those with Stage I ulcers.

- Assess bed- and chair-bound clients as well as those who are unable to reposition themselves.
- Assess clients on admission to acute-care and rehabilitation hospitals, nursing homes, home care programs, and other health care facilities.
- Use a validated risk assessment tool.
- Conduct a systematic skin inspection at least once a day, paying particular attention to the bony prominences.
- Clean the skin at the time of soiling and at routine intervals, as frequently as the client's needs dictate. Use lukewarm water, a mild cleansing agent, and gentle pressure.
- Minimize environmental factors leading to skin drying, such as low humidity and exposure to cold or dry heat. Treat dry skin with moisturizers.
- Avoid massage over bony prominences.
- Minimize skin exposure to moisture due to incontinence, perspiration, or wound drainage.
- To minimize skin injury due to friction and shearing forces, use proper positioning, transferring, and turning techniques. Lubricants, protective films, protective dressings, and protective padding may also reduce friction injuries.
- Assess factors involved in inadequate dietary intake of protein or kilocalories. Offer nutritional supplements.

- Maintain the client's current level of activity, mobility, and range of motion.
- For the client who is on bed rest or is immobile, reposition every 2 hours; use positioning devices such as pillows or foam wedges to protect bony prominences; maintain the head of the bed at the lowest degree of elevation consistent with the client's medical condition; and place any at-risk client on a pressure-reducing device, such as a foam, static air, alternating air, gel, or water mattress.
- For chair-bound clients, use pressure-reducing devices and reposition the client every hour. Teach clients who can do so to shift their weight every 15 minutes.

CLIENT TEACHING

- Teach the client and significant others the importance of position changes and range-of-motion (ROM) exercises. Encourage the client to participate in each as much as possible.
- Teach significant others the proper technique for prescribed dressing changes.
- Teach the client about general nutrition and how to maintain a well-balanced diet.
- Teach the client and significant others to recognize signs of healing as well as signs of further skin breakdown.

HOME CARE CONSIDERATIONS

- Referral to a home health agency can help the family through the lengthy healing process.
- Referral to a wound care center for treatment of non-healing wounds with growth factor may be appropriate.

For more information on Decubitus Ulcers, see Medica-Surgical Nursing *by LeMone and Burke,* *p. 618.*

Dehydration

OVERVIEW

- Dehydration is excessive water loss from body tissues.
- The term dehydration often is used interchangeably with *fluid volume deficit*, which results when both water and electrolytes (isotonic body fluids) are lost.
- Left unchecked, extracellular fluid volume deficit will result in hypovolemia and possibly shock.

CAUSES

- *Fluid volume deficits* (isotonic) may be due to excessive fluid losses, insufficient fluid intake, or a combination of both. Common causes of fluid volume deficit include:
  1. blood loss, hemorrhage
  2. vomiting, nasogastric (NG) tube suction
  3. diarrhea, frequent enemas
  4. draining fistulas or abscesses
  5. ileostomy, colostomy
  6. burns, severe wounds
  7. diuretic therapy
  8. sweating
  9. third-space shifts
- *Hypotonic (pure water) losses* create a hypertonic dehydration because water loss is greater than solute loss. Disorders causing dehydration by this mechanism are uncommon:
  1. water unavailable
  2. comatose or paralyzed patients
  3. impaired thirst mechanism
  4. fever with hyperventilation
  5. profuse diaphoresis
  6. diabetes insipidus

Signs & Symptoms

- Cardiovascular: increased heart rate, decreased blood pressure, postural hypotension, thready pulses, flat veins
- Renal: oliguria, dark urine, increased specific gravity (except in diabetes insipidus)
- Skin/mucous membranes: poor skin turgor, tenting; dry, sticky tongue; sunken eyeballs; pale, if in shock
- Neuromuscular: lethargy, confusion, coma
- Gastrointestinal: anorexia, decreased motility and bowel sounds; nausea, vomiting, constipation (unless dehydration is due to diarrhea)
- General: fever, thirst (if alert and thirst mechanism intact), weakness, dizziness, weight loss

Diagnostics

- Blood urea nitrogen (BUN) may be elevated due to fluid deficit.
- Hematocrit (HCT) may be elevated due to fluid deficit.
- Serum electrolyte levels vary related to the cause of dehydration.
- Serum osmolarity is elevated.
- Urine specific gravity is elevated (but reduced with diabetes insipidus).

MEDICAL INTERVENTIONS

- Intravenous fluids are often prescribed to correct fluid volume deficit:
  1. Isotonic electrolyte solutions are used to expand plasma volume in hypotensive clients or to replace abnormal losses.
  2. Five percent dextrose in water (D5W) is given to treat total body water deficits.
  3. Hypotonic saline solutions or hypotonic mixed electrolyte solutions are used as maintenance solutions.

SELECTED NURSING DIAGNOSES WITH INTERVENTIONS

Fluid Volume Deficit

- Assess for factors contributing to abnormal fluid losses such as excessive losses from the GI tract, wounds, decreased intake, and so on.
- Assess intake and output accurately at scheduled intervals (e.g., hourly). A urine output of less than 30 mL per hour should be reported. Measure urine specific gravity.
- Assess vital signs, including orthostatic BP, central venous pressure (CVP), and volume of peripheral pulses at least every 4 hours.
- Assess for indicators of dehydration: thirst; poor skin turgor; dry, sticky mucous membranes; coated tongue.
- Weigh client under standard conditions daily.
- Administer and monitor the intake of oral fluids as prescribed.
- Administer IV fluids as prescribed using an electronic infusion pump. Assess for indicators of fluid overload from excessively rapid replacement: dyspnea, tachypnea, tachycardia, increased CVP, jugular vein distention, and edema.
- Assess laboratory values.

Risk for Altered Tissue Perfusion

- Assess for restlessness, anxiety, and agitation, as well as changes in muscle strength.
- Assess for hypotension and tachycardia when the client is in the supine position. Assess for orthostatic hypotension.

Risk for Injury

- Institute safety precautions, including keeping the bed in a low position, using side rails, and slowly raising the client from supine to sitting or sitting to standing position.
- Teach the client and significant others to avoid dehydration by replacing lost fluids, avoiding alcohol and caffeine, and avoiding prolonged exposure to intense heat.

- Teach the client and significant others how to avoid orthostatic hypotension, for example, by moving from one position to another in stages, using a walker, avoiding prolonged standing, resting in a recliner, and using assistive devices to pick up objects from the floor.

CLIENT TEACHING

- Emphasize the importance of maintaining adequate fluid intake, and teach the signs and symptoms of fluid imbalance, the steps to take to prevent fluid deficit, and the importance of following the prescribed medication regimen.
- Provide both verbal and written instructions, including:
  1. Amount and type of fluids to take each day.
  2. Avoidance of overexposure to heat and exercise.
  3. Eating three meals a day.
  4. Increase fluid intake in hot weather.
  5. Decrease activity during hot weather.
  6. If vomiting, take frequent small amounts of ice chips or clear liquids such as ginger ale.
  7. Coffee, tea, alcohol, and large amounts of sugar increase urine output and can cause fluid loss.
  8. Replace fluids lost through diarrhea with fruit juices, bouillon or a balanced electrolyte solution such as Gatorade or Pedialyte, rather than large amounts of tap water.

HOME CARE CONSIDERATIONS

- A referral to a home health agency may be appropriate for the client needing continued evaluation and monitoring.
- A referral to a social worker may be appropriate to evaluate the home environment, or to assess the need to place the client in an assisted-living or a long-term-care facility.

For more information on Dehydration, see Medical-Surgical Nursing *by LeMone and Burke, p. 106.*

Diabetes Insipidus (DI)

OVERVIEW

- Diabetes insipidus (DI) is a deficiency of, or reduced sensitivity to, antidiuretic hormone (ADH), also known as arginine vasopressin.
- ADH is made in the hypothalamus; it is stored and secreted from the posterior pituitary gland.
- ADH release is increased with stimulation of osmoreceptors (hyperosmolality); volume receptors (hypovolemia); baroreceptors (decreased blood pressure).
- ADH normally promotes the reabsorption of pure water in distal renal tubules (distal convoluted and collecting tubules).
- DI is characterized by excessive diuresis of very dilute urine (hypotonic polyuria).
- Untreated, DI can result in dehydration, hypo-volemia, and possibly shock.

CAUSES

Central (Neurogenic) DI:

- A deficiency of ADH secretion
- Genetic defect: autosomal recessive Wolfram syndrome
- Neoplasms of hypothalamus or pituitary gland
- Hypothalamic or pituitary trauma secondary to head injury or surgery
- Hypoxia or ischemia (cardiopulmonary arrest, shock, hemorrhage)
- Pregnancy/postpartum Sheehan's syndrome
- Idiopathic

Nephrogenic DI

- A reduced response (sensitivity) to ADH at the renal tubules
- Genetic defect: X-linked recessive defect in ADH receptors in renal tubules
- Electrolyte disturbance
- Drugs: lithium, demeclocycline, methoxyflurane

- Other medical conditions: amyloidosis, post-renal obstruction, sickle-cell anemia

Signs & Symptoms

- Polyuria: 3 to 20 L/day; the greater the volume, the more dilute the urine
- Polydipsia/thirst: usually matches polyuria
- Almost colorless urine
- Dehydration, hypovolemia: if unable to meet fluid needs

Diagnostics

- Plasma osmolality >300 mOsm/L.
- Urine osmolality <50–200 mOsm/L.
- Urine specific gravity <1.005.
- ADH challenge test: response to ADH (antidiuresis) will be negative if nephrogenic; positive if central.

MEDICAL INTERVENTIONS

- Primary treatment is correction of the underlying cause.
- Other medical interventions include administering IV hypotonic fluids, increasing oral fluids, and replacing ADH for neurogenic diabetes insipidus.

SELECTED NURSING DIAGNOSES

- Fluid Volume Deficit
- Risk for Injury
- Risk for Altered Health Maintenance
- Sleep Pattern Disturbance
- Altered Urinary Elimination: Polyuria

SELECTED NURSING INTERVENTIONS

- Institute safety precautions if the client is dizzy and/or weak.
- Ensure access to bathroom, urinal, or bedpan.
- Provide meticulous skin and mouth care with alcohol-free emollient products after bath, and a soft toothbrush.
- Encourage verbalization of feelings and assist in development of coping strategies.

- Monitor fluid intake and output hourly.
- Monitor vital signs frequently.
- Weigh the client daily, in the same clothes and at the same time each day.
- Monitor urine specific gravity.
- Monitor serum electrolytes and blood urea nitrogen (BUN).
- Monitor laboratory values for hypernatremia.

CLIENT TEACHING

- Teach the client how to maintain adequate fluid intake to prevent dehydration.
- Stress the importance of reporting immediately to the physician signs of dehydration and hypovolemia.
- Encourage the client to keep a record of daily weights, intake and output, and urine specific gravity. Teach the client how to use a hydrometer to measure urine specific gravity.
- Stress the need for long-term hormone therapy, the importance of taking medications as prescribed, and the importance of not stopping medications abruptly. Describe the effects and side effects of the medications.
- Teach the client and significant others how to give subcutaneous and IM injections of ADH and how to use nasal applicators.

HOME CARE CONSIDERATIONS

- Stress the importance of long-term medical follow-up care.
- Explain to clients the importance of carrying medications with them at all times.
- Provide information on how to obtain a Medic-Alert bracelet or necklace and stress the need to wear it at all times.
- Refer the client to social services or a psychologist if appropriate.

For more information on Diabetes Insipidus, see Medical-Surgical Nursing *by LeMone and Burke,* *p. 714.*

Diabetes Mellitus (DM)

OVERVIEW

- Diabetes mellitus (DM) is a group of chronic metabolic disorders, all characterized by inappropriate hyperglycemia.
- It results from a deficiency of, or resistance to, the hormone insulin.
- Insulin is normally secreted from the beta islet cells of the pancreas in response to increased blood glucose levels.
- Adequate insulin effect is necessary for glucose transport into insulin-dependent cells (muscle, adipose tissue); anabolic synthesis of glycogen (liver, muscle), cellular proteins (muscle), and triglycerides (adipose tissue); and maintenance of normal blood glucose (sugar) concentration (normal blood glucose is 70–110 mg/dL).
- Inadequate insulin effect leads to chronic hyperglycemia, with acute and chronic complications.
- Acute complications of Type 1 DM include hypoglycemia (diabetics on exogenous insulin); and diabetic ketoacidosis (DKA).
- An acute complication of Type 2 DM is hyperosmolar nonketotic coma (HNKC).
- Chronic complications of DM include vasculopathy (nephropathy, retinopathy, peripheral) and neuropathy (sensory, motor, autonomic).
- About 5% of the U.S. population is diabetic.

CAUSES

- There are two primary types of DM: Type 1 and Type 2.

Type 1 DM:

- Results from destruction of pancreatic islet beta cells due to an autoimmune process.
- Precipitating factors include a genetic predisposition, an environmental trigger such as a viral infection (mumps, rubella, or coxsackievirus B4), or chemical toxin. An abnormal immune response that targets normal islet beta cells follows, destroying them.

- Produces an absolute insulin deficiency, necessitating exogenous insulin therapy.
- Affects approximately 5% to 10% of people with DM.

Type 2 DM:

- Results from insufficient insulin to maintain normal blood glucose levels.
- Exact cause unknown; theories include limited beta cell response to hyperglycemia, peripheral insulin resistance, and abnormalities of insulin receptors.
- Associated with obesity that decreases number of available insulin receptor sites in skeletal muscle and adipose tissues.
- Unlike Type 1 DM, there is sufficient insulin present to prevent fat breakdown.
- Higher incidence among Hispanics, Native Americans, and African Americans.

Other Types:

- Genetic beta-cell defects
- Genetic insulin-action defects
- Exocrine pancreatic disorders
- Drug or chemical induced
- Infections
- Gestational DM

Signs & Symptoms

Short-Term S/S

- Hyperglycemia
- Polyuria
- Polydipsia
- Polyphagia (Type 1)
- Fatigue, weakness
- Weight loss (Type 1)
- Blurred vision, frequent skin infections (Type 2)

Long-Term S/S

- Angiopathy of small vessels (microangiopathy) or large vessels (macroangiopathy)
- Microangiopathy:
  1. retinopathy, may progress to blindness
  2. nephropathy, may progress to renal failure

- Macroangiopathy:
  1. coronary artery disease (CAD), may result in myocardial infarction
  2. cerebral vascular disease, may result in stroke
  3. peripheral vascular disease (PVD), may progress to gangrene/amputation
- Neuropathy: conduction is slowed in peripheral and autonomic nerves
  1. peripheral neuropathy with numbness, tingling, hypesthesia, paresthesias, reduced reflexes
  2. autonomic neuropathy resulting in orthostatic hypotension, slowed digestion, urinary bladder incontinence or retention, male impotence

Acute Complications

- Type 1:
  1. S/S of hypoglycemia (insulin shock) due to excess insulin or lack of food intake
  2. S/S of ketoacidosis due to insufficient insulin
- Type 2:
  1. S/S of HNKC with significant hyperglycemia and a plasma osmolarity of 340 mOsm/L or higher

Diagnostics

- Fasting plasma glucose (FPG) ≥126 mg/dL at least two times.
- Random plasma glucose ≥200 mg/dL at least two times.
- Glucose tolerance test (GTT) ≥200 mg/dL during 2-hour testing period.
- Urine glucose/ketones positive (none normally present in urine).
- Glycosylated hemoglobin (Hgb) >7% (normal, 4%–7%); assesses degree of hyperglycemia and compliance over past 2- to 3-month period.
- Renal function tests (BUN, creatinine, creatinine clearance) and urine protein to detect nephropathy.
- Serum cholesterol and triglyceride levels to evaluate risk of CAD.

MEDICAL INTERVENTIONS

- Clients with Type 1 DM require a lifelong exogenous source of the insulin hormone to maintain life. Oral hypoglycemic agents may be used to treat clients with Type 2 DM.
- The goals of dietary management include restoring normal blood glucose and optimal lipid levels; attaining and maintaining reasonable body weight; staying consistent in timing of meals and snacks; and improving overall health through optimal nutrition. The diet should be high in fiber and low in saturated fat and cholesterol. Nonnutritive sweeteners and fructose, sorbitol, and xylitol may be used. Alcohol may be consumed only in restricted amounts: no more than two drinks at one time and only with a meal.
- Regular exercise reduces glucose levels by increasing the uptake of glucose by muscle cells, potentially reducing the need for insulin. Exercise also reduces cholesterol and triglyceride levels, decreasing the risk of CAD.
- Surgical management of DM involves replacing or transplanting the pancreas, pancreatic cells, or beta cells.

SELECTED NURSING DIAGNOSES WITH INTERVENTIONS

Altered Skin Integrity

- Conduct baseline and ongoing assessments of the feet, as clients with diabetes are at significant risk for lower extremity gangrene due to the effects of peripheral neuropathy and angiopathy.
- Teach foot hygiene.
- Stress the importance of well-fitting shoes and avoiding barefoot walking.
- Discuss the importance of not smoking.
- Discuss the importance of maintaining blood glucose levels through prescribed diet, medication, and exercise.

Risk for Infection

- Use and teach meticulous hand washing.
- Monitor for clinical manifestations of infection in clients at high risk.

- Discuss the importance of skin care. Keep the skin clean and dry, using lukewarm water and mild soap.
- Teach dental health measures.
- Teach women with diabetes the symptoms of and preventive measures for vaginitis caused by *Candida albicans*.

Risk for Injury

- Assess for the presence of contributing or causative factors that increase the risk of injury, including blurred vision, cataracts, decreased adaptation to dark, decreased tactile sensitivity, hypoglycemia, hyperglycemia, hypovolemia, joint immobility, and unstable gait.
- Reduce environmental hazards in the health care facility, and teach the client about safety in the home.
- Monitor for, and teach the client with Type 1 DM and significant others to recognize and seek care for, the manifestations of DKA, including hyperglycemia, thirst, headaches, nausea and vomiting, abdominal pain, increased urine output, ketonuria, dehydration, and decreasing level of consciousness.
- Monitor for, and teach the client with Type 2 DM and significant others to recognize and seek care for, the manifestations of HNKC, including extreme hyperglycemia, increased urinary output, thirst, dehydration, hypotension, seizures, and decreasing level of consciousness.
- Monitor for, and teach the client and significant others to recognize and treat the manifestations of, hypoglycemia, including low blood glucose, anxiety, headache, uncoordinated movements, sweating, rapid pulse, drowsiness, and visual changes.
- Recommend that the client wear a MedicAlert bracelet or necklace identifying self as a person with diabetes.

Ineffective Individual Coping

- Assess the client's psychosocial resources.
- Explore with the client and significant others the effects (actual and perceived) of the diagnosis and treatment on finances, occupation, energy levels, and relationships.

- Teach constructive problem-solving techniques:
  1. Identify the problem.
  2. Find the cause of the problem.
  3. Determine the options.
  4. List the advantages and disadvantages of each option.
  5. Choose an option and make a plan.
- Provide information about support groups and resources, such as suppliers of products, journals, cookbooks, and so on.

CLIENT TEACHING

- Teach the client and significant others the importance of strict compliance with treatment regimens, including diet, exercise, medications, and blood glucose monitoring techniques and injection of insulin.
- Provide the client with information on the role of blood glucose levels on long-term health.
- Teach the rationale for and importance of regular foot care.
- Stress the importance of reading nutritional labels for hidden sugar content, and provide the client with a list of terms that indicate sugar content as well as those that are safe to consume.

HOME CARE CONSIDERATIONS

- A referral to a social worker or home health nurse may be appropriate. Consider the client's income level, as money to purchase medications and supplies often must be taken out of a fixed income.
- Provide the client with information on how to purchase supplies, and how to obtain a MedicAlert bracelet or necklace.
- Encourage regular eye examinations.
- Provide the client with a list of community resources such as the American Diabetes Asssociation.

For more information on Diabetes Mellitus, see Medical-Surgical Nursing *by LeMone and Burke, p. 716.*

Diabetic Ketoacidosis (DKA)

OVERVIEW

- Diabetic ketoacidosis (DKA) is a form of metabolic acidosis that results when insulin deficit causes fat stores to break down, releasing fatty acids and ketones.

CAUSES

- Occurs in untreated Type 1 diabetes mellitus
- May occur in people with diagnosed Type 1 DM when energy requirements increase during stress, causing release of gluconeogenic hormones that stimulate carbohydrate formation from protein or fat
- Lack of insulin causes hyperglycemia, hyperosmolarity, and resulting osmotic diuresis
- Ketoacids accumulate, causing metabolic acidosis

Signs & Symptoms

- Fatigue, confusion, coma
- Polyuria secondary to high blood glucose
- Poor skin turgor/dry mucous membranes secondary to fluid losses
- Fever secondary to fluid volume deficit
- Hypotension
- Kussmaul's (deep, rapid, labored) respirations
- Anorexia, nausea, vomiting, abdominal pain
- Altered levels of consciousness: confusion, stupor, coma

Diagnostics

- ABGs show plasma pH <7.3; plasma HCO_3 (bicarbonate) <15 mEq/L, decreased $Paco_2$.
- Blood glucose levels >300 mg/dL.
- Ketones present in blood and urine; glycosuria.

MEDICAL INTERVENTIONS

- DKA requires immediate medical attention. Fluids are administered for dehydration, and insulin is given to reduce hyperglycemia and acidosis.

- Potassium replacement is begun early in the course of treatment.

SELECTED NURSING DIAGNOSES

- Risk for Injury
- Altered Nutrition: More than Body Requirements
- Fluid Volume Deficit
- Ineffective Individual Coping
- Knowledge Deficit

SELECTED NURSING INTERVENTIONS

- Administer fluids, insulin, and potassium as prescribed.
- Monitor blood sugars using the fingerstick method.
- Encourage resumption of diabetic diet, oral fluid intake, and insulin self-administration as soon as possible.

CLIENT TEACHING

- Teach client and significant others "sick day" management.
- Teach the client and significant others the signs and symptoms of impending diabetic ketoacidosis and ways to prevent condition.
- Assess the client's knowledge of his or her individual diabetes management plan and reinforce teaching where needed.

HOME CARE CONSIDERATIONS

- Stress the need for long-term follow-up care with the physician, diabetic clinical nurse specialist, and dietitian.
- A referral to a social worker or psychologic counselor for assistance in coping with chronic diabetes may be appropriate.

For more information on Diabetic Ketoacidosis, see Medical-Surgical Nursing *by LeMone and Burke, p. 723.*

Disseminated Intravascular Coagulation (DIC)

OVERVIEW

- Disseminated intravascular coagulation (DIC) is usually an acute disorder of the coagulation system secondary to a precipitating event that releases thromboplastic substances and triggers the clotting cascade.
- Accelerated rates of clotting produce diffuse fibrin deposition within the microcirculation of multiple body organs; most commonly the extremities, kidneys, adrenal glands, lung, brain, pituitary gland, and GI system.
- Red blood cells (RBCs) become trapped in the fibrin clot and hemolyze.
- As fibrin deposits rapidly form, both platelets and coagulation factors are consumed.
- As platelets and clotting factors become depleted, fibrinolysis of previously formed clots begins.
- Because clotting factors have become depleted and fibrinolysis digests previously formed clots, abnormal and excessive bleeding occurs in the final stages.
- A chronic type may be seen with malignant neoplastic disease.

CAUSES

Precipitating events include:

- Burns, especially extensive ones
- Embolism: pulmonary, fat
- Infection: especially bacterial septicemia, but possible with any organism
- Hemolysis: transfusion reaction, sickle cell crisis
- Obstetric complications: abortion (second trimester), abruptio placenta, amniotic fluid embolus, endometritis with sepsis, fetal demise, hemorrhage, toxemia of pregnancy

- Necrotizing disorders, such as frostbite, gunshot wounds, head injury, trauma, transplant rejection, liver necrosis
- Neoplastic disease, especially leukemias, lymphomas, metastatic carcinoma
- Other: acute respiratory distress syndrome (ARDS), cardiac arrest, cardiopulmonary bypass, diabetic ketoacidosis (DKA), drug reactions, shock, heat stroke, snakebite, cirrhosis

Signs & Symptoms

S/S can be rapidly fulminating or mild. They include:

- Spontaneous bleeding without a prior history of bleeding disorder and with known or suspected precipitating event
- Epistaxis (nosebleed)
- Cutaneous S/S: ecchymosis, hematoma, petechiae, purpura, oozing of blood from surgical incisions or venipuncture sites
- Respiratory S/S: dyspnea, tachypnea, hemoptysis
- Cardiovascular S/S: shock, reduced amplitude of pulses, chest pain
- Gastrointestinal S/S: nausea, vomiting, abdominal pain, hematemesis, rectal bleeding/melena
- Renal S/S: hematuria, oliguria, flank pain
- Central nervous system (CNS) S/S: decreased level of consciousness (LOC), seizures
- Pain: severe muscle, back, abdominal, chest
- S/S of multiple organ dysfunction syndrome (MODS) possible

Diagnostics

- Prothrombin time (PT) is increased (>15 seconds).
- Partial thromboplastin time (PTT) is increased (>60–80 seconds).
- Plasma fibrinogen levels are decreased (<150 mg/dL).
- Fibrin degradation products (FDPs) or fibrin split products (FSPs) are increased (>10 μg/mL).
- Platelet count is decreased (<100,000/μL).
- D-dimer test is positive at <1:8 dilutions.

MEDICAL INTERVENTIONS

- Fresh frozen plasma and platelet concentrates are administered to control bleeding.
- Heparin may be administered to prevent the consumption of clotting factors that occurs with uncontrolled clotting. It is used when bleeding is not controlled by plasma and platelets, as well as for manifestations of thrombotic problems such as acrocyanosis and possible gangrene.

SELECTED NURSING DIAGNOSES WITH INTERVENTIONS

Altered Tissue Perfusion

- Assess the client's extremities for pulses, warmth, and capillary refill. Assess LOC and mental status.
- Report to the physician promptly any changes in mental status, extremities, GI function, and urinary output.
- Carefully turn the client from side to side every 2 hours.
- Discourage the client from crossing his or her legs, and do not use the knee gatch on the bed.
- Minimize the use of adhesive tape on the skin.

Impaired Gas Exchange

- Administer oxygen as prescribed.
- Position the client in the semi-Fowler's or high-Fowler's position.
- Maintain bed rest.
- Encourage deep breathing and effective coughing.
- If the client is unable to cough effectively, careful nasotracheal suctioning may be instituted.
- Monitor pulse oximetry and arterial blood gas (ABG) results, and report abnormal results to the physician.
- Take measures to reduce pain and fear.

Fear

- Allow the client and significant others to verbalize concerns.
- Answer questions truthfully.
- Identify coping strategies the client and significant others may be able to use.

- Provide emotional support to the client and significant others.
- Maintain a calm environment.
- Respond promptly when the client calls for help.
- Instruct the client in relaxation techniques.

CLIENT TEACHING

- Teach the client and significant others the pathophysiology of the disorder, its treatment, including medications, and how to prevent further bleeding.

HOME CARE CONSIDERATIONS

- Referral to a home health nurse may be appropriate.

For more information on Disseminated Intravascular Coagulation, see Medical-Surgical Nursing *by LeMone and Burke, p. 1292.*

Diverticular Disease

OVERVIEW

- Diverticular disease is the formation of abnormal herniations, called *diverticula*, of mucosal tissue through the muscle layers in the walls of the gastrointestinal (GI) tract.
- Any portion of the tubular GI tract can form diverticula, but they are most commonly found in the colon, especially the sigmoid portion.
- It is thought to be due to high intraluminal pressures.
- *Diverticulosis* is the presence of diverticula; most are asymptomatic.
- *Diverticulitis* refers to inflamed diverticula that occur when fecal material becomes trapped in a diverticulum and forms a hard mass (or fecalith); it may result in obstruction, infection, perforation, hemorrhage, or fistula formation.

- It is mostly seen in adults in the United States: 5% of people in their 40s and 50% or more of those over 80 have diverticula.

CAUSES

- Risk factors include a low-fiber diet: diverticular disease is almost unknown in undeveloped countries where unrefined (high-fiber) diets are consumed
- Decreased activity levels and postponement of defecation may be contributing factors

Signs & Symptoms

Diverticulosis

- Usually asymptomatic but may produce abdominal cramping, decreased stool caliber, constipation, and occult blood in the stool.

Diverticulitis

- S/S may occur in paroxysmal attacks
- Pain: mild to severe left-lower-quadrant (LLQ) abdominal; crampy; often relieved upon defecation; rebound tenderness
- Nausea, vomiting, anorexia; gas; flatus
- Irregular bowel habits; alternating constipation, diarrhea
- S/S of infection: fever, chills, leukocytosis

Diagnostics

- Barium enema is used to illustrate the diverticula.
- Sigmoidoscopy or colonoscopy is used to detect diverticulosis.
- Abdominal x-rays detect presence of gas; degree of obstruction; and presence of air in the abdominal cavity, which may indicate perforation.
- Computed tomography (CT) scan is appropriate for those not able to tolerate barium enema; it can identify diverticula, wall changes, abscesses, and fistulas.
- A complete blood count (CBC) with differential is done: the white blood cell (WBC) count may be elevated, with an increased number of immature WBCs.

- Guaiac testing of the stool often reveals the presence of occult blood.

MEDICAL INTERVENTIONS

- Pharmacologic agents include systemic broad-spectrum antibiotics effective against usual bowel flora. Pentazocine may be prescribed for pain relief. A stool softener such as docusate sodium may be prescribed. Laxatives are avoided.
- Bowel rest is prescribed for the client with acute diverticulitis. A high-residue diet with fiber is recommended following recovery.
- Resection of the affected bowel segment, with anastomosis of the proximal and distal portions, may be elected for clients with acute diverticulitis; temporary colostomy may be a possibility.

SELECTED NURSING DIAGNOSES WITH INTERVENTIONS

Impaired Tissue Integrity: Gastrointestinal

- Monitor blood pressure, rate and rhythm of pulse, and respiratory rate at least every 4 hours.
- Take temperature every 4 hours.
- Perform an abdominal assessment every 4 to 8 hours, or more often as indicated.
- Assess for evidence of lower intestinal bleeding by visual examination and guaiac testing of stools for occult blood.
- Maintain IV fluids, total parenteral nutrition, and accurate intake and output records.

Pain

- Ask the client to rate pain on a scale of 0 to 10. Document the level of pain, and note any changes in the location or character of the client's pain.
- Administer prescribed analgesic, assessing its effectiveness one half hour after administration. Avoid morphine administration.
- Maintain bowel rest and total body rest as prescribed.
- Reintroduce oral foods and fluids slowly, providing a soft, low-fiber diet, followed by a high-fiber diet with bulk-forming agents after recovery.

Anxiety

- Assess and document the client's level of anxiety.
- Demonstrate empathy and awareness of the perceived threat to the client's health.
- Attend to the client's physical care needs.
- Spend as much time as possible with the client.
- Assess the client's level of understanding about his or her condition.
- Encourage supportive significant others to remain with the client as much as possible.
- Assist the client to identify and use appropriate coping mechanisms.
- Involve the client and significant others (as appropriate) in care decisions.

CLIENT TEACHING

- For the client with acute diverticulitis, explain all diagnostic and therapeutic procedures. Discuss oral food and fluid limitations, and explain the rationale for a low-residue diet initially.
- Teach the client with chronic diverticular disease the importance of maintaining a high-fiber diet for the remainder of his or her life. Discuss means of increasing dietary fiber, and refer the client to a dietitian as needed.
- Discuss the complications of diverticular disease and how to recognize their manifestations.

HOME CARE CONSIDERATIONS

- Clients undergoing surgery will require instructions in home care, including information on where to purchase additional supplies, if appropriate.
- Clients with a colostomy will need information on management, as well as referral to the United Ostomy Association.
- A referral to a home health agency may be appropriate.

For more information on Diverticular Disease, see Medical-Surgical Nursing *by LeMone and Burke, p. 869.*

Dysfunctional Uterine Bleeding

OVERVIEW

- Dysfunctional uterine bleeding is defined as abnormal uterine bleeding patterns.
- It is due to abnormal hormonal patterns, especially when estrogen is secreted unopposed by progesterone, producing endometrial hyperplasia.
- It accounts for a significant amount of gynecologic surgery.

CAUSES

- Polycystic ovary syndrome
- Anovulatory cycles: perimenopausal
- Obesity
- Immature hypothalamic-pituitary function (adolescents)

Signs & Symptoms

- Menorrhagia: excessive bleeding with menses
- Hypermenorrhea: prolonged menstrual periods (> 8 days)
- Polymenorrhea: frequent menstrual periods (<18 days)
- Metrorrhagia: bleeding in the middle of the cycle
- Postmenopausal bleeding
- S/S of anemia

Diagnostics

- Dilation and curettage (D&C) to obtain endometrial tissue for biopsy.
- Biopsy can reveal endometrial hyperplasia.
- Hemoglobin and hematocrit will be low if anemia is present.

MEDICAL INTERVENTIONS

- Dysfunctional uterine bleeding in some clients can be corrected with hormonal agents. Progesterone or medroxyprogesterone may be prescribed. Oral iron supplements may be used to replace iron lost through bleeding.
- Surgical options include therapeutic D&C, endometrial ablation, and hysterectomy.

SELECTED NURSING DIAGNOSES WITH INTERVENTIONS

Ineffective Individual Coping

- Discuss the results of tests and examinations with the client face to face.
- Involve the client in developing the treatment plan.
- Assist the client in identifying personal strengths and coping strategies.
- Encourage the client to be involved in care activities, demonstrate feelings, express concerns, and request the attention and involvement of significant others.

Sexual Dysfunction

- Offer information about engaging in sexual intercourse during menstruation.
- Provide an opportunity for the client to express concerns related to alterations in lifestyle and sexual functioning.
- Encourage frequent rest periods.
- Provide information about alternative methods of sexual expression.

Decreased Cardiac Output

- Monitor vital signs, hemoglobin, and hematocrit to determine severity of blood loss.
- Monitor bleeding pattern, including duration and amount of bleeding.
- Administer prescribed medications and monitor response to therapy.

CLIENT TEACHING

- Teach the client about her disorder and the therapeutic interventions indicated.
- Discuss medication regimen, including oral contraceptives, iron supplements, and other agents, including dosage, effects, and side effects.
- Nutritional teaching should center on the need to maintain a balanced diet, increasing iron-rich foods such as beans, liver, beef, and shrimp.

HOME CARE CONSIDERATIONS

- Encourage the client to document her menstrual cycles on a calendar to assist in diagnosis and to monitor the effectiveness of treatment.
- Emphasize the need to report recurring episodes of dysfunctional uterine bleeding, particularly in postmenopausal women.

For more information on Dysfunctional Uterine Bleeding, see Medical-Surgical Nursing *by LeMone and Burke, p. 2009.*

Emphysema

OVERVIEW

- Emphysema is a progressive type of chronic obstructive pulmonary disease (COPD).
- It is characterized by destruction of alveolar walls that causes enlargement of distal air spaces and loss of surface area for gas exchange.
- About 65% of clients with emphysema are male.
- Most lungs at autopsy have some degree of emphysematous change.

CAUSES

- Genetic defects: alpha$_1$-antitrypsin deficiency causes excessive interalveolar tissue, elasticity loss
- Smoking releases inflammatory mediators that break down alveolar walls

Signs & Symptoms

- Shortness of breath (SOB), progresses from dyspnea on exertion to dyspnea at rest
- Chronic cough (expectorations not excessive)
- Pursed-lip breathing (slow, deep, with prolonged expiratory phase)
- Auscultation reveals reduced breath sounds, rales, wheezing, grunting, distant heart sounds
- Percussion reveals hyperresonance
- Anorexia, weight loss
- Barrel chest (increased AP diameter)
- Hypertrophy of accessory muscles of respiration
- Clubbing of fingernails
- Pink color usually; known as "pink puffers"
- Cyanosis indicates respiratory failure
- If PaCO_2 is >50 mm Hg: occipital headache, drowsiness, decreased ability to concentrate
- If PaCO_2 is >75 mm Hg: asterixis (hand-flapping tremor), confusion, coma

Diagnostics

- Chest x-rays show hyperinflation with flattened diaphragm, reduced vascular markings and enlarged AP diameter.
- Pulmonary function tests show increased residual volume, total lung capacity, and inspiratory flows.
- Arterial blood gases show decreased Pao_2 with $Paco_2$ normal or near normal (early); $Paco_2$ rises later.

MEDICAL INTERVENTIONS

- Pharmacologic agents include antibiotics, bronchodilators, and $alpha_1$-antitrypsin replacement therapy.
- Smoking cessation is vital.
- Pulmonary hygiene measures include hydration, effective cough, percussion, and postural drainage.
- The client may require oxygenation and inspiratory positive-pressure assistance with a face mask or intubation and mechanical ventilation.
- Lung transplantation may be an option.

SELECTED NURSING DIAGNOSES

(Also see COPD)

- Ineffective Breathing Pattern
- Ineffective Airway Clearance
- Impaired Gas Exchange
- Activity Intolerance
- Fatigue

SELECTED NURSING INTERVENTIONS

(Also see COPD)

- Monitor respiratory status, including atertial blood gases (ABGs), pulmonary function tests, and red blood cell (RBC) count for increase, which may indicate lung or vascular congestion.
- Provide chest physiotherapy and postural drainage every 4 hours or as needed.

- Schedule respiratory treatments at least 1 hour before or after meals.
- Encourage fluid intake of 2 to 3 L per day.
- Provide a calm, quiet environment and encourage frequent rest periods.
- Administer prescribed medications, including inhalers and nebulizers, and monitor response.
- Encourage verbalizations of concerns and fears, and answer questions honestly.

CLIENT TEACHING

- Explain to the client the importance of smoking cessation. Also teach the client to avoid respiratory irritants such as second-hand smoke and pollution, and to avoid crowds and people with known infections.
- Teach the client and significant others chest physiotherapy and postural drainage techniques, as well as effective coughing and breathing techniques.
- Review medication regimen, including proper use of inhalers and nebulizers.
- Encourage a high-kilocalorie, protein-rich diet.
- Encourage the client to avoid cold, windy weather and to cover the mouth and nose when outdoors in cold weather.
- Tell the client to report sudden, sharp chest pain that is exacerbated by chest movement, breathing, and coughing.

HOME CARE CONSIDERATIONS

- A referral to a smoking cessation program may be appropriate.
- A home health care referral may be appropriate for oxygen therapy needs.
- Stress the need for lifelong medical care.

For more information on Emphysema, see Medical-Surgical Nursing *by LeMone and Burke, p. 1434.*

Empyema

OVERVIEW

- Empyema is a collection of pus in the pleural space that is thick and foul-smelling.
- Purulent material is retrievable by thoracentesis.
- Atelectasis of lung tissue is proportional to the size of the collection of pus.
- It usually occurs secondary to another respiratory problem.
- Chest tubes or thoracotomy may be needed to remove pus.

CAUSES

- Pulmonary infection, usually lung abscess
- Thoracic surgery, chest trauma

Signs & Symptoms

- Fever, chills, night sweats
- Anorexia, weight loss
- Chest pain
- Dyspnea
- Cough
- Decreased chest wall movement on affected side
- Auscultation: decreased breath sounds over area
- Percussion: flat
- Palpation: diminished or absent fremitus

Diagnostics

- Chest x-ray reveals visible opaque effusion if volume is sufficient.
- Thoracentesis allows for removal of fluid for analysis (culture and sensitivity).

MEDICAL INTERVENTIONS

- Thoracentesis is performed to drain the pus from the pleural cavity.
- An open thoracotomy and surgical debridement of the pleural space may be used in severe cases.

- Antibiotics are the primary pharmacologic treatment.

SELECTED NURSING DIAGNOSES

- Impaired Gas Exchange
- Ineffective Breathing Pattern
- Pain

SELECTED NURSING INTERVENTIONS

- Assess respiratory status, including rate and depth of respirations, breath sounds, and so on, frequently.
- Monitor arterial blood gases (ABGs) if the client is hypoxic.
- Prepare the client for thoracentesis and chest tube insertion. If required, prepare the client for surgery.
- Exercise standard precautions. Maintain strict aseptic technique when caring for chest tubes, including on air-occlusive dressing around tube insertion site.
- Administer antibiotics and oxygen as prescribed and monitor responses.

CLIENT TEACHING

- Explain all tests and procedures, medications, and their effects and side effects.
- Discuss home management of the drainage tube, if indicated.
- Encourage yearly vaccinations against influenza and pneumonia.

HOME CARE CONSIDERATIONS

- Referral to a smoking cessation program may be appropriate.
- Home health care referral may be required for tube management and oxygen therapy.
- Stress the importance of long-term medical follow-up care.

For more information on Empyema, see Medical-Surgical Nursing *by LeMone and Burke, p. 1393.*

Encephalitis

OVERVIEW

- Encephalitis is an inflammation of the brain parenchyma (functional tissue) and meninges (covering membranes).

- It is most frequently due to viral organisms; however, any organism is possible.
- Viral infections are characterized by infiltration of lymphocytes; bacterial types by polymorphonuclear leukocytes (PMNs).
- Brain tissues are inflamed; edema formation increases intracranial pressure.
- Cerebral edema can be mild or severe enough to cause brain stem herniation, a medical emergency.
- Brain cells are destroyed; the number and type varies with the cause.
- Residual neurologic deficits may follow.
- The prognosis depends on the specific offending organism and the client's resistance.

CAUSES

- Most frequently due to viral infections; prognosis varies with type:

  1. Common viruses include arboviruses (epidemic type), enteroviruses, herpes simplex virus-1 (HSV-1), mumps
  2. Less common viruses are cytomegalovirus (CMV), Epstein-Barr virus (EBV), human immunodeficiency virus (HIV), varicella-zoster virus (VZV), and measles
  3. Rare viruses include Colorado tick-fever virus (CTFV), lymphocytic choriomeningitis virus (LCMV), adenoviruses, influenza A, rubella, and rabies

- Other, nonviral organisms that can cause encephalitis are:

  1. Bacteria (*Listeria monocytogenes, Mycobacterium tuberculosis*)
  2. Mycoplasma
  3. Fungi (*Cryptococcus*)

4. Protozoa (*Toxoplasmosis*)
5. Rickettsia
- Other, noninfectious causes are neoplasms, vascular disease, abscess, toxins, Reye's syndrome, subdural hematoma, and systemic lupus erythematosus

Signs & Symptoms

- S/S of infection: fever, chills, malaise
- S/S of meningeal irritation: nuchal rigidity (stiff neck), neck pain, positive Brudzinski's sign, positive Kernig's sign
- S/S of increased intracranial pressure: headache; changes in level of consciousness such as irritability, confusion, drowsiness, stupor, coma, and declining Glascow coma scale; vital sign changes such as bradycardia, hypertension, increased pulse pressure, and altered respiratory patterns; pupillary changes such as inequality or dilation; brain stem herniation is rapidly fatal
- Focal S/S: vary widely but may include photophobia, aphasia, sensory deficits (blindness, deafness, loss of taste/smell), motor deficits (ataxia), psychosis, or seizures

Diagnostics

- Lumbar puncture and cerebrospinal fluid (CSF) analysis may reveal elevated CSF pressure, increased white blood cells (WBCs), increased protein, but normal glucose; fluid is usually clear.
- Electroencephalogram (EEG) may show focal or general electric slowing.
- Compute tomography (CT) scanning or magnetic resonance imaging (MRI) can rule out other neurologic conditions or show areas of swelling.
- Brain biopsy collects brain tissue specimens to identify specific virus.

MEDICAL INTERVENTIONS

- Pharmacologic agents include antiviral drugs to treat the infection and osmotic diuretics and corticosteroids to control cerebral edema.

SELECTED NURSING DIAGNOSES

- Pain
- Altered Tissue Perfusion: Cerebral
- Sleep Pattern Disturbance
- Risk for Altered Skin Integrity
- Risk for Injury

SELECTED NURSING INTERVENTIONS

- Assess for fever, malaise, headache, listlessness, joint pain, nausea, vomiting, change in level of consciousness, hemiparesis, tremors, seizures, stiff neck, aphasia, and cranial nerve dysfunction.
- Maintain a quiet, calm environment and organize care to minimize unnecessary stimulation.
- Maintain the bed in the low position, with side rails up and padded and the head of the bed elevated 30° to 45°.
- Assess vital signs frequently and administer analgesics/antipyretics as prescribed to reduce temperature.
- Monitor nutritional and fluid balance status and report any abnormalities.
- Institute measures to prevent complications resulting from immobility (e.g., turn the client every 2 hours, use an air mattress to reduce pressure, provide range-of-motion [ROM] exercises, change wet linens promptly).
- Assess client and family support and coping skills and intervene to assist in coping with potential long-term rehabilitation and possible neurologic deficits.

CLIENT TEACHING

- Teach the client and significant others about the disease process and its treatments, medication regimen, prognosis, and any necessary restrictions or precautions.
- Teach significant others necessary procedures for caring for the client at home if appropriate. These include techniques for communicating if the client has aphasia, preventing seizures, assisting with self-care, and so on.

- Refer the client and significant others to a social worker and/or spiritual counselor if appropriate to assist with developing coping skills and planning for long-term care.
- The client with permanent neurologic deficits that result from encephalitis is usually discharged to a rehabilitation setting or a long-term-care facility.

For more information on Encephalitis, see Medical-Surgical Nursing *by LeMone and Burke, p. 1748.*

Endocarditis

OVERVIEW

- Endocarditis is an inflammation of the endo-cardium, the membrane lining the heart chambers and covering the valves.
- It is usually due to a bacterial infection that produces vegetations, each of which is a matrix of fibrin, blood cells, and organisms, that adhere to the endocardium, usually on the heart valves.
- It occurs more frequently in the left heart, affecting the mitral and aortic valves.
- Vegetations on the valves can result in regurgitation (inadequate closure) or stenosis (narrowing).
- It can also affect the mural portions of the endo-cardium and produce inflammation and degeneration of the myocardium.
- There is a high risk for the formation of vegetative emboli that can be released to the systemic circulation; most frequently to the coronary vessels, brain, kidney, spleen, liver, extremities, or lung (right-sided vegetation).
- Depending on the specific organism, the course can be subacute, or acute, fulminating, and rapidly fatal.
- Infective endocarditis is almost always fatal if untreated.

CAUSES

- Can be caused by infectious or noninfectious sources
- Almost any bacteria can cause endocarditis; other types of organisms are also possible
- Infective endocarditis can be classified into three categories, each with its own specific organisms and course:

  1. *Native valve endocarditis* can affect normal or damaged heart valves. Streptococci, endococci, and staphylococci account for the majority of cases. Men are affected more frequently; most are over 50; 60% to 80% have pre-existing valve disease. Dental procedures, surgery, or instrumentation of the gastrointestinal or genitourinary tracts are common portals of entry for bacteria.
  2. *Intravenous drug abuse (IVDA) endocarditis* produces right-heart vegetation in about 50% of patients and a high rate of pulmonary emboli. The course is often acute; skin organisms such as *S. aureus* (>50% of cases), streptococci, enterococci, fungi, and gram-negative bacilli cause the majority of cases.
  3. *Prosthetic valve endocarditis* accounts for about 20% of all cases. Intracardiac and/or vascular sutures, pacemaker wires, or silastic tubing can be foci of infection.

Signs & Symptoms

- S/S may develop rapidly or insidiously; they usually appear within 2 weeks of the precipitating event
- Early, nonspecific S/S include intermittent fever, night sweats, malaise, anorexia, weight loss, arthralgia
- Heart murmur (usually loud and regurgitative)
- Splenomegaly
- Lesions of abnormal bleeding, such as petechiae (conjunctiva, oral mucosa, skin); splinter hemorrhages (subungual); Roth's spots (retina); Janeway lesions (palms and soles)

- Ostler nodes (small tender nodules on the fingers and toes)
- Normocytic, normochromic anemia
- S/S of embolism (pulmonary, cerebral, or peripheral arterial, depending on location of vegetation)
- Organ failure if destroyed by embolic vegetation

Diagnostics

- Blood culture: usually three are drawn within a 24-hour period; usually identifies organism.
- White blood cell (WBC) count is elevated.
- Erythrocyte sedimentation rate (ESR) is elevated.
- Red blood cell (RBC) count, hemoglobin (Hgb), and hematocrit (HCT) are reduced and reveal a normocytic, normochromic anemia.
- Rheumatoid factor (autoantibody) is positive in 50% of clients.
- Echocardiograms may show vegetation and valvular damage.
- EKG may show atrial fibrillation.

MEDICAL INTERVENTIONS

- Antibiotic therapy is the mainstay of treatment for infective endocarditis.
- Surgical intervention is used to replace severely damaged valves, remove large vegetations, or remove a valve that is a continuing source of infection.

SELECTED NURSING DIAGNOSES WITH INTERVENTIONS

Risk for Altered Body Temperature

- Record the client's temperature every 2 to 4 hours. Notify the physician if it rises above 101.5 F (39.4 C). Assess the client for complaints of discomfort.
- Obtain blood cultures as prescribed before giving the first dose of antibiotics.
- Administer anti-inflammatory or antipyretic agents as prescribed.
- Administer antibiotics as prescribed; obtain peak and trough drug levels as indicated.

Risk for Altered Tissue Perfusion

- Assess for and document any manifestations of decreased perfusion to major organ systems:
  1. Neurologic system: decreased level of consciousness, numbness or tingling in extremities, hemiplegia, visual disturbances.
  2. Renal system: decreased output, hematuria, elevated blood urea nitrogen (BUN) or creatinine.
  3. Pulmonary system: dyspnea, hemoptysis, shortness of breath, diminished breath sounds, restlessness, sudden chest or shoulder pain.
  4. Cardiovascular system: complaints of chest pain radiating to jaw or arms, tachycardia, anxiety, tachypnea, hypotension.
- Assess and document skin color and temperature, quality of peripheral pulses, and capillary refill.

CLIENT TEACHING

- Teach the client about the disease process, manifestations, treatment, and prognosis.
- Stress the importance of promptly reporting to the physician any unusual manifestation, such as change in vision, sudden pain, or weakness.
- Discuss the use of prophylactic antibiotics, the time period required, and procedures that may require them in the future.
- Clients who contract infective endocarditis as a result of IV drug abuse require additional teaching about the risks associated with the intravenous injection of drugs.

HOME CARE CONSIDERATIONS

- Provide the client with educational materials from the American Heart Association.
- Stress the need for lifelong follow-up and prophylactic antibiotics as appropriate.
- Refer clients who contract infective endocarditis as a result of IV drug abuse to a susbstance abuse treatment facility.

For more information on Endocarditis, see Medical-Surgical Nursing *by LeMone and Burke, p. 1159.*

Endometrial (Uterine) Cancer

OVERVIEW

- Endometrial (uterine) cancer is the most common invasive malignancy of the female reproductive tract.
- It is a fairly slow-growing neoplasm, usually discovered during the postmenopausal period.
- It arises from glandular endometrial tissues to produce an adenocarcinoma.
- Initially cancer affects only the superficial uterine lining; later it invades the cervix and underlying myometrium.
- Cancer eventually invades the vagina, uterine tubes, ovaries, and local lymphatics.
- It metastasizes via both blood and lymph to lungs, liver, bones and also intra-abdominally.
- The prognosis depends on stage at diagnosis.

CAUSES

The cause is unknown. Risk factors include:

- Early menarche/late menopause
- Nulliparity/infertility (especially anovulatory)
- Diabetes
- Hypertension
- High-fat diet, obesity
- Unopposed estrogen replacement therapy (i.e., estrogen without progestin)

Signs & Symptoms

- Dysfunctional uterine bleeding (DUB)
- Palpable mass on pelvic examination

Diagnostics

- Aspiration curettage/endometrial biopsy (an office procedure) can identify dysplastic or neoplastic cells.
- Dilation and curettage (D&C) with biopsy (a surgical procedure) collects endometrial cells for biopsy, which can identify neoplastic cells.

- Hysteroscopy visualizes the uterine lining; may show malignant growth areas.
- Metastatic work-up includes chest x-ray, intravenous urography, sigmoidoscopy, and CT or MRI scans.

MEDICAL INTERVENTIONS

- Surgery includes a total abdominal hysterectomy and bilateral salpino-oophorectomy.
- Radiation therapy may be used as a preoperative measure, postoperatively to reduce the incidence of recurrence, or as adjuvant treatment in advanced cases.
- Progesterone agents and the antiestrogen tamoxifen are used to treat invasive disease.

SELECTED NURSING DIAGNOSES WITH INTERVENTIONS

Pain

- Assess the client's level of pain on a scale of 0 to 10 before and after administering medications.
- Administer analgesics as prescribed and monitor for effects and side effects.
- Insert a rectal tube if ordered to relieve flatus.
- Apply heat to the abdomen and recommend that the client use a heating pad at home.

Body Image Disturbance

- Actively listen to the client and acknowledge her concerns about the disease prognosis, treatment, and effects.
- Assist the client in identifying personal strengths, and develop with her a plan of care that identifies coping mechanisms and acknowledges limitations.
- Encourage the client to maintain her usual daily grooming routine as far as possible and to dress in a way that enhances her self-esteem.
- Allow time and the opportunity for the client to verbalize her concerns about her body image and to grieve.

Altered Sexuality Patterns

- Encourage the client and her partner to express their feelings about the impact of cancer on their lives and sexual relationship.

- Tell the client that sexual intercourse may be resumed 3 weeks after a vaginal hysterectomy and 6 weeks after an abdominal hysterectomy.
- Suggest that the couple explore alternative sexual positions and coordinate sexual activity with rest periods and with periods that are relatively free from pain.

CLIENT TEACHING

- Provide the client with information about the specific treatment and prognosis for her cancer.
- Explain the expected side effects of radiation implant therapy.
- Discuss the medication regimen and alternative methods of pain control, including relaxation, guided imagery, distraction, and so on.
- Tell the client that it is normal to experience feelings of weakness, fatigue, emotional lability, and depression at this time.
- Teach the client to avoid tub baths for 2 to 3 weeks, to avoid sitting for prolonged periods, and to avoid jogging, fast walking, horseback riding, and douching for several months.
- Tell the client to avoid heavy lifting and strenuous activity for 6 to 8 weeks.
- Tell the client to report to the physician any signs of bleeding or temperature elevation.

HOME CARE CONSIDERATIONS

- For clients receiving radiation therapy, emphasize the importance of keeping appointments and, if necessary, help them arrange for transportation to and from the facility.
- Refer the client to a local cancer support group and to a psychologic counselor if appropriate for assistance with sexual and body image adjustment.
- Home care may be necessary to assist clients with maintaining activities of daily living (ADLs).
- Refer clients with terminal cancer to hospice services.

For more information on Endometrial (Uterine) Cancer, see Medical-Surgical Nursing *by LeMone and Burke, p. 2033.*

Endometriosis

OVERVIEW

- Endometriosis is the growth of endometrial tissue in ectopic locations such as the uterine tubes, or on pelvic organs such as the ovaries, external surface of the uterus, bladder, or bowel.
- Endometrial tissue located within the myometrium is called *adenomyosis*.
- Occasionally, endometrial tissue may implant in distant locations, anywhere in the body.
- It is usually diagnosed in women 30 to 40 years old; it is uncommon before 20 years of age.
- Lesions are hormone dependent, and they proliferate and bleed during the menstrual cycle just like uterine tissue. However, bleeding in ectopic locations produces inflammation with subsequent formation of fibrous tissue adhesions.
- Endometriosis is a major cause of uterine-tube obstruction, resulting in infertility, ectopic pregnancy, or spontaneous abortion.
- Signs and symptoms worsen during the menstrual years and abate following menopause.

CAUSES

- No direct cause is known.
- Theories have suggested that it may be due to:
  1. reflux of endometrial cells through the uterine tubes
  2. metastasis via lymph or blood
  3. incomplete regression of embryonic mesenchyme
- Risk factors include:
  1. early menarche
  2. short cycles (<27 days)
  3. long flow (>7 days)
  4. heavy flow
  5. dysmenorrhea
  6. delayed childbearing
  7. residence in Western countries

Signs & Symptoms

- Acquired dysmenorrhea: constant (i.e., not crampy) vaginal, pelvic, back pain; begins 5 to 7 days prior to menses, lasts until 2 to 3 days after
- Dyspareunia
- May also be painful urination, defecation
- Infertility

Diagnostics

- Pelvic examination may reveal tenderness at characteristic cycle times, ovarian enlargement, or thickened adnexa.
- Hysterosalpingogram may show obstruction of oviduct; can be therapeutic.
- Laparoscopy allows visualization of pelvic lesions and ablation treatment.

MEDICAL INTERVENTIONS

- Pharmacologic agents include oral contraceptives for women who do not desire pregnancy, danazol for women who wish to become pregnant, and analgesics to control pain.
- Surgical resection of any visible implants of endometrial tissue is often accomplished during laparoscopy.
- Laser vaporization may be used for all but the deepest implants.
- In advanced cases in which childbearing is not an issue, a hysterectomy may be performed.

SELECTED NURSING DIAGNOSES

- Pain
- Ineffective Individual Coping
- Anticipatory Grieving
- Risk for Fluid Volume Deficit

SELECTED NURSING INTERVENTIONS

- Explain the condition, its symptoms, treatment alternatives, and prognosis. Help the client evaluate treatment options and make choices appropriate for her.
- If medication is begun, review the dosage, schedule,

possible side effects, and any warning signs.

- Provide comfort measures such as back rubs and position changes to assist with pain relief.
- Assess the client's vital signs, pad count, complete blood count (CBC), abdominal distention, and abdominal pain for indications of severe bleeding.
- Assess the client's stage in the grieving process for loss of reproductive ability. Be a nonjudgmental listener: accept the client's emotional state, encourage her to discuss her feelings about her potential loss of fertility, and provide support.
- Assess the couple's coping mechanisms and assist them in identifying additional strategies for coping with loss. Provide a private, empathetic environment to allow them to openly discuss their feelings.

CLIENT TEACHING

- Give verbal and written instructions about medications, including drug name, dosage, schedule, purpose, precautions, potential side effects, and warning signs.
- Stress the importance of reporting signs and symptoms of excessive blood loss and, if surgery has been performed, of caring for the wound and reporting indications of infection.

HOME CARE CONSIDERATIONS

- Suggest the client and her partner try alternative positions to reduce pain associated with sexual intercourse.
- Discuss the advantages of having children soon and in rapid succession, using oral contraceptives between pregnancies to reduce bleeding.
- Discuss the possible risks and benefits of long-term oral contraceptive therapy for the client with endometriosis.
- Emphasize the importance of follow-up visits to the physician for continuing care.
- A referral to a support group such as RESOLVE may be appropriate.

For more information on Endometriosis, see Medical-Surgical Nursing *by LeMone and Burke, p. 2026.*

Epilepsy

OVERVIEW

- Epilepsy is a chronic, idiopathic condition with recurrent episodes of seizure activity.
- A seizure (convulsion) is an abnormal, excessive electric discharge within the brain.
- It may be primary or secondary to another condition.
- Epilepsy occurs in approximately 0.5% to 2.0% of the general population, usually in persons less than 20 years of age; most are well controlled with medication.
- Large amounts of glucose and oxygen are consumed by neurons during a seizure.
- Status epilepticus is prolonged seizure activity that may result in neuron death due to lack of glucose and/or oxygen; it is usually precipitated by anticonvulsant withdrawal or noncompliance, metabolic disturbances, drug toxicity, or CNS pathology such as infection, tumor, or injury.
- Epileptic seizures can be classified as generalized or local.

CAUSES

- Primary, idiopathic: cause not known
- Secondary causes of seizures include fever, infection (meningitis, encephalitis, brain abscess); cerebrovascular disease; head injury, brain tumor, metabolic conditions (electrolyte/blood sugar derangements), and toxins (carbon monoxide, mercury, ethyl alcohol)

Signs & Symptoms

- Seizures are classified as *partial* (focal) or *generalized*.
- *Partial seizures* occur within discrete regions of the brain; the client may remain conscious (simple-partial seizures) or consciousness may be impaired (complex-partial seizures). In some instances, partial seizures may spread to involve

the entire cerebral cortex (partial seizures with generalization).

- *Generalized seizures* involve both cerebral hemispheres of the brain simultaneously.

Partial (Focal) Seizures

- Simple-partial seizures cause motor, sensory, autonomic, or psychic manifestations without impaired consciousness. Partial motor seizures cause symptoms such as involuntary movements of a hand or the face; in some cases, the movements may spread from a very restricted focus (such as the fingers) to involve a larger portion of the extremity (Jacksonian march). Other forms of simple-partial seizures may cause changes in sensation (parethesias), vision, hearing, smell, equilibrium, autonomic function (flushing, sweating, piloerection), or psychic manifestations.
- Complex-partial seizures are characterized by focal seizure activity with transient alteration in consciousness. The client is unable to respond to commands and may exhibit involuntary, automatic behaviors such as chewing, lip smacking, swallowing, picking movements, a display of emotion, or running. A period of confusion usually follows the seizure activity.

Generalized Seizures

- Absence seizures (petit mal) are characterized by sudden, brief lapses of consciousness without loss of posture; duration typically in seconds. Nearly always begin in childhood or early adolescence; 60% to 70% of affected children will experience spontaneous remission during adolescence.
- Atypical absence seizures usually involve a longer lapse of consciousness and are associated with diffuse or multifocal structural brain abnormalities.
- Generalized, tonic-clonic seizures (grand mal) usually begin abruptly without warning, although some clients may experience an aura, or abnormal sensation (smell, flashing lights, or vague premonition), prior to the seizure. Sequence of seizure is: tonic contraction of muscles throughout the body

that interferes with breathing and increases heart rate, BP, and pupil size; clonic phase with alternating muscle relaxation and contraction; postictal period, during which client is unresponsive, with flaccid muscles and excessive salivation that may impair airway and breathing. Bowel and bladder incontinence may occur. Consciousness gradually returns over minutes to hours, with confusion common.

- Atonic seizures are characterized by sudden, very brief loss of postural muscle tone.
- Myoclonic seizures involve sudden, brief muscle contraction of a part or the whole body.

Status Epilepticus

- Continuous seizure activity or repetitive discrete seizures with impaired consciousness between seizures. A medical emergency; cardiorespiratory dysfunction, hyperthermia, and metabolic disruptions can lead to irreversible neuronal injury after approximately 2 hours.

Diagnostics

- Electroencephalogram (EEG) performed during a seizure will reveal excessive electric discharge; may also reveal abnormal patterns of discharge; may be normal during periods between seizures.
- Positron emission tomography (PET) locates areas of neural glucose depletion, indicative of excessive discharge; especially useful in identifying focal disease.
- Magnetic resonance imaging (MRI) and computed tomography (CT) scan are used to rule out space-occupying lesions.
- Lumbar puncture and cerebrospinal fluid (CSF) analysis can rule out infection or increased intracranial pressure (ICP).
- Serum chemistry and electrolytes may reveal electrolyte or metabolic causes.

MEDICAL INTERVENTIONS

- Most seizure activity can be reduced or controlled through the use of anticonvulsant medications.
- Status epilepticus is a medical emergency that

requires immediate intervention to preserve life. Interventions include establishing and maintaining an airway, IV administration of dextrose to prevent hypoglycemia, and IV administration of diazepam to stop seizure activity. Phenytoin is also administered intravenously for longer term control of seizures.

- When all attempts to control the client's seizures fail, surgical excision of the tissue involved in the seizure activity may be an effective and safe treatment alternative.

SELECTED NURSING DIAGNOSES WITH INTERVENTIONS

Risk for Ineffective Airway Clearance

- Provide interventions during a seizure to maintain a patent airway:
  1. Loosen clothing around neck.
  2. Turn the client on the side.
  3. Do not force anything into the client's mouth.
  4. If prescribed and available, administer oxygen by mask.
- Teach significant others how to care for the client during a seizure.

Risk for Injury

- Obtain information about past seizures, including most recent seizure, precipitating factors, and so on.
- Provide interventions during a seizure to reduce the risk of injury:
  1. Maintain the bed in low position and keep the side rails up and padded.
  2. If the client is sitting or standing, ease to the floor.
  3. Place a folded towel or pillow under the client's head.
- Teach the client and significant others measures to prevent injury at home:
  1. Avoid smoking when alone or in bed.
  2. Avoid alcohol.
  3. Avoid becoming excessively tired.
  4. Install grab bars in the shower and tub area.
  5. Do not lock bedroom or bathroom doors.
  6. Avoid excessive caffeine.

CLIENT TEACHING

- Teach the client and significant others seizure management, especially how to maintain a patent airway and prevent client injury (see above).
- Explain anticonvulsant medication protocols, including dosage, effects, and side effects. Stress the importance of maintaining dosage as prescribed even when no seizures are experienced. Emphasize the importance of avoiding alcohol and limiting caffeine.
- Discuss factors that may trigger a seizure, such as abrupt withdrawal from medication, constipation, fatigue, excessive stress, fever, menstruation, and sights and sounds such as television, flashing video and computer screens, and so on.

HOME CARE CONSIDERATIONS

- Provide the name and location of community and national resources such as the Epilepsy Foundation of America.
- Stress the importance of follow-up care and keeping medical appointments.
- Review state and local laws regarding operation of a motor vehicle that apply to people with seizure disorders.
- Stress the importance of wearing a MedicAlert bracelet or necklace at all times, and provide information on how to obtain one.

For more information on Epilepsy, see Medical-Surgical Nursing *by LeMone and Burke, p. 1719.*

Fibrocystic Breast Disease (Mammary Dysplasia)

OVERVIEW

- Fibrocystic breast changes are common breast lesions, primarily affecting women between the ages of 30 and 50.
- Cysts, fibrosis, and ductal epithelial hyperplasia are common microscopic findings.
- Cysts form from ductal epithelium and are responsive to female hormones.
- Signs and symptoms wax and wane with the menstrual cycle.
- In those clients with proliferative types, there is a greater risk of breast cancer.

CAUSES

The exact cause is unknown. May be due to:

- Imbalance of estrogen and progesterone with excessive tissue response
- Increased sensitivity of the glandular epithelium to hormones
- Incomplete resolution of hormonal effect within the glandular epithelium
- Dysplastic cell changes

Signs & Symptoms

- Multiple breast masses, "shotty" (multiple tiny lumps) feeling or dense
- Masses enlarge during the premenstrual period; regress with onset of menses
- Pain and breast heaviness accompanies enlargement

Diagnostics

- Mammography can identify malignant masses; will show cystic structure of lumps; shows calcified tissue; false-positive and false-negative results occur frequently.

F

- Ultrasonography can reliably identify cysts and/or enlarged ducts.
- Magnetic resonance imaging (MRI) can image and rule out large breast cancers.
- Aspiration with Pap smear is used to assess cells for dysplasia or neoplasia.
- Incisional/excisional biopsy secures tissue for microscopic study to rule out malignancy.

MEDICAL INTERVENTIONS

- Hormonal therapy is controversial due to the benign nature of the disease. Danazol, a synthetic androgen, may relieve severe pain.
- Eliminating caffeine and chocolate, which both contain methylxanthines, has been reported to be helpful for some women.
- Aspirin, mild analgesics, and local heat or cold are recommended.

SELECTED NURSING DIAGNOSES

- Pain
- Anxiety
- Risk for Body Image Disturbance
- Knowledge Deficit

SELECTED NURSING INTERVENTIONS

- Teach breast self-examination (BSE) and encourage monthly BSE, annual physician examinations, and mammography as per the physician's recommendations. Stress the importance of becoming aware of the normal feeling of breast tissue, and the need to be aware of any changes in the size, consistency, or mobility, of lumps.
- Encourage the client to verbalize her feelings of discomfort and her fears.
- Explain that fibrocystic breast changes are not a disease but are normal changes, probably influenced by hormonal cycles and aging, that are common in premenopausal women.
- Review available prescription and nonprescription medication options, their effects, and side effects.

CLIENT TEACHING

- Teach the client to eliminate caffeine and chocolate from her diet, especially right before her menstrual period. Limiting salt premenstrually may also help. Tell her that taking vitamin E supplements (400 IU) may offer relief from the swelling and tenderness.
- Encourage the client to wear a well-fitting, supportive brassiere.
- Tell the client that the application of heat or cold may relieve her discomfort.

HOME CARE CONSIDERATIONS

- Emphasize the benign nature of the disease, and reassure the client that manifestations are rare after menopause.
- Provide or suggest pamphlets, books, and other resources for the client to learn about fibrocystic breast changes.
- Give the client written instructions for performing monthly breast self-examination.

For more information on Fibrocystic Breast Disease, see Medical-Surgical Nursing *by LeMone and Burke, p. 2051.*

Flail Chest

OVERVIEW

- Flail chest is an instability of the chest wall caused by fracture of three or more ribs in two or more places.
- When several contiguous ribs are fractured, producing a flail portion of chest wall, the flail segment of the chest is unsupported.
- Lack of support in the flail section of the chest causes paradoxical chest movements.

- On inspiration, the flail portion retracts inward while the rest of the chest rises; on expiration, when the rest of the chest falls, the flail portion bulges outward.
- Alveoli under the flail segment collapse, making that portion of lung tissue stiff; gas exchange is impaired.
- Work of breathing is greatly increased, resulting in fatigue.
- Pulmonary contusion with edema and bleeding into lung tissue is common underlying the flail segment and can further compromise ventilation and gas exchange.
- Respiratory failure may result.

CAUSES

- Blunt trauma (motor vehicle crash, fall) to the chest wall

Signs & Symptoms

- Obvious paradoxical chest motion
- Severe dyspnea
- Rapid, shallow breathing
- Rales, decreased breath sounds
- Grunting
- Cyanosis
- Severe chest pain, especially with inspiration

Diagnostics

- Arterial blood gases (ABGs) show degree of hypoxia, hypercapnia, and acidosis.
- Chest x-rays identify the area and extent of chest wall injury.

MEDICAL INTERVENTIONS

- The preferred treatment for flail chest is intubation and mechanical ventilation using positive pressure.
- Intercostal nerve blocks or continuous epidural analgesia may be employed to manage pain.
- In some cases, internal or external fixation of the flail segment may be done.

SELECTED NURSING DIAGNOSES

- Pain
- Ineffective Breathing Pattern
- Altered Tissue Perfusion

SELECTED NURSING INTERVENTIONS

- Administer prescribed analgesics on a schedule to maintain pain control rather than on an as-needed basis that allows pain to become severe between doses.
- Assess the client frequently for adequate pain control.
- Assess the client frequently for possible respiratory depression resulting from narcotic analgesia.
- Assess lung sounds and respiratory rate, depth, and effort frequently. Have the client cough, deep breathe, and change position every 1 to 2 hours, and encourage the client to use the incentive spirometer.
- Teach the client how to splint the affected area when coughing.
- Suction the client's airway as indicated. Elevate the head of the bed to facilitate lung expansion.
- Promptly report to the physician signs of complications such as diminished breath sounds, increasing crackles (rales) or rhonchi, dull or hyper-resonant percussion tones, unequal chest movement, hemoptysis, chills, or fever, or changes in vital signs.
- For severe flail chest with respiratory failure, prepare for intubation and mechanical positive-pressure ventilation.

CLIENT TEACHING

- If intubation and mechanical ventilation are required, teach the client communication strategies. Reassure the client and significant others that mechanical ventilation generally is required for no more than 2 to 3 weeks.
- Teach the client the importance of coughing and deep breathing, and demonstrate to the client how to splint the affected area when coughing.

- Explain the reasons for not taping or wrapping the chest continuously.
- Review the client's prescribed pain management and its relationship to preventing respiratory complications.

HOME CARE CONSIDERATIONS

- List the complications that should be reported to the physician, including chills and fever, productive cough, purulent or bloody sputum, shortness of breath or difficulty breathing, and increasing chest pain.
- Emphasize the importance of avoiding respiratory irritants such as cigarette smoke.

For more information on Flail Chest, see Medical-Surgical Nursing *by LeMone and Burke, p. 1478.*

Fracture

OVERVIEW

- A fracture is a broken bone.
- Local soft tissue is always damaged to some extent with a fracture.
- Bone can fracture in an infinite number of ways. Some general categories are:
  1. *Closed (simple):* fracture line in bone is well opposed; skin intact over fracture; minimal soft-tissue injury.
  2. *Compound (open):* skin over fracture site is lacerated; increased possibility of infection.
  3. *Complete:* fracture line extends through entire bone.
  4. *Incomplete (greenstick):* fracture line through bone is incomplete; occurs more often in children.
  5. *Comminuted:* bone is shattered into multiple fragments at fracture site.

6. *Displaced:* fractured ends of bone are widely separated from each other.
7. *Telescoped:* a displaced fracture in which the broken segments of bone are parallel to each other.
8. *Impacted (compression):* a fracture produced when bones are forcefully driven into each other.
9. *Complicated:* any fracture that results in a large degree of soft-tissue, blood vessel, or nerve damage.
10. *Pathologic:* a fracture of any bone with a pre-existing disease that has weakened the bone; only small forces are necessary to induce fracture.

CAUSES

- Any force directed to the bone that is greater than the bone can withstand.
  1. A normal bone subjected to an unusually large force
  2. An intrinsically weakened bone subjected to a small force

Signs & Symptoms

- Pain: point tenderness, increased with movement
- Swelling: due to inflammation at fracture site
- Deformity: bulging at fracture site; increase or decrease in limb length
- Decreased function/paralysis
- Crepitus: a grinding noise made when bone edges rub together
- Bruising: due to subcutaneous bleeding
- Decreased pulses: signal impaired arterial perfusion
- Color changes: due to arterial perfusion disruption; pallor, mottling, cyanosis
- Coolness: signals impaired perfusion
- Muscle spasm
- Paresthesias: numbness, tingling
- Complications: hemorrhagic shock, fat embolus, aseptic necrosis, renal calculi, permanent deformity or reduced function

Diagnostics

- X-ray reveals fracture line.
- A bone scan may be necessary to determine whether a fracture is present.
- Blood tests are performed to assess blood loss, renal function, muscle breakdown, and risk of excessive bleeding or clotting.
- Urine myoglobin is measured to assess muscle breakdown.

MEDICAL INTERVENTIONS

- Pharmacologic agents include narcotics for pain relief, nonsteroidal anti-inflammatory drugs, and antibiotics.
- Traction is applied to return or maintain the fractured bones in normal anatomic position.
- Casts are applied on clients who have relatively stable fractures.
- Electric bone stimulation is the application of electric current at the fracture site. It is used to treat fractures that are not healing properly.
- Surgery is required for fractures that require direct visualization for repair, fractures with long-term complications, and fractures that are severely comminuted and threatening vascular supply.

SELECTED NURSING DIAGNOSES WITH INTERVENTIONS

Pain

- Monitor baseline vital signs, since some analgesics decrease respiratory effort and blood pressure.
- Ask the client to rate the pain on a scale of 0 to 10 before and after any intervention.
- Splint and support the injured area.
- Elevate the injured extremity 2 inches above the heart.
- Apply ice.
- Move the client gently and slowly.
- Encourage distraction.
- Administer pain medications as prescribed.
- Encourage deep breathing and relaxation exercises.

Impaired Physical Mobility

- Assist client with range of motion (ROM) exercises of the unaffected limbs.
- Teach isometric exercises, and encourage the client to perform them every 4 hours.
- Encourage the client to ambulate when he or she is able to do so. Provide assistance as needed.
- Teach and observe the client's use of assistive devices in conjunction with the physical therapist, as appropriate.
- Encourage flexion and extension exercises of the feet, ankles, elbows, shoulders, and knees.
- Turn the client on bed rest every 2 hours. If the client is in traction, teach the client to shift his or her weight every hour.
- Observe the client's ambulation.

Risk for Altered Tissue Perfusion

- Assess pain, pulses, and pallor.
- Assess the cast for tightness.
- If the cast is tight, be prepared to assist the physician with bivalving (splitting the cast down both sides to alleviate pressure on the injured extremity).
- Promptly report to the physician manifestations of compartment syndrome: unrelenting pain, paresthesias, color and pulse changes.
- Maintain skeletal traction weight and alignment at all times.
- Administer heparin per physician's prescription.
- Apply antiembolism stockings or pneumatic compression boots.

CLIENT TEACHING

- Teach the client the use of all assistive devices.
- Teach the client measures to prevent complications from immobility.
- Review care of the cast, splint, brace, external fixator, or wound, as appropriate.
- Teach the client how to recognize signs of infection.
- Teach the client how to walk on crutches, if appropriate.
- Review medication regimen, including dosage, effects, and side effects.

HOME CARE CONSIDERATIONS

- Referrals to a home health agency and community services are appropriate, especially for the older client.
- Evaluate the client's living situation for possible hazards to safety and mobility.
- Emphasize the importance of appropriate cast care, including keeping the cast dry, avoiding putting any objects into the cast to relieve itching, padding cast edges as needed.
- Discuss with the client the importance of follow-up care with the physician and physical therapists, as needed.

For more information on Fracture, see Medical-Surgical Nursing *by LeMone and Burke, p. 1573.*

Gastritis (Gastropathy)

OVERVIEW

Gastritis is an acute or chronic inflammation of the gastric mucosa.

Acute Gastritis

- Acute gastritis may either be infectious or erosive.
  1. *H. pylori* infection may cause acute gastritis associated with a transient increase in gastric acid secretion followed by hypochlorhydria. Acute *H. pylori* gastritis may precede chronic gastritis.
  2. Erosive gastritis is commonly caused by drugs, especially NSAIDs, alcohol, or stress related to severe medical or surgical illness (stress gastritis). Other causes are ingestion of a caustic substance and radiation.
     a. Stress-related mucosal erosions and hemorrhages develop in the majority of critically ill clients. Trauma, burns, hypotension, sepsis, head injury, coagulopathy, mechanical ventilation, and organ system(s) failure are major risk factors. Overt bleeding is uncommon.
     b. NSAID gastritis affects about half of all clients taking NSAIDs on a regular basis, but frequently is asymptomatic. Associated bleeding usually is not severe.
     c. Alcoholic gastritis accounts for about 20% of upper GI bleeds in chronic alcoholics.

Chronic Gastritis

- A progressive irreversible disorder that results in gastric mucosal atrophy, loss of hydrochloric acid (HCL), and gastric ulceration. Two types of inflammatory chronic gastritis have been described:
  1. *Type A*: an autoimmune process directed at parietal cells within the stomach, leading to their continuous destruction; secretion of HCL and

G

intrinsic factor (IF) is reduced; associated with pernicious anemia due to inability to absorb vitamin B_{12}

2. *Type B*: much more common than Type A; is usually due to chronic infection of the stomach with *H. pylori*.

CAUSES

Acute gastritis
- Ingestion of gastric irritants such as aspirin, NSAIDS, or alcohol; acute *H. pylori* infection; severe physiologic stress

Chronic gastritis
- *H. pylori* infection; autoimmune process

Signs & Symptoms

Acute and Chronic Gastritis
- May be asymptomatic (erosive)
- Epigastric discomfort, tenderness, cramping
- Eructation
- Nausea and vomiting
- Malaise
- Hematemesis, "coffee-grounds" emesis
- Melena

Diagnostics

- Gastroscopy reveals red, inflamed gastric mucosa and/or ulceration.
- Hematest: of vomitus or stool may be positive for blood.
- Hematocrit may be low due to bleeding.
- Serum vitamin B_{12} levels are measured to evaluate the client with chronic gastritis for possible pernicious anemia.

MEDICAL INTERVENTIONS

- Sucralfate or H_2 receptor antagonists such as cimetidine, ranitidine, or famotidine are used to prevent stress gastritis.

- Acute gastritis (erosive, NSAID- or alcohol-induced) is treated with the above drugs or proton-pump inhibitors such as omeprazole (Prilosec) or lansoprazole (Prevacid). Discontinuing alcohol consumption or the offending drug also are important treatment measures.
- Chronic atrophic gastritis may be treated with antacids or histamine$_2$-receptor antagonists. Sucralfate may also be used.
- Chronic autoimmune atrophic gastritis may be treated with anticholinergic drugs and/or corticosteroids. Vitamin B$_{12}$ injections are necessary when there is no remaining intrinsic factor.

SELECTED NURSING DIAGNOSES WITH INTERVENTIONS

Fluid Volume Deficit

- Assess, monitor, and record vital signs at least every 2 hours until the client is stable, then every 4 hours. Check for orthostatic hypotension.
- Assess, monitor, and record intake and output carefully every 1 to 4 hours. Weigh the client daily.
- Assess and record skin turgor and condition and status of oral mucous membranes frequently. Provide frequent skin and mouth care.
- Monitor laboratory values for electrolytes and acid-base balance.
- Administer fluids as prescribed.
- Administer medications as prescribed.
- Take measures to ensure the safety of clients with orthostatic hypotension.

Altered Nutrition: Less than Body Requirements

- Monitor and record food and fluid intake and any abnormal losses (such as vomiting).
- Weigh the client daily at the same time.
- Monitor laboratory values.
- Arrange for consultation with dietitian, and consider client food preferences.
- Provide nutritional supplements between meals, or frequent small feedings as needed.
- Maintain tube feedings or parenteral nutrition as prescribed.

CLIENT TEACHING

- Help the client to identify causative factors, and teach avoidance of these factors in the future.
- Emphasize the importance of taking NSAIDs or aspirin with food to decrease the risk of gastritis.
- Teach the client and significant others management of acute symptoms and reintroduction of fluids and solid foods.
- Tell the client and significant others to watch for indicators of the need for further medical interventions, such as intractable vomiting, signs of dehydration, and signs of electrolyte imbalance.
- Provide clients with chronic gastritis with information on maintenance of nutritional status, use of prescribed medications, and avoidance of known irritants, such as aspirin, alcohol, and cigarette smoke.

HOME CARE CONSIDERATIONS

- Discuss treatment plans for *H. pylori* infection and their potential benefit.
- Clients with chronic gastritis may need long-term care, including referral to a home health nurse.
- Referral to smoking-cessation classes or programs to treat alcohol abuse may be indicated.

For more information on Gastritis, see Medical-Surgical Nursing *by LeMone and Burke, p. 478.*

Gastroenteritis (Enteritis, Food Poisoning, Cholera, Traveler's Diarrhea)

OVERVIEW

- Gastroenteritis is an inflammatory process of the stomach and bowel (usually the small intestine).

- When the large intestine is primarily affected, the condition is called *dysentery.*
- Bacterial or viral infection of the GI tract produces inflammation, tissue damage, and clinical manifestations by the following mechanisms:
  1. exotoxins excreted by bacteria damage and inflame gastrointestinal mucosa, impairing intestinal absorption and drawing fluids and electrolytes into the bowel lumen
  2. direct invasion and ulceration of bowel mucosa by the organism, causing bleeding, fluid exudate formation, and water and electrolyte secretion
- Distension of the upper GI tract by unabsorbed chyme and excess water can lead to nausea and vomiting; inflammation and fermentation of undigested food causes abdominal pain and cramping; and excess fluid and electrolytes secreted into the bowel result in diarrhea with possible secondary fluid, electrolyte, and acid-base disruptions.
- Gastroenteritis is a major cause of morbidity and mortality in undeveloped countries.
- Gastroenteritis is a major cause of morbidity in the United States, and can be life-threatening in children, the elderly, or the immunocompromised.

CAUSES

- Bacteria: *Staphylococcus aureus, Salmonella, Shigella, Clostridium botulinum, C. perfringes, Escherichia coli*
- Viruses: rotavirus, enteric calcivirus (Norwalk virus), enteric adenovirus, ECHOvirus, Coxsackie viruses
- Amoebae: especially *Entamoeba histolytica*
- Parasites: *Ascaris, Enterobius, Trichinella spiralis*
- Immune reactions: food allergy, drug reactions
- Enzyme deficiencies

Signs & Symptoms

- Diarrhea: copious, foul smelling, watery/mucoid; possibly bloody
- Abdominal discomfort: from mild cramps to severe crampy pain
- Borborygmi
- Nausea and vomiting
- Fever: low-grade to 103F

- Malaise
- S/S of dehydration: poor skin turgor, dry mucous membranes, orthostatic hypotension, oliguria
- S/S of viral infection: headache, myalgia

Diagnostics

- Stool culture may identify offending organism.
- Blood culture may show offending organism, if blood borne.
- Serum osmolality, serum electrolytes, and arterial blood gases (ABGs) are used to assess the client's fluid, electrolyte, and acid-base balance.
- Sigmoidoscopy helps to differentiate infectious processes from ulcerative colitis.

MEDICAL INTERVENTIONS

- Antibiotics may be used for clients with cholera, salmonellosis, or shigellosis.
- Antidiarrheal drugs may be prescribed for infections in which diarrhea predominates.
- Botulism antitoxin is administered to clients with suspected botulism. Antidiarrheals are *not* used for these clients.
- Oral rehydration is the preferred route for administering physiologic fluids. Intravenous rehydration may be necessary for the client with severe diarrhea and fluid loss.
- Gastric lavage may be ordered to remove unabsorbed toxin from the GI tract. Plasmapheresis may be used to remove circulating antigen in clients with botulism or hemorrhagic colitis caused by *E. coli*.

SELECTED NURSING DIAGNOSES

- Diarrhea
- Activity Intolerance
- Altered Nutrition: Less than Body Requirements
- Fluid Volume Deficit
- Bowel Incontinence
- Risk for Impaired Skin Integrity (in anal area with copious diarrhea)

SELECTED NURSING INTERVENTIONS

- Replace fluids as prescribed with oral rehydration solutions such as Resol or IV solutions such as Ringer's solution and others.
- Encourage client to take small amounts of clear liquids with electrolytes and to progress slowly to diet as tolerated.
- Administer antibiotics and antidiarrheal medications as prescribed.
- Apply repellent cream such as zinc oxide, Desitin, A&D ointment, or moisture barriers to protect skin in the anal area.

CLIENT TEACHING

- Teach the client proper hand-washing techniques, especially after toileting, to minimize transmission of bacteria to others.
- Stress the importance of not sharing utensils, glasses, and so on, and of washing soiled garments separately in hot water and detergent.
- Encourage the client to maintain adequate fluid intake.
- Provide written and oral instructions for medications.

HOME CARE CONSIDERATIONS

- Provide the client and significant others with information about the proper cooking, refrigeration, and freezing of foods. Emphasize the importance of following instructions when home-canning foods.
- Encourage clients traveling out of the country to consume only bottled water or to use water purification tablets.
- Tell the client to return to the physician for follow-up care if diarrhea, vomiting, or dizziness returns.

For more information on Gastroenteritis, see Medical-Surgical Nursing *by LeMone and Burke, p. 804.*

Glaucoma

OVERVIEW

- Glaucoma is a group of ocular disorders characterized by increased intraocular pressure (IOP).
- Increased IOP, left untreated, reduces blood flow to the retina and optic nerve, eventually causing blindness.
- Glaucoma is responsible for about 10% of all cases of blindness.
- It may be congenital, primary, or secondary.
- *Congenital glaucoma* is the result of abnormal development of the trabecular network.
- *Primary glaucoma* results from intrinsic pathologic processes in the circulation and/or reabsorption of aqueous humor. There are two forms:
  1. *Open angle (chronic) glaucoma* is usually due to degeneration of the trabecular network or canal of Schlemm, which results in obstruction to aqueous humor flow.
  2. *Closed, or narrow, angle (acute) glaucoma* can occur in a single eye and is due to narrowing of the angles between the iris and the cornea (i.e., the anterior chamber).
- *Secondary glaucoma* appears as a result of extrinsic factors (see below).

CAUSES

- Congenital glaucoma is an autosomal dominant trait
- Primary glaucoma has no identified precipitating cause
- Secondary glaucoma results from trauma, hemorrhage into the anterior chamber, surgery, infection, tumor, prolonged steroid use, or vessel occlusion secondary to neovascularization seen with diabetes mellitus

Signs & Symptoms

S/S may develop in clients with little or no increase in eye tension, and clients with high IOPs may show no S/S.

- Increased IOP (usually)
- Chronic open angle glaucoma is bilateral and develops insidiously; S/S are late:
  1. mild ache in eyes
  2. peripheral field vision loss
  3. loss of visual acuity
  4. reduced night vision
  5. halos around lights
- Acute closed (narrow) angle glaucoma can occur in one eye and usually develops rapidly; it is considered an ocular emergency:
  1. pressure-like eye pain
  2. non-reactive/dilated pupil
  3. cloudy cornea
  4. blurred vision
  5. halos around lights
  6. nausea, vomiting
  7. photophobia

Diagnostics

- Tonometry measures IOP.
- Slit-lamp ophthalmic examination can show changes in anterior chamber structures.
- Gonioscopy measures the anterior chamber angles; distinguishes open angle from closed angle.
- Perimetry establishes degree of peripheral field loss.
- Ophthalmoscopy reveals changes in the fundus such as cupping, pallor, and/or atrophy of optic disk.
- Serial photographs of the fundus can be used to monitor changes over time.

G

MEDICAL INTERVENTIONS

- Pharmacologic agents include timolol, a beta-adrenergic blocking agent that reduces aqueous humor production and increases outflow; epinephrine, which also reduces aqueous humor production; and miotics such as pilocarpine that cause pupil contraction and facilitate aqueous humor outflow. Dorzolamide, a topical carbonic anhydrase inhibitor that decreases aqueous humor production and reduces intraocular pressure, may be used when beta-blockers are contraindicated. Acetazolamide, a systemic carbonic anhydrase inhibitor, also may be used.
- Surgical intervention is indicated for clients with glaucoma that is not controlled with medications and for clients with acute closed angle glaucoma.

SELECTED NURSING DIAGNOSES WITH INTERVENTIONS

Risk for Sensory-Perceptual Alteration: Visual

- Address the client by name and identify yourself with each interaction. Orient the client to time, place, person, and situation as indicated. Tell the client the purpose of your visit.
- Provide any visual aids that the client routinely uses. Keep them in close proximity, making sure that the client knows where they are and can reach them easily.
- Orient the client to the environment. Explain the location of the call bell, personal items, and the furniture in the room. If the client is able to ambulate, provide a walking tour of the client's room and immediate facilities, including the toilet and sink.
- Provide other tools or items that can help compensate for diminished vision, such as bright, non-glare lighting, large-print books and magazines, books on tape, telephones with oversize pushbuttons, and a clock with large numbers that can be felt.
- Assist the client with meals by reading menu selections and marking choices, describing the position of foods on the meal try, placing utensils in or near the client's hands, removing lids from containers, and so on.

- Assist the client with mobility and ambulation by having the client hold your arm or elbow, describing the surroundings as you proceed, and advising the client to feel the chair, bed, or commode with the hands and the backs of the legs before sitting.

Risk for Injury

- Assess the client's ability to provide for self-care in activities of daily living (ADLs).
- Provide for a safe environment by removing furniture and other objects from traffic pattern areas. Orient the client to the environment. Be sure that frequently used items are readily accessible.
- Notify housekeeping and place a sign on the client's door to alert all personnel not to change the arrangement of the client's room.
- Raise the side rails on the client's bed.
- Work with the client and significant others to identify changes in the home environment to help the client remain as independent as possible and prevent falls or other injuries.

Anxiety

- Assess the client for verbal and nonverbal indicators of level of anxiety and for normal coping mechanisms. Repeated expressions of concern or denial that the vision change will affect the client's life are indicators of anxiety. Nonverbal indicators include tension, difficulty concentrating, restlessness, poor eye contact, rapid speech, voice quivering, tremors, tachycardia, and dilated pupils.
- Encourage the client to verbalize fears, anger, and feelings of anxiety.
- Listen actively.
- Discuss the client's perception of the eye condition and its effects on lifestyle and roles.
- Help the client identify coping strategies that have been useful in the past and to adapt these strategies to the present situation.
- Provide diversional activities and relaxation strategies.
- Identify and enlist the client's support system.

CLIENT TEACHING

- Teach the client about the medications prescribed, dosage, effects, side effects, and the proper way to instill eye drops. Tell the client that certain medications, including nonprescription drugs, can increase intraocular pressure and should not be taken without consulting the physician.

- Tell the client to report to the physician immediately any signs of complications of surgery, including brow pain, severe eye pain, nausea, changes in vital signs, and so on.
- Instruct the postoperative client to avoid bending from the waist, lifting heavy objects, straining with bowel movements, and coughing, per the physician's instructions.

HOME CARE CONSIDERATIONS

- Emphasize to all clients, particularly those over 40, the need for regular eye examinations.
- Provide referral to community, state, and national agencies and resources specializing in information and assistive devices for the visually impaired.
- A referral to home health care may be appropriate.
- Emphasize the importance of lifetime therapy and periodic eye examinations to prevent blindness.

For more information on Glaucoma, see Medical-Surgical Nursing *by LeMone and Burke, p. 1911.*

Glomerulonephritis

Acute
Chronic

OVERVIEW

- Glomerulonephritis is an inflammatory disorder in which the structure and function of the glomerulus are altered, disrupting glomerular filtration.
- Glomerulonephritis may be a primary disorder or occur secondarily to multisystem disease or a hereditary condition.

- Acute glomerulonephritis, rapidly progressive glomerulonephritis, chronic glomerulonephritis, and nephrotic syndrome are the most common primary forms; diabetic nephropathy and lupus nephritis are the most common secondary forms.
- Acute post-streptococcal glomerulonephritis is the predominant form of acute glomerulonephritis. Circulating immune complexes trapped in the glomerular membrane lead to an inflammatory response, with damage to the capillary endothelium and basement membrane. While primarily a disease of children, most of whom recover completely, adults also may be affected and have a poorer prognosis.
- Rapidly progressive glomerulonephritis (RPG) may be either idiopathic or secondary to infectious disease or multisystem diseases such as systemic lupus erythematosus or Goodpasture's syndrome. In RPG, glomerular cells proliferate forming crescent-shaped lesions that obliterate Bowman's space. Most people with RPG eventually develop renal failure.
- Chronic glomerulonephritis may be idiopathic or the end-stage of disorders such as RPG, lupus nephritis, or diabetic nephropathy. Chronic glomerulonephritis results in progressive destruction of glomeruli and loss of entire nephrons with increasing impairment of renal function.
- Nephrotic syndrome, characterized by massive proteinuria, hypoalbuminemia, hyperlipidemia, and edema, has several forms. *Minimal change disease* is the most common cause in children and has a good prognosis. In adults, *membranous glomerulonephropathy* may cause idiopathic nephrotic syndrome and also occurs with some systemic diseases, such as systemic lupus erythematosus and hepatitis B, and with drugs such as gold or penicillamine. *Focal sclerosis* and *membranoproliferative glomerulonephritis* also are forms of nephrotic syndrome.

CAUSES

- Idiopathic
- Immunologic
  1. post streptococcal—group A beta-hemolytic streptococci

2. following other bacterial and viral infections such as staphylococcal infection, hepatitis B, mumps, varicella
3. systemic lupus erythematosus
4. bacterial endocarditis

- Metabolic
  1. diabetes mellitus
- Hemodynamic
  1. hypertension
- Toxic
  1. *E. coli* toxin
  2. drugs such as gold, penicillamine, captopril, NSAIDs, probenecid, trimethadione, chlormethi-azole, mercury
- Malignancy
  1. leukemias, lymphomas
  2. carcinoma of the breast, lung, colon, other organs
- Miscellaneous
  1. sickle cell disease, Crohn's disease, Fanconi's syndrome, sarcoidosis
  2. heroin use

Signs & Symptoms

- Azotemia: increased blood urea nitrogen (BUN), creatinine, and uric acid
- Hematuria: gross; smokey, cola-/coffee-colored urine; may be occult; red cell casts may be present
- Proteinuria
- Edema: mild to moderate; peripheral, including eyelids
- Hypertension: mild to severe
- Oliguria
- Fatigue
- Possible S/S of pulmonary congestion/edema: dyspnea, shortness of breath (SOB), orthopnea, paroxysmal nocturnal dyspnea (PND)
- Possible ascites

Diagnostics

- Venous blood sample reveals altered electrolytes (decreased sodium, elevated chloride, elevated

potassium), increased blood urea nitrogen (BUN), increased creatinine, increased uric acid, increased erythrocyte sedimentation rate (ESR), increased anti-streptolysin (ASO) titer.
- Hematology reveals decreased red blood cell (RBC) count secondary to decreased erythropoietin.
- Arterial blood gas (ABG) analysis reveals metabolic acidosis.
- Urinalysis is positive for protein, RBCs, white blood cells (WBCs), casts.
- Creatinine clearance may show reduced GFR.
- X-rays of the kidneys, ureters, and bladder reveal enlarged kidneys.
- Renal biopsy may be necessary to assess the degree of renal tissue damage.

MEDICAL INTERVENTIONS

- Penicillin or other broad-spectrum antibiotics may be prescribed for the client with poststreptococcal glomerulonephritis. Antihypertensives may be prescribed to maintain the blood pressure within normal levels. Clients with an acute inflammatory process may be placed on corticosteroids and cytotoxic agents.
- Plasmapheresis, the removal of harmful components in the plasma, may be used to treat rapidly progressive glomerulonephritis and Goodpasture's syndrome.
- When edema is significant or the client is hypertensive, sodium intake may be restricted.
- The client who experiences renal failure as a result of a glomerular disorder may require dialysis to restore fluid and electrolyte balance and remove waste products from the body.

SELECTED NURSING DIAGNOSES WITH INTERVENTIONS

Fluid Volume Excess
- Monitor the client's vital signs, including blood pressure, apical pulse, respirations, and breath sounds, at least every 4 hours.
- Record fluid intake and output at least every 4 to 8 hours.

- Weigh the client daily at the same time each day.
- Assess for the presence, location, and degree of edema.
- Monitor the serum electrolytes, hemoglobin and hematocrit, blood urea nitrogen, and creatinine.
- Maintain fluid restriction as prescribed, offering ice chips in limited and measured amounts and frequent mouth care to relieve thirst.
- Monitor and regulate IV infusions, including as intake any fluid used for dilution of medications.
- Arrange for consultation with a dietitian to plan the diet when sodium is restricted and proteins are either restricted or increased.
- Administer prescribed medications such as diuretics, monitoring for desired and adverse effects.
- Provide frequent position changes and good skin care.

Fatigue

- Assess and document the client's energy level.
- Provide for adequate rest and energy conservation through activity and procedure scheduling. Prevent unnecessary fatigue.
- Assist the client with activities of daily living (ADLs) as needed.
- Educate the client and significant others about the relationship between fatigue and the disease process.
- Reduce the client's energy demands by scheduling more frequent, small meals and short periods of activity. Limit the number of visitors and visit length.
- Provide a diet with complete proteins and adequate calories, iron, and minerals.
- Assist the client to cope with reduced energy by providing support, understanding, and active listening.

Altered Protection

- Monitor and record the client's vital signs, including temperature and mental status, every 4 hours.
- Assess the client frequently for other signs of infections such as purulent wound drainage, productive cough, adventitious breath sounds, and red or inflamed lesions. Monitor for signs of urinary tract infection.

- Monitor the complete blood count (CBC), paying particular attention to the WBC count and differential.
- Use good hand-washing technique and protect the client from cross-infection by providing a private room and limiting ill visitors.
- Avoid or minimize invasive procedures.
- If the client requires catheterization, use intermittent straight catheterization or maintain a closed drainage system for an indwelling catheter. Prevent reflux of urine from the drainage system to the bladder or the bladder to the kidneys by ensuring a patent, gravity system.
- Provide support and education to the client and family.

CLIENT TEACHING

- Provide information about the disease process and prognosis; the use, effects, and side effects of medications; activity and diet restrictions; and the risks, manifestations, prevention, and management of complications such as edema and infection.
- Teach the signs, symptoms, and implications of improving or declining renal function.
- Teach self-care of peritoneal or vascular access devices and self-dialysis if appropriate.

HOME CARE CONSIDERATIONS

- Stress the importance of long-term follow-up medical care.
- Discuss measures to avoid further glomerular injury such as maintaining hydration and avoiding nephrotoxic drugs.
- A referral for a home health nurse is appropriate for optimal long-term self-management of the disease.

For more information on Glomerulonephritis, see Medical-Surgical Nursing by LeMone and Burke, p. 953.

Gonorrhea

OVERVIEW

- Gonorrhea is a sexually transmitted disease caused by *Neisseria gonorrhoea*, a gram-negative diplococcus.
- Symptoms appear 3 to 10 days after unprotected intercourse with an infected partner.
- Persons, especially women, may be asymptomatic.
- In males, the most commonly infected site is the urethra, producing urethritis. The genital tract may also become infected, causing prostatitis, seminal vesicle inflammation, and/or epididymitis.
- In females, the cervix and urethra are the most commonly infected sites. Upper genital tract infections (endometritis, salpingitis, oophoritis, peritonitis, pelvic inflammatory disease) are not as common, but are much more serious.
- In both males and females, a systemic form exists in about 1% of those infected, and sterility is a complication.
- In both males and females the oral mucous membranes can be infected via oral sex and the rectal mucous membranes via anal sex.

CAUSES

- Infection with *N.gonorrhoeae* is acquired through intimate sexual contact such as vaginal intercourse, oral or anal sex
- Neonates may acquire the disease in utero or during the birth process
- Hand to eye transmission is possible

Signs & Symptoms

In the male:

- Dysuria, frequency
- Discharge, penile or anal—profuse yellow-green, or scant clear

In the female:

- Dysuria, frequency

- Discharge (vaginal, urethral, or anal)—profuse, purulent
- Pruritius of vulva
- Signs and symptoms of pelvic inflammatory disease (PID)

In both males and females:

- Anal itching, inflammation, pain, bleeding
- Painful defecation
- Pharyngitis
- Conjunctivitis
- Arthritis, if systemic
- Rash

Diagnostics

- Culture of infectious site (penis, cervix, throat, anus/rectum, conjunctiva), grown on Thayer-Martin culture medium.
- Scrapings of conjunctiva.

MEDICAL INTERVENTIONS

- The antibiotic ceftriaxone is recommended for the treatment of gonorrhea.
- Erythromycin or doxycycline is also usually given to treat any coexisting chlamydial infection.

SELECTED NURSING DIAGNOSES WITH INTERVENTIONS

Noncompliance

- Help the client understand the need for taking all medications as directed and keeping follow-up appointments to be sure no reinfection has occurred. Explain the prevalence of gonorrhea and the potential complications if it is not cured.
- Discuss with the client the importance of sexual abstinence until the infection is cured, referral of partner(s) for treatment, and condom use to prevent reinfection.

Impaired Social Interaction

- Provide privacy, confidentiality, and a safe, nonjudgmental environment for the client to express concerns.

- Help the client understand that gonorrhea is a consequence of sexual behavior, not a "punishment," and that it can be avoided in the future.

CLIENT TEACHING

- Discuss the importance of taking any and all prescribed medication.
- Tell the client to refer the sexual partner(s) for evaluation and treatment.
- Stress the importance of abstaining from all sexual contact until the client and partner(s) are cured, and of using a condom to avoid infection in the future.

HOME CARE CONSIDERATIONS

- Teach all sexually active clients safer sex practices to reduce the risk of STDs.
- Explain the need for a follow-up visit 4 to 7 days after treatment is completed.
- Provide a list of systemic symptoms: fever, chills, skin lesions, arthritis, and meningitis.

For more information on Gonorrhea, see Medical-Surgical Nursing *by LeMone and Burke, p. 2087.*

Gout (Gouty Arthritis)

OVERVIEW

- Gout is a metabolic disorder characterized by elevated serum uric acid levels and deposition of urate crystals in synovial fluid and surrounding tissues.
- It may be due to primary or secondary hyperuricemia.

CAUSES

- *Primary gout* is caused by one of several X-linked genetic disturbances in purine metabolism. Uric acid production is greater than renal excretion, producing hyperuricemia. The increased uric acid levels set the stage for precipitation of urate crystals in the tissues, especially synovial tissue.

- *Secondary gout* accompanies other disorders, especially those associated with excess breakdown of nucleic acids, which results in excess uric acid production. Such disorders include malignancies, leukemia, multiple myeloma, polycythemia, and sickle cell anemia. Chronic renal disease, hypertension, starvation, DKA, and some drugs cause hyperuricemia by reducing the amount of uric acid secreted by the kidneys.

Signs & Symptoms

Four stages have been recognized:

- *Asymptomatic hyperuricemia,* with elevated uric acid levels but no S/S
- *Acute gout,* with acute S/S:
  1. arthritis of a single joint, usually the big toe; may affect foot, ankle, heel, knee, elbow, or hand
  2. pain, severe in affected joints
  3. possible low-grade fever
- *Intercritical periods,* during which pathology continues but S/S are absent
- *Chronic gout (tophaceous gout),* an unremitting stage with:
  1. polyarthritis, with joint stiffness, limited ROM, and deformity
  2. subcutaneous tophi in cartilage, synovial membranes, tendons, and soft tissue
  3. possible ulceration at tophi

Diagnostics

- Needle aspiration of synovial fluid reveals intracellular crystal via polarized light microscopy.
- Serum uric acid levels are increased.
- Urine uric acid levels are decreased.

MEDICAL INTERVENTIONS

- Pharmacologic agents include nonsteriodal anti-inflammatory drugs (NSAIDs) for pain and inflammation. If NSAIDs are contraindicated, colchicine may be prescribed, or a corticosteroid may be injected into the affected joint. Drugs that inhibit the formation of uric acid (such as allopurinol) or increase renal excretion of uric acid (such as probenecid and sulfinpyrazone) also may be prescribed for recurrent attacks.

SELECTED NURSING DIAGNOSES

- Pain
- Activity Intolerance
- Impaired Physical Mobility
- Knowledge Deficit

SELECTED NURSING INTERVENTIONS

- Counsel the client to avoid alcohol and to drink 3000 mL of fluids per day. Foods high in purine, such as organ meats and shellfish, should be consumed in moderation.
- Assess the client's level of pain on a scale of 0 to 10 before and after treatment is begun. Also assess the location of the pain and its characteristics and duration. Encourage the client to report activities that increase pain and fatigue.
- Administer prescribed medications for pain and inflammation and monitor effects and side effects.
- Position the client to provide comfort, reduce the risk of skin breakdown, promote skin integrity, and promote healing. During an acute attack, even the weight of the bedclothes on the affected joint may cause tremendous pain.

CLIENT TEACHING

- Teach the client about the disease process, its causes, treatment, and prevention. The client with secondary gout needs information about the primary disease process and its relationship to the client's gout.

- Teach the client about the prescribed medication regimen, including dosage, effects, and side effects.

HOME CARE CONSIDERATIONS

- Stress the importance of avoiding alcohol (which is high in purines and interferes with uric acid excretion) and maintaining a liberal fluid intake to prevent future attacks.
- Emphasize the need for long-term medical treatment and to continue prescribed medication even when asymptomatic.

For more information on Gout, see Medical-Surgical Nursing *by LeMone and Burke, p. 1632.*

Guillain-Barré Syndrome (Acute Demyelinating Polyneuropathy)

OVERVIEW

- Guillain-Barré syndrome (GBS) is an acute polyneuropathy characterized by inflammation and demyelinization.
- It results in areflexic motor paralysis with possible sensory deficits.
- Approximately 3500 cases develop each year in North America.
- Both sexes are affected equally.
- About 30% of people with GBS require ventilatory support at some point during the illness.
- Recovery is spontaneous and complete in 80% to 90% of affected persons.
- Neurologic deficits such as weakness may persist, especially in the lower extremities.

CAUSES

- Most frequently follows a viral infection by about 1 to 3 weeks; most often with Epstein-Barr virus (EBV) or cytomegalovirus (CMV)
- May also be triggered by other infectious agents, such as *Campylobacter jejuni* gastroenteritis, immunization, or trauma, including surgery
- Probably an autoimmune response to the original trigger; exact mechanism is unknown
- Incidence is higher in those with a pre-existing lymphoma, including Hodgkin's disease, and systemic lupus erythematosus (SLE)

Signs & Symptoms

- Muscle weakness progressing to flaccid paralysis that begins distally and progresses in a proximal pattern; legs usually precede arms or cranial nerves
- Paresthesias are a common symptom
- Areflexia
- Other possible S/S depend on area of involvement, and include:
    1. dysarthria
    2. dysphagia
    3. ophthalmoplegia

Diagnostics

- Cerebrospinal fluid (CSF) analysis reveals clear fluid with elevated total protein and normal white blood cell (WBC) count; pressure may be slightly elevated.
- Complete blood count (CBC) shows leukocytosis with a left shift; it returns to normal rapidly.
- Electromyography (EMG) often shows repetitive firing of single motor units rather than normal diffuse stimulation.
- Nerve conduction velocities are slower than normal following the onset of symptoms.

MEDICAL INTERVENTIONS

- There are no pharmacologic agents available for the specific treatment of Guillain-Barré syndrome;

however, high-dose immunoglobulin may be pre-scribed during the acute phase.

- Ventilatory support with endotracheal intubation and mechanical ventilation may be necessary if respiratory muscle paralysis develops.
- Plasma exchange (plasmapheresis) may be beneficial, particularly when performed within the first 2 weeks of the syndrome's development.
- Nutritional support and physical and occupational therapy are important for recovery.

SELECTED NURSING DIAGNOSES WITH INTERVENTIONS

Impaired Verbal Communication

- Choose alternative methods of communication while the client is able to participate. With full progression of paralysis, the client may only be able to click the tongue or blink his or her eyes. Cognitive abilities, however, are retained throughout the course of the disease.
- Use therapeutic communication techniques even when the client is unable to respond verbally. Maintain eye contact and talk directly to the client rather than to others in the room.
- Involve the client in decisions regarding care and daily routines to reduce the sense of isolation and powerlessness caused by the inability to talk.
- Develop a regular schedule of visits to the client's room to identify care needs; remember that the client may be unable to use call devices to signal for help.

Risk for Impaired Skin Integrity

- Inspect bony prominences and provide skin care at least every 2 hours. Reposition the client and clean, dry, and lubricate the skin as needed.
- Pad bony prominences such as sacral areas, heels, and elbows.
- Use an alternative-pressure mattress or water bed.
- Monitor for incontinence and provide thorough skin care following any episode of incontinence.

G

CLIENT TEACHING

- Teach the client and significant others about the disease process and the long-term effects.
- Discuss the medication regimen, including dosage, effects, and side effects.
- Review the use of adaptive and assistive devices, especially for ambulation.
- Teach the client how to prevent and assess for skin breakdown.
- Provide instruction in range-of-motion (ROM) exercises.

HOME CARE CONSIDERATIONS

- A home care referral may be appropriate for evaluation of needs and hazards in the home environment.
- Referral to a rehabilitation facility may be required.
- The client and significant others may benefit from referral to social services for help with coping strategies.

For more information on Guillain-Barré Syndrome, see Medical-Surgical Nursing *by LeMone and Burke, p. 1860.*

Heart Failure (Congestive Heart Failure, CHF)

Left Ventricular Failure (LVF)
Right Ventricular Failure (RVF)

OVERVIEW

- Heart failure is defined as failure of the heart to pump adequate blood to meet the metabolic demands of tissues.
- Ineffective pumping results in accumulation of blood and fluid in a backward direction.
- The left ventricle more often fails first, inducing right ventricular failure (RVF).
- Eventually biventricular failure occurs with left (LVF) or right (RVF) ventricular failure.

Left Ventricular Failure

- Reduced cardiac output to the general systemic circulation with inadequate tissue perfusion and hypoxia (forward effect).
- Pulmonary edema results when excess blood accumulates in the pulmonary circulation, causing pulmonary hypertension and eventually pulmonary edema (backward effect).

Right Ventricular Failure

- Reduced cardiac output to the lungs, which compromises left ventricular cardiac filling and output (forward effect).
- Inability to pump blood forward reduces venous return, producing peripheral edema (backward effect).

CAUSES

General

- Congenital heart or vascular defects
- Myocardial disease: coronary artery heart disease (CAD), myocardial infarction (MI), cardiomyopathies, myocarditis

- Pericarditis
- Secondary conditions: anemia, fluid volume overload, thyrotoxicosis

Major Causes of LVF
- Myocardial infarction
- Coarctation of the aorta
- Hypertension
- Aortic and/or mitral valve disease

Major Causes of RVF
- LVF is the most common cause
- Cor pulmonale is RVF due to pulmonary disease: chronic obstructive pulmonary disease (COPD), adult repiratory distress syndrome (ARDS), pulmonary embolism (PE), pulmonary hypertension, pulmonary edema (see Cor Pulmonale)
- Right-heart valve disease

Signs & Symptoms

Of LVF
- Dyspnea, initially on exertion; later at rest
- Orthopnea and paroxysmal nocturnal dyspnea (PND)
- Cough: dry, frothy, or with blood-tinged sputum
- Bibasilar rales
- Tachypnea
- Central cyanosis secondary to inadequate oxygenation in lungs and peripheral tissues, due to poor cardiac output and tissue perfusion
- Hypotension
- Elevated pulmonary capillary wedge pressure (PCWP)
- Tachycardia, dysrhythmias
- Heart sounds: S_3, S_4, ventricular gallop at apex
- Fatigue, muscle weakness
- CNS symptoms: difficulty concentrating, irritability, restlessness

Of RVF
- Fatigue
- Peripheral edema, initially dependent and pitting; later anasarca
- Weight gain
- Elevated central venous pressure (CVP)

- Distended neck veins
- Hepatomegaly, splenomegaly
- Ascites
- Anorexia, GI distress
- Peripheral cyanosis, secondary to insufficient perfusion

Diagnostics

- EKG shows tachycardia and extrasystoles, and may reflect heart ischemia or enlargement.
- Chest x-ray shows ventricular dilatation. In LVF, pulmonary vascular markings are enlarged; interstitial pulmonary edema or pleural effusion is seen.
- Pulmonary artery monitoring in LVF shows elevation of PCWP.
- Central venous pressure (CVP) monitoring in RVF shows elevation.
- Cardiac catheterization may show increased ventricular volumes, CAD, or valve defects.

MEDICAL INTERVENTIONS

- The main drugs used to treat heart failure are the angiotensin converting enzyme (ACE) inhibitors, diuretics, direct vasodilators, and digitalis glycosides.
- If the cause of the client's heart failure is a valve problem, surgery may be performed. In addition, dynamic cardiomyoplasty, which attempts to improve function in the existing heart, and cardiac transplantation may be options.

SELECTED NURSING DIAGNOSES WITH INTERVENTIONS

Decreased Cardiac Output
- Monitor and record vital signs as indicated.
- Auscultate heart and breath sounds regularly.
- Note and report manifestations of decreased cardiac output: changes in mentation; decreased urine output; cool, clammy skin; diminished pulses; pale or cyanotic coloring; dysrhythmias.
- Administer supplemental oxygen as needed.
- Administer medications per physician's prescription.
- Encourage the client to rest, explaining the rationale for bed rest. Keep the head of the bed elevated to

reduce the work of breathing. Provide a bedside commode, and assist the client with personal needs. Instruct the client to avoid the Valsalva maneuver and isometric exercises.

Fluid Volume Excess

- Assess the client's respiratory status, including respiratory rate, effort, any shortness of breath, dyspnea, cough, orthopnea, or PND. Auscultate lung sounds at least every 4 hours.
- Notify the physician immediately if the client develops air hunger, an overwhelming sense of impending doom or panic, tachypnea, the need to sit straight up in bed, or a cough productive of large amounts of pink, frothy sputum.
- Monitor and record intake and output. Notify the physician if the urine output drops to less than 30 mL/hour.
- Weigh the client daily.
- Maintain bed rest, with the head of the bed elevated to 45°.
- Assess for other manifestations of fluid volume excess, including jugular venous distention, peripheral edema, and cardiac rhythm changes.
- Monitor and record hemodynamic parameters. Note changes in pulmonary artery pressures and systemic vascular resistance and decreases in cardiac output and blood pressure.
- Administer diuretics and other medications as prescribed.
- Restrict fluids as instructed. Encourage the client to choose the time and type of fluid consumed, scheduling the majority of the intake during the morning and afternoon. Offer ice chips and frequent mouth care.

Activity Intolerance

- Assess vital signs and cardiac rhythm before and after the client engages in activity. Teach the client to rest if signs of activity intolerance are noted.
- Assess the client for signs of decreasing activity tolerance.
- Organize nursing care to allow for rest periods.
- Assist the client as needed with self-care activities. Encourage the client to perform activities of daily living (ADLs) independently within prescribed limits.

- Plan and implement a progressive activity plan. Employ passive and active range-of-motion (ROM) exercises as appropriate. Consult with a physical therapist on the activity plan.
- Provide written and verbal information about activity after discharge.

CLIENT TEACHING

- Reinforce the need for, and provide information on, following a low-sodium, high-potassium diet. The American Heart Association has guidelines and recipes that may make following the prescribed diet easier.
- Stress the need for each medication, and teach medication dosage, actions, and side effects.
- Explain the purpose of and preparation for diagnostic examinations.
- Explain the rationale for activity restriction and methods to conserve energy. Encourage prescribed exercises within prescribed limits to strengthen the heart muscle and increase aerobic capacity.
- Review with the client the warning signals of cardiac decompensation that require physician notification.

HOME CARE CONSIDERATIONS

- Advise the client and significant others to report to the physician immediately any of the following: weight gain greater than 3 to 5 lbs per week or increased swelling; dizziness or blurred vision; shortness of breath or cough; palpitations; decreased urine output.
- Stress the importance of lifelong follow-up medical care.
- A referral to home health care may be appropriate. Additionally, the client may require assistance with shopping, transportation, cleaning, and so on.
- Identify for the client and significant others community organizations that supply information and/or psychosocial support.

For more information on Heart Failure, see Medical-Surgical Nursing *by LeMone and Burke, p. 1118.*

Hemophilia

OVERVIEW

- Hemophilia is an X-linked hereditary bleeding disorder caused by a deficiency of one of several plasma clotting factors.
- *Hemophilia A* (classic hemophilia), a lack of factor VIII, accounts for most (80%) of all hemophilias; about 1 in 10,000 males is born with this defect.
- *Hemophilia B* (Christmas disease), a deficiency of factor IX, accounts for about 20% of all hemophilias; incidence is 1 in 100,000 males.
- Both forms result in abnormal bleeding into muscles, joints, and/or body cavities following an injury. Chronic disability usually results.
- Von Willebrand's disease, another type of hemophilia, is a common hereditary bleeding disorder that results from a deficiency of vW factor and is often accompanied by a deficiency of factor VIII and platelet dysfunction.

CAUSES

- An X-linked recessive hereditary disease that almost always affects males
- Females are carriers and have a 50% chance of passing the gene to each child
- A son receiving this gene from the mother would have hemophilia; a daughter would be a carrier
- A daughter can acquire both defective genes only if her father has the disease and her mother is a carrier

Signs & Symptoms

- Abnormal bleeding, which may be mild to severe in any given individual
- Spontaneous bleeding may occur
- Hematoma formation, following even slight injury
- Pain, tenderness
- Swelling
- Deformity, may follow repeated bleeding bouts
- Shock, possibly leading to death

Diagnostics

- Factor assays: reveal decreased factor VIII in hemophilia and von Willebrand's disease, and decreased factor IX in hemophilia B.
- Activated partial thromboplastin time (APTT) is prolonged
- Thrombocyte count, function, bleeding time, and prothrombin time are all normal.

MEDICAL INTERVENTIONS

- People with hemophilia A and B require replacement of the deficient clotting factors for maintenance, as a prophylactic measure, and to control bleeding.
- Von Willebrand's disease may be treated with regular IV administration of cryoprecipitate, which contains the vW factor.

SELECTED NURSING DIAGNOSES WITH INTERVENTIONS

Risk for Impaired Skin Integrity

- Use safety measures in personal care. For example, use an electric razor rather than a razor blade to shave a client.
- Avoid activities that place the client at risk, and minimize safety hazards. Avoid intramuscular injections, rectal temperatures, and enemas.
- Monitor for signs of bleeding, including hematomas, ecchymoses, and purpura, as well as surface oozing or bleeding.
- If surface bleeding occurs, control blood loss: Apply gentle pressure until bleeding stops; apply ice; apply a topical hemostatic agent.
- Notify the physician at the first sign of bleeding.

Risk for Ineffective Management of Therapeutic Regimen: Individual

- Assess the client's knowledge of the disorder and the related treatments.
- Provide information about the bleeding disorder and the home medications and treatments.
- Provide emotional support to the client, and express confidence in the client's self-care abilities.

H

- Provide opportunities for the client to learn and practice administering clotting factors and topical hemostatic agents under supervision.

CLIENT TEACHING

- Teach the client to recognize the manifestations of internal bleeding, including pallor, weakness, restlessness, headache, disorientation, pain, and swelling. Tell the client to report these immediately.
- Tell the client to apply cold packs and immobilize the joint for 24 to 48 hours if hemarthrosis occurs.
- Stress that the client should not take aspirin. Tell the client to request a prescription for medications if pain is severe.
- Encourage the client to maintain a safe home environment. For example, the client should not keep razor blades in the home (use an electric razor for shaving), should pad sharp edges of furniture, leave a light on at night, avoid using scatter rugs, and wear protective gloves when working in the house or yard.
- Stress the importance of good dental hygiene to decrease potential tooth decay and extractions. If dental procedures are necessary, tell the client to discuss with the dentist and physician the need for prophylactic clotting factor administration.
- Teach the client to prepare and administer IV medications.

HOME CARE CONSIDERATIONS

- Provide information to the client on obtaining and wearing a MedicAlert bracelet or necklace.
- Referral to a home health nurse may be appropriate to evaluate the client's home environment and to review with the client the administration of IV medications.

For more information on Hemophilia, see Medical-Surgical Nursing *by LeMone and Burke, p. 1297.*

Hemorrhoids

OVERVIEW

- Hemorrhoids are dilated, torturous veins of the superior (above pectinate line), or inferior (below pectinate line) hemorrhoidal plexus.
- Varicosities of the superior plexus produce internal hemorrhoids; those of the inferior plexus cause external hemorrhoids.
- They are very common, affecting nearly all adults in the United States.
- Hemorrhoids occur mainly in middle-aged individuals (30 to 50 years).
- They affect both sexes, and are common among childbearing women.

CAUSES

- Probably due primarily to an increase in rectal pressure, such as occurs when straining to defecate
- Risk factors include:
  1. pregnancy, labor
  2. frequent constipation or diarrhea
  3. frequent coughing or vomiting
  4. heart failure, especially right congestive failure
  5. hepatic disease, especially with portal hypertension
  6. low-fiber diet
  7. obesity

Signs & Symptoms

- May be asymptomatic
- External hemorrhoids, which are red and fleshy lesions, may protrude from the rectum
- Anal discomfort, mild to severe
- Bleeding, with bright red blood, especially following defecation
- Anal pruritis
- Sensation of incomplete evacuation

Diagnostics

- Rectal examination confirms clinical signs and symptoms.
- Proctoscopy confirms diagnosis and rules out polyps or other neoplasms.
- Additional tests include testing of stool for occult blood, barium enema, and sigmoidoscopy to rule out cancer of the colon or rectum.

MEDICAL INTERVENTIONS

- A high-fiber diet and increased water intake may be prescribed to relieve constipation.
- Stool softeners or laxatives also may be prescribed to relieve constipation.
- Anesthetic suppositories and creams may reduce discomfort.
- Sclerotherapy, rubber band ligation, hemorrhoidectomy, or cryosurgery may be used for hemorrhoids that are permanently prolapsed, thrombosed, or produce significant symptoms.

SELECTED NURSING DIAGNOSES

- Constipation
- Pain
- Risk for Infection
- Impaired Skin Integrity

SELECTED NURSING INTERVENTIONS

The client who has undergone a hermorrhoidectomy will require appropriate surgical management:

- Maintain side-lying position.
- Apply ice to the dressing.
- Use a sitz bath three to four times in the first 12 hours postoperatively.
- Administer opioid analgesic prior to first bowel movement as prescribed.
- After the first defecation postoperatively, ensure adequate cleaning, usually with a sitz bath.
- Administer stool softeners as prescribed.
- Assess for urinary retention.

CLIENT TEACHING

- Teach the client to respond to the urge to defecate, rather than delaying defecation.
- Stress the importance of drinking plenty of fluids, avoiding caffeine, and eating a high-fiber diet.
- Discuss the proper use of over-the-counter stool softeners, laxatives, and hemorrhoidal suppositories and creams.
- If necessary, teach clients how to reduce prolapsed hemorrhoids digitally.

HOME CARE CONSIDERATIONS

- Review the signs of possible hemorrhoidal complications such as chronic bleeding, prolapse, and thrombosis.
- Discuss the link between manifestations of hemorrhoids and colorectal cancer. Stress the need to seek medical evaluation if symptoms persist.
- For clients who have had surgery, stress the importance of returning to the physician for postoperative care.

For more information on Hemorrhoids, see Medical-Surgical Nursing *by LeMone and Burke, p. 875.*

Hepatitis

OVERVIEW

- Hepatitis is inflammation of the liver, usually caused by a viral infection.
- The chronic form produces necrosis and scarring of liver tissue.
- Six known viruses can produce hepatitis. All produce a similar illness and all may range in severity from asymptomatic, to subclinically progressive, to rapidly fatal.

- Four types of hepatitis are recognized:
  1. viral hepatitis
  2. alcoholic hepatitis
  3. toxic hepatitis
  4. hepatobiliary hepatitis

CAUSES

Viral Hepatitis

- *Hepatitis A virus (HAV):* Fecal–oral spread; highly contagious; acute onset; usually mild course; no chronic or carrier state; no relevance to liver cancer; prognosis excellent
- *Hepatitis B (HBV) virus:* Parenteral, perinatal, sexual spread; acute or insidious onset; severe course, 1% fulminant; chronic state; carrier state; progression to cancer possible; prognosis guarded, worse if client is very young, old, or debilitated
- *Hepatitis C virus (HCV):* Usually parenterally spread, perinatal, sexual spread possible; insidious onset; moderately severe course, rarely fulminant; commonly converts to chronic, rarely to carrier state; progression to cancer possible; prognosis guarded
- *Hepatitis D virus (HDV):* Parenteral, perinatal, sexual spread; insidious or acute onset; occasionally severe course, 5% to 20% fulminant; progression to chronic state common; to carrier state variable; possibly related to development of liver cancer; prognosis for acute form is good; for chronic, poor
- *Hepatitis E virus (HEV):* Fecal–oral spread; acute onset; mild course; few fulminant cases; no chronic or carrier state; no progression to cancer; prognosis good
- *Hepatitis G virus (HGV):* Parenteral spread; possible perinatal and sexual spread; acute or insidious onset; rarely causes clinical hepatitis; accounts for less than 0.5% of community-acquired cases of hepatitis.

Alcoholic Hepatitis

- Chronic alcohol abuse or an acute toxic reaction to alcohol

Toxic Hepatitis

- Ingestion of acetaminophen, benzene, carbon tetrachloride, halothane, chloroform, poisonous mushrooms, or other agents

Hepatobiliary Hepatitis

- Cholestasis—the interruption of the normal flow of bile

Signs & Symptoms

Preicteric phase

- Low-grade fever
- Fatigue, malaise
- Arthralgia, myalgia
- Nausea, vomiting, anorexia
- Upper right quadrant abdominal pain and tenderness
- Headache, photophobia
- Cough, coryza
- Altered taste/smell

Icteric Phase (1–2 weeks)

- Jaundice
- Weight loss
- Clay-colored stools
- Liver tender, enlarged

Posticteric Phase (2–12 weeks; longer with HBV or HCV)

- Continued fatigue
- Abdominal pain or tenderness
- Indigestion
- Flatulence

Diagnostics

- Diagnosis is mainly by clinical history.
- Specific antibody tests as follows: for HAV, anti-HAV; for HBV, anti-HBsAg, anti-Hbe, anti-Hbc, and IgM; for HCV, anti-HCV; for HDV, anti-HBs and anti-HDV; for HEV, anti-HEV.

- Liver enzymes are elevated, including alkaline phosphatase (ALP), GGT, ALT, AST, and LDH.
- Both conjugated and unconjugated bilirubin levels may be elevated in viral hepatitis.
- Prothrombin time may be prolonged.

MEDICAL INTERVENTIONS

- Preexposure prophylaxis with hepatitis A vaccine or immunoglobulin and hepatitis B vaccine is recommended for people at risk for hepatitis A and B, such as travelers and health care workers.
- Postexposure prophylaxis with immunoglobulin is recommended for people exposed to HAV and HBV.
- Vitamin supplementation may be indicated during hepatitis.

SELECTED NURSING DIAGNOSES WITH INTERVENTIONS

Risk for Infection (Transmission)

- Use standard precautions and meticulous hand washing.
- Use contact isolation precautions in addition to standard precautions for clients with hepatitis A who are diapered or have fecal incontinence.

Activity Intolerance

- Facilitate the client's self-direction of activities as determined by the client's feeling of fatigue.
- Encourage the client to resume activities gradually.
- Provide progressive ambulation and simple exercises, in consultation with a physical or occupational therapist.
- Promote rest, and incorporate safety and fall-prevention techniques.

Altered Nutrition: Less than Body Requirements

- Help clients with acute viral hepatitis select a diet that provides a high-kilocalorie intake.
- Since many clients with hepatitis are nauseated later in the day, encourage the client to consume the majority of kilocalories in the morning.
- Encourage a low-fat diet.

- If nausea and vomiting persist, use IV supplementation as prescribed, and encourage smaller, more frequent meals. Monitor fluids and electrolytes and assess for dehydration.

CLIENT TEACHING

- Teach the modes of hepatitis transmission and the methods for preventing transmission. For instance, instruct the client and significant others not to share towels or eating utensils. Explain that until the client's serologic indicators return to normal, sexual and close personal contact with others should be avoided.
- Tell the client to avoid hepatotoxic substances, such as alcohol and acetaminophen.

HOME CARE CONSIDERATIONS

- Encourage clients in high risk groups to obtain hepatitis A and/or hepatitis B immunizations.
- Emphasize the importance of childhood immunizations.
- Stress the need for long-term follow-up care with the physician.
- Review the health habits needed to prevent further liver damage, such as avoidance of hepatotoxic substances. Clients with alcoholic hepatitis may require referral to a support group such as Alcoholics Anonymous. Stress that without continued abstinence, progression to cirrhosis is common.
- Teach safer sex practices to clients with hepatitis B, C, or D and discuss other important measures to prevent its spread, such as avoiding sharing needles, syringes, and razors.
- Referral to a home health nurse may be appropriate for some clients.

For more information on Hepatitis, see Medical-Surgical Nursing *by LeMone and Burke, p. 520.*

Herniated Intervertebral Disk

OVERVIEW

- A herniated disk is the rupture of the soft, internal portion (nucleus pulposus) of a vertebral disk through the tough outer portion (annulus fibrosis).
- The extruded disk material impinges upon spinal nerve roots and/or the spinal cord.
- Most occur in the lumbar vertebrae; cervical vertebrae are the second most common site; thoracic, the least common.
- They are more common in males under 45 years of age.

CAUSES

- Severe trauma or lumbar strain
- Improper body mechanics, especially with lifting
- Disk degeneration, especially in elderly

Signs & Symptoms

- Pain:
    1. lower back
    2. severe
    3. usually unilateral
    4. radiates in sciatic pattern (buttock, leg, foot)
    5. exacerbated by movement
- Paresthesias such as numbness or tingling
- Possible motor deficits/muscle wasting

Diagnostics

- X-rays are taken of vertebrae to rule out other causes (e.g., fracture); not diagnostic for herniated intervertebral disk.
- Myelography reveals spinal canal compression.
- Computed tomography (CT) scan and magnetic resonance imaging (RMI) reveal spinal cord compression.

MEDICAL INTERVENTIONS

- Pain is managed with nonsteroidal anti-inflammatory drugs. Muscle spasms are treated with muscle relaxants.
- Transcutaneous electrical nerve stimulation (TENS) may be used for pain relief.
- Surgery is indicated for clients who do not respond to conservative management.

SELECTED NURSING DIAGNOSES WITH INTERVENTIONS

Pain

- Encourage discussion of pain. Assess degree of pain and identify contributing and relieving factors.
- Maintain bed rest and activities as prescribed. Teach client how to logroll when changing positions.
- Use a firm mattress or place a board under the mattress.
- Teach the client to avoid turning or twisting the spinal column and to assume positions that decrease stress on the vertebral column.
- Provide analgesic medications on a regular basis around the clock.

Chronic Pain

- Treat the client's reports of pain with respect.
- Do not refer to the client as being addicted to pain medication. Tolerance to medications does not imply addiction.
- Monitor the client carefully for any changes in condition.
- Ensure that the client understands the reason for the pain experienced.
- Do not withdraw pain medications abruptly. Suggest a gradual withdrawal for clients who have been taking narcotic or sedative medications for longer than 3 weeks.
- Follow recommended guidelines for administering pain medications.
- Maintain written plans of care for pain management that are individualized and ensure continuity of care.

- Teach the client alternative methods of pain management. Consider the client's coping style when recommending methods.
- Encourage the client to take part in regular physical and mental activities.
- Include significant others in the care plan.
- Identify client support systems and encourage their use.
- Refer the client to a physical therapist for an exercise program if appropriate.
- Assess the need for referrals (and make them if necessary) for the client who is depressed or anxious.

Constipation

Reduced mobility, bed rest, and pain medications increase the client's risk for developing constipation.

- Assess the client's usual bowel routine, including diet, fluid intake, and the use of laxatives or enemas.
- Encourage a fluid intake of 2500 to 3000 mL per day, unless contraindicated by the presence of renal or cardiac disease.
- Increase fiber and bulk in the diet. Consult with the physician about the use of stool softeners or bulk-forming agents.
- Place the client on the bedpan or (if allowed) help the client to the bathroom or bedside commode at the usual time of bowel movements. Provide privacy.

CLIENT TEACHING

- Teach the client about pain control, including medications, positioning the body, use of proper body mechanics, and nonpharmacologic methods of pain management, including relaxation, guided imagery, distraction, hypnosis, and music.
- Discuss with the client scheduling of analgesics. Although many people believe that the use of analgesic medications causes addiction, it is now widely accepted that providing medications on a routine schedule is the preferred administration method.

HOME CARE CONSIDERATIONS

- Encourage the client to remain physically active and maintain weight within the desired range.

- A referral to a support group for people with chronic pain may be appropriate.
- A referral to a psychologic counselor may be appropriate for helping the client cope with the chronic pain.

For more information on Herniated Intervertebral Disk, see Medical-Surgical Nursing *by LeMone and Burke, p. 1802.*

Herpes Simplex Virus (HSV)

Herpes Labialis (Cold Sores, Fever Blisters)
Herpes Genitalis
Herpetic Whitlow
HSV Keratitis

OVERVIEW

- Infection with HSV I and/or HSV II.
- Each strain is highly contagious.
- HSV I usually affects mucous membranes of the lips, oral mucosa, and/or facial skin.
- HSV II usually affects mucous membranes and skin of the genital/rectal area; it is considered a sexually transmited disease (STD).
- Cross-infection is possible.
- Herpetic whitlow is an HSV infection of the fingers with either strain of the virus.
- HSV keratitis is a corneal infection and is the most common cause of corneal blindness in the United States.
- Infection in early pregnancy may result in spontaneous abortion.
- In immunocompromised patients, including infected neonates, HSV disseminates widely to skin, central nervous system (CNS), and viscera.

- During the primary, or initial, infection, peripheral sensory or autonomic nerves are colonized by the herpes virus.
- Following the primary infection, the virus moves by axonal transport to the cell body of the neurons contained in ganglia.
- Secondary infection (reinfection) of peripheral mucous membranes/skin occurs episodically.
- Secondary attacks may be precipitated by other infections, stress, sunlight, menses, fever, or exposure to excess heat or cold.

CAUSES

- Herpes virus hominis (HVH); strain HSV I or HSV II; enveloped DNA viruses
- Acquired through intimate contact: kissing, sexual intercourse; maternal-to-fetal spread by transplacental or vaginal routes
- Autoinoculation of eye via finger
- Spreads to contiguous area upon reactivation

Signs & Symptoms

- Vesicles develop in clusters and initially are small, inflamed, and fluid-filled; later, vesicle rupture produces ulceration, oozing, and the formation of a crust
- Pain, burning in nature, is characteristic of early and late lesions
- Itch may precede or accompany pain
- A prodrome of itching or tingling may signal an impending secondary attack
- Lymphadenopathy may be present with primary infection

Diagnostics

- Viral culture of lesions reveals HSV I or II.
- Biopsy also confirms presence of herpes virus infection.
- A general rise in Ig titers and white blood cell (WBC) count supports the diagnosis.

MEDICAL INTERVENTIONS

- The antiviral drug acyclovir is the treatment of choice for most types of HSV infections.
- Other antiviral medications include vidarabine, idoxuridines, and trifluorothymidine.
- Aspirin and other nonprescription analgesics may reduce the pain of herpes lesions.
- Clients with AIDS may require prophylactic treatment.

SELECTED NURSING DIAGNOSES WITH INTERVENTIONS

Pain

- Teach the client to keep herpes blisters clean and dry. A solution of warm water, soap, and hydrogen peroxide can be used to cleanse the lesions two or three times daily. The client should wear loose cotton clothing that will not trap moisture.
- For clients experiencing dysuria, suggest pouring water over the genitals while urinating, or urinating in the tub or shower. Drinking additional fluids also helps dilute the acidity of the urine. Fluids that increase acidity, such as cranberry juice, should be avoided.
- Nonpharmacologic measures to reduce pain include application of heat or cold and sitz baths.

Sexual Dysfunction

- Provide a supportive, nonjudgmental environment for the client to discuss feelings and ask questions about what this diagnosis means to future sexual relationships.
- Discuss the disease process and factors that may contribute to recurrent infections.
- Offer information about support groups and other resources for people with herpes such as the National Herpes Information Hotline.

Anxiety

- Advise the client about the need for regular Pap smears, as appropriate. Some authorities suggest Pap smears every 6 months for women with genital herpes.

- Discuss with women of childbearing age that cesarean delivery can prevent transmission of infection to the neonate. In women without signs or symptoms of recurrence, vaginal delivery is possible.

CLIENT TEACHING

- Teach the client about the disease process and factors that affect it. Discuss how to recognize prodromal symptoms of recurrence and factors that seem to trigger recurrences (such as emotional stress, acidic food, sun exposure).
- Instruct the client to abstain from sexual contact from the time the prodromal symptoms appear until 10 days after all lesions have healed.
- Stress the importance of using latex condoms and careful hygiene practices (such as not sharing towels) even during latency periods.
- Share with the client strategies for discussing the condition with current or future sexual partners.

HOME CARE CONSIDERATIONS

- Emphasize the need for lifelong follow-up care to manage recurrences.
- Refer the client to local support groups and information services such as the National Herpes Information Hotline.

For more information on Herpes Simplex Virus, see Medical-Surgical Nursing *by LeMone and Burke, p. 584.*

Hiatal Hernia

OVERVIEW

- A hiatal or diaphragmatic hernia is a defect in the esophageal hiatus of the diaphragm that allows herniation of the stomach into the chest cavity.

- Hernias are classified as sliding (axial) or rolling (paraesophageal).
- A sliding hernia is the most common type; both the stomach and esophagogastric junction rise through the herniated diaphragm.
- A rolling hernia occurs when only a portion of the stomach rises through the diaphragm; the esophagogastric junction remains fixed.
- Sliding herniations are very common, affecting about 50% of the adult population; the incidence rises with age.

CAUSES

- Sliding hernias represent a weakening of the esophageal-diaphragm junction. Risk factors include:
  1. congenital malformation
  2. age greater than 60 years
  3. esophageal carcinoma
  4. kyphoscoliosis
  5. trauma/surgery
- Rolling hernias are associated with increased abdominal pressure, as with:
  1. pregnancy
  2. ascites
  3. obesity
  4. constrictive clothing
  5. movement, such as like bending, coughing, straining, Valsalva maneuver
  6. severe physical exertion

Signs & Symptoms

- May be asymptomatic
- Heartburn/retrosternal chest pain, from gastro-esophageal reflux; usually follows meals by about 1 to 4 hours; aggravated by reclining, belching, straining
- Regurgitation and/or vomiting
- Dysphagia
- Dyspnea
- Bleeding, usually occult
- Incarcerated hiatal hernia presents abruptly with severe sharp pain; S/S of shock

H

Diagnostics

- Chest x-ray may reveal a retrocardiac shadow.
- Barium swallow reveals diaphragmatic pouch outline.
- Endoscopy/biopsy is used to rule out varices and neoplasms.
- Esophageal motility test shows motor anomalies.
- Hematest of gastric contents or stool may be positive for blood.

MEDICAL INTERVENTIONS

- Treatment for most hiatal hernias is based on the symptoms of gastroesophageal reflux. Pharmacologic agents may include antacids, histamine$_2$-receptor antagonists, and antisecretory agents.
- If complications occur, surgery—most commonly a Nissen fundoplication—may be performed.

SELECTED NURSING DIAGNOSES

- Altered Nutrition: Less than Body Requirements
- Pain

SELECTED NURSING INTERVENTIONS

- Encourage the client to consume frequent small meals throughout the day rather than three large meals, and to avoid bedtime snacks.
- Encourage weight reduction and smoking cessation as appropriate.
- Keep the head of the client's bed elevated 8 to 12 inches.
- Ensure that the client remains upright for at least 2 hours after eating.
- Administer antacids, histamine$_2$-receptor antagonists, and antisecretory agents as prescribed.
- Postoperatively, assess for complications of surgery; elevate the head of the bed 30°, and supervise the client's first food or fluid intake by mouth.
- Teach the client to support the incision when turning, coughing, and deep breathing.
- Encourage the client to change position frequently, and encourage early ambulation.

CLIENT TEACHING

- Teach the client to avoid straining at stools, heavy lifting, heavy manual labor, and climbing stairs for at least 3 weeks postoperatively.
- Encourage the client to follow a diet low in fat, and to avoid caffeine, alcohol, acidic foods, carbonated beverages, and gas-producing foods such as cabbage, bananas, and nuts, and to refrain from chewing gum.
- Encourage the client to drink with a straw.
- Encourage small meals throughout the day rather than three large meals.

HOME CARE CONSIDERATIONS

- Refer the client to smoking cessation and/or weight reduction programs as necessary.
- A home health referral may be appropriate for wound care.
- Stress the importance of follow-up care with the physician. Tell the client to report immediately any signs of infection such as elevated temperature.

For more information on Hiatal Hernia, see Medical-Surgical Nursing *by LeMone and Burke, p. 471.*

Hodgkin's Disease

OVERVIEW

- Hodgkin's disease is a malignant neoplastic disease of lymphoid tissues.
- It occurs worldwide, in all races, but is slightly more common in European Americans.
- In the United States it shows a bimodal peak incidence; first peak at age 15 to 35, second after age 50.
- It is more prevalent in males, particularly among children and young adults.
- It tends to cluster in families.

- The incidence of Hodgkin's disease is increased in immunocompromised individuals.
- It is highly treatable in the early stages, but without treatment is ultimately fatal.
- The 5-year survival rate is about 90% for all stages.

CAUSES

- The exact cause is unknown but certain risk factors have been identified:
  1. genetic predisposition, e.g., an identical twin or sibling with Hodgkin's
  2. certain human leukocyte antigen (HLA) types
  3. possible male hormonal influence
  4. possible viral infection, particularly Epstein-Barr virus (EBV)
  5. immunodeficiency or autoimmune disease

Signs & Symptoms

- Lymphadenopathy, painless swelling of a single node, usually cervical; progresses to other areas
- Palpation of involved nodes reveals enlarged, nontender, rubbery feeling mass; size increases during fevers
- History of persistent fever, night sweats
- Anorexia, weight loss
- Fatigue, malaise
- Pruritis
- Advanced cases show:
  1. increased incidence of infection
  2. edema of face or neck
  3. jaundice

Diagnostics

- Biopsy shows typical Reed-Sternberg cells; large bilobular cells with obvious nuclear inclusions.
- Lymphangiography determines the extent of lymphatic involvement.
- Bone marrow, spleen, and liver biopsies help to stage the disease.
- Lung, bone, liver scans assist in staging the disease

- Blood tests may reveal normocytic anemia, variable white blood cell (WBC) counts (high, normal, low), increased serum alkaline phosphatase, increased calcium levels, increased lactic acid, increased lysozyme, increased C-reactive protein.

MEDICAL INTERVENTIONS

- Radiation therapy usually involves extensive external radiation of the involved lymph node region.
- Multiple-drug chemotherapy is used to treat advanced disease.
- Surgery is conducted primarily to obtain biopsy specimens or to obtain tissue for staging.
- If the spleen is enlarged, a therapeutic splenectomy may be performed.

H

SELECTED NURSING DIAGNOSES WITH INTERVENTIONS

Altered Protection

- Assess the onset, sites, precipitating factors, and methods of relieving pruritis.
- Provide and teach the client and significant others interventions to enhance comfort and relieve itching: use cool water and mild soap to bathe; blot skin dry; apply cornstarch or nonperfumed powder or lotion; use lightweight blankets and clothing; maintain adequate humidity and a cool room temperature; wash bedding and clothes in mild detergent and put them through the second rinse cycle.

Altered Nutrition: Less than Body Requirements

- Provide small feedings of high-kilocalorie, high-protein foods and fluids.
- Assist the client with oral care, general hygiene, and environmental control of temperature, appearance, and odors.
- Identify and provide foods the client prefers.
- Place the client in a sitting position during and immediately after meals.
- Assess factors that precipitate nausea and/or vomiting, the frequency and type of vomiting, and relief measures used by the client.
- Administer prescribed antiemetics before chemotherapy is started.

Body Image Disturbance

- Assess body image perception by collecting subjective data through such questions as: What do you like most/least about your body? Has the illness changed the way you feel others will respond to you?
- Assess the client for risk of developing alopecia.
- Provide interventions to enable client to cope with alopecia:
  1. Encourage verbalization of feelings.
  2. Teach the client the effects of chemotherapy on hair follicles and the potential for regrowth of hair.
  3. Discuss use of wigs, scarves, hats and so on.
  4. If eyebrows and eyelashes are lost, discuss measures to protect the eyes such as eyeglasses and hats with wide brims.
  5. Teach proper scalp care: Use mild shampoo, soft brush, and sunscreen.
- Provide interventions to enable the client to cope with actual or potential sexual dysfunction or sterility.

CLIENT TEACHING

- Teach the client about the disease process, prognosis, treatment, and side effects of treatments.
- Teach the importance of proper skin care, and to avoid scratching to prevent skin breakdown.
- Tell the client to plan activities of daily living (ADLs) to ensure adequate rest and exercise, and to eat a well-balanced diet.
- Provide teaching to prevent or relieve nausea and vomiting: eat soda crackers or hard candy; eat food cold or at room temperature; eat soft, bland foods; avoid unpleasant odors and get fresh air; do not eat immediately before chemotherapy; use distraction or progressive muscle relaxation when nauseated; do not eat for several hours if vomiting occurs.
- Teach the client to monitor the side effects of radiation and chemotherapy treatments, including infection, bleeding, anemia, nausea and vomiting, skin irritation and breakdown in area of radiation, and impaired liver function.
- Males who receive radiation to the pelvic region may become sterile. Encourage the client to discuss

with the physician and with significant others the possibility of storing sperm in a sperm bank before treatment.

HOME CARE CONSIDERATIONS

- Discuss the need to avoid exposure to people with contagious infections or diseases.
- Emphasize the need for long-term follow-up care with the oncologist.
- Refer the client to the local chapter of the American Cancer Society for information, financial assistance, and counseling.
- A home care referral may be appropriate.

For more information on Hodgkin's Disease, see Medical-Surgical Nursing *by LeMone and Burke,* *p. 1317.*

Human Immunodeficiency Virus (HIV) Disease (HIV, AIDS)

OVERVIEW

- Acquired immune deficiency syndrome (AIDS) is a syndrome of immunodeficiency seen in the final phase of infection with HIV (human immunodeficiency virus).
- HIV primarily infects helper T cells of the immune system with CD_4 cell-surface receptors.
- HIV is a retrovirus that contains an RNA genome and reverse transcriptase enzyme that converts RNA to DNA.
- HIV is slow-growing; the median time from initial infection to the appearance of S/S of AIDS is 8 to 10 years.
- Generally, HIV infection follows the following course:

Primary Infection

- Lasts about 12 weeks, during which an acute viremia with widespread lymphatic seeding occurs.
- Virus titers peak at about the eighth week, as CD_4 counts fall to approximately 500 cells/μL (50% normal).
- During the primary infection 50% to 70% of clients show an acute HIV syndrome, which resembles an acute bout of mononucleosis.
- By the end of this stage the CD_4 count has rebounded to about 700 cells/μL.
- The primary infection is the window period, a time at which the virus is present but undetectable by standard tests that measure antibodies to the virus.
- Detectable antibodies are usually found by the end of this stage (seroconversion). However, some clients may not display adequate measurement levels for a year.

Clinical Latency

- Follows the primary infection and is characterized by:
  1. the presence of detectable HIV antibodies
  2. reduced viremia
  3. lymphoid sequestration of virus
  4. a steady decline in the CD_4 count from about 700 to 200 cells/μL over the next 8 to 10 years
- Some clients may display persistent generalized lymphadenopathy (PGL), oral lesions, shingles, or other minor opportunistic diseases.

Clinically Apparent Disease (AIDS)

- Heralded when the CD_4 count reaches about 200 cells/μL.
- The client may develop constitutional S/S or may present with an opportunistic infection or neoplasm.
- Neurologic disease, such as aseptic meningitis, HIV encephalopathy, and peripheral neuropathies is common.
- Death usually occurs as the result of overwhelming infection or cancer.

CAUSES

- HIV is acquired:
  1. during sexual intercourse, especially anal sex
  2. via blood transfusion
  3. via use of contaminated needles
  4. via perinatal transmission from mother to fetus
- Risk factors include a history of:
  1. unprotected sex between men
  2. unprotected sex with multiple partners
  3. unprotected sex with an infected partner
  4. injection drug use or unprotected sex with an injection drug user
  5. infection with a sexually transmitted disease
  6. transfusion with blood or pooled blood products, especially prior to 1985
  7. pre/perinatal exposure to an HIV-infected mother
  8. postnatal exposure, via breast milk, to an infected mother
  9. occupational accidents, such as needle sticks, cuts or puncture wounds during surgery, or human bites

Signs & Symptoms

Primary Stage
- Fever, lymphadenopathy
- Malaise, fatigue
- Arthralgia, myalgia
- Headache, pharyngitis
- Rash, urticaria
- Abdominal cramps, diarrhea

Latent Stage
- Persistent generalized lymphadenopathy (PGL)
- Persistent fever, night sweats
- Chronic diarrhea, weight loss
- Fatigue
- Candidiasis of mouth (thrush)

Clinically Apparent Stage (AIDS)
Specific S/S of AIDS indicator conditions
- Candidiasis of bronchi/lung
- Candidiasis of esophagus

H

- Coccidioidomycosis, extrapulmonary
- Cryptococcosis, extrapulmonary
- Cryptosporidiosis, intestinal >1 month
- Cytomegalovirus (CMV)
- CMV retinitis with loss of vision
- HIV encephalopathy/dementia
- Herpes simplex virus (HSV) >1 month
- HSV, disseminated
- Invasive cancer of the cervix
- Isoporiasis with diarrhea >1 month
- Kaposi's sarcoma
- Lymphoma: immunoblastic, Burkitt's
- *Mycobacterium avium,* or any species
- Tuberculosis (*M. tuberculosis*), any site
- *Pneumocystis carinii* pneumonia (PCP)
- Pneumonia, any species/recurrent
- Progressive leukoencephalopathy
- Salmonella septicemia, recurrent
- Toxoplasmosis of brain
- HIV wasting syndrome

Diagnostics

Primary Stage (End of)
- Positive ELISA and Western blot (HIV antibody tests). (Negative ELISA and Western blot until end of stage.)
- CD_4 >500 cells/μL.

Latent Stage
- Positive ELISA and Western blot (HIV antibody tests).
- CD_4 = 200–700 cells μL.
- Decreased red blood cells (RBCs), hemoglobin (Hgb), hematocrit (HCT), white blood cells (WBCs), lymphocytes, and platelets.

Clinically Apparent Stage
- Positive ELISA and Western blot (HIV antibody tests).
- CD_4 <200 cells/μL.
- Decreased RBCs, Hgb, HCT, and WBCs.
- Lymphocytes <14%.
- Blood chemistry abnormalities.

MEDICAL INTERVENTIONS

- Treatment for HIV infection includes antiretroviral therapy to suppress the HIV infection, prophylaxis and treatment for opportunistic infections and malignancies, and hematopoetic stimulating factors.

SELECTED NURSING DIAGNOSES WITH INTERVENTIONS

Ineffective Individual Coping

- Assess client's social support network.
- Promote interaction between the client, significant others, and family.
- Encourage client to obtain information and make care decisions.
- Support positive coping behaviors, client decisions, actions, and achievements.
- Provide referrals to counselors, support groups, and agencies.

Impaired Skin Integrity

- Assess skin frequently.
- Monitor lesions.
- Turn client at least every 2 hours.
- Use pressure-relieving devices.
- Keep skin clean and dry.
- Massage around but not over affected pressure sites.
- Caution client against scratching.
- Encourage ambulation.

Altered Nutrition: Less than Body Requirements

- Assess the client's nutritional status.
- Assess for oral or esophageal lesions, fever, nausea, or diarrhea.
- Administer medications as prescribed.
- Provide a diet high in protein and kilocalories.
- Offer soft foods and serve small portions.
- Provide food that the client likes, and encourage significant others to bring favorite foods from home.
- Assist the client with eating as needed.
- Provide supplementary vitamins and enteral feedings, such as Ensure.
- Provide or assist client with frequent oral hygiene.

Altered Sexuality Patterns

- Examine your own feelings about sexuality.
- Establish a trusting, therapeutic relationship with the client.
- Provide the client and significant others with factual information about HIV infection.
- Discuss safe sex practices.
- Encourage the client and significant others to discuss fears and concerns.
- Refer client and significant others to local support groups.

CLIENT TEACHING

- Provide information about transmission of HIV and any coexisting infections, and how to avoid transmission of HIV through safe-sex practices and avoidance of sharing injection drug paraphernalia.
- Instruct the client to inform any sexual partners of HIV status.
- Teach the importance of maintaining optimal level of health through proper nutrition, exercise, smoking cessation, stress reduction, rest, regular check-ups, Mantoux testing, and avoidance of illegal drugs.
- Provide information about medications, effects, and side effects. Stress the importance of precisely following the prescribed medication regimen.
- Teach client proper care of central or peripheral IV lines and venous access devices.
- Teach the importance of regular self-assessment for early signs of opportunistic infections, and to report any signs of infection or any changes in neurologic status.

HOME CARE CONSIDERATIONS

- Ensure access to follow-up care.
- Provide the names, locations, and phone numbers of local support groups for clients and significant others, including local visiting nurses associations, home health agencies, Meals-on-Wheels, and so on, as well as national information resources such as the National AIDS Information Clearinghouse.

- Discuss assessment of safety of the home environment.
- Discuss the availability of hospice care as appropriate.

For more information on Human Immunodeficiency Virus Disease, see Medical-Surgical Nursing *by LeMone and Burke, p. 291.*

Hyperglycemia

OVERVIEW

- Hyperglycemia is defined as a rise in blood glucose levels to >120 mg/dL, usually due to diabetes mellitus (DM).
- It results when glucose cannot enter insulin-dependent cells (skeletal muscle and adipose tissue) or when glucose is released from hepatic stores (glycogenolysis and gluconeogenesis).
- It may be attributable to an absolute lack of insulin, as in Type 1 (formerly known as insulin-dependent diabetes mellitus), or to insulin resistance, as in Type 2 (formerly known as non–insulin-dependent diabetes mellitus).
- Secondary hyperglycemia is associated with disorders of insulin target tissue and with pancreatic disorders.
- Hyperglycemia represents a hyperosmolar state that causes cellular dehydration.
- When blood glucose rises to >180 mg/dL, glucose spills into the urine, producing an osmotic diuresis.
- In Type 1 DM, severe hyperglycemia may cause diabetic ketoacidosis (DKA), possibly progressing to diabetic coma.
- In Type 2 DM, severe, profound hyperglycemia causes hyperosmotic nonketotic coma.

CAUSES

- Diabetes mellitus: Type 1 or Type 2
- Endocrine disorders causing excess production of growth hormone, glucocorticoids, catecholamines, glucagon, or somatostatin
- Medications such as thiazide diuretics, phenytoin, niacin, and high-dose corticosteroids
- Chronic pancreatitis
- Cirrhosis
- Stress

Signs & Symptoms

- Polyuria (if blood sugar >180 mg/dL), due to osmotic diuresis
- Polydipsia, secondary to increased blood osmolarity
- Abdominal pain
- Warm, dry, flushed skin
- Poor skin/eye turgor
- Hypotension
- Tachycardia
- Altered level of consciousness (LOC), confusion, stuporous to coma

Diagnostics

- Serum glucose >120 mg/dL.
- Serum osmolality is elevated in proportion to blood glucose level.
- Serum sodium and potassium levels vary.
- Blood urea nitrogen (BUN) and creatinine levels may be elevated.
- Glycosuria when blood glucose exceeds 180 mg/dL.

MEDICAL INTERVENTIONS

- Insulin replacement therapy as indicated by underlying cause.
- Fluid and electrolyte replacement therapy.

SELECTED NURSING DIAGNOSES

- Risk for Injury
- Altered Nutrition: More than Body Requirements
- Risk for Altered Thought Processes
- Risk for Sensory/Perceptual Alteration: Visual
- Ineffective Management of Therapeutic Regimen: Individual

SELECTED NURSING INTERVENTIONS

- Administer insulin as prescribed.
- Monitor blood glucose levels.
- Encourage fluid intake.
- Encourage adherence to prescribed diet.
- Following insulin treatment, monitor for signs of hypoglycemia: change in mental status, diaphoresis, cool, clammy skin. If observed, provide a source of glucose (orange juice, hard candy, glucagon, or 50% glucose).
- Assess for signs of skin breakdown and for decreased urine output.
- Encourage the client to have baseline ophthalmic examination and regular follow-up care.

CLIENT TEACHING

- Teach diet and medication management and the correlation between the two.
- Teach self-monitoring of blood glucose and prevention of hyper- and hypoglycemia.
- Review self-administration of insulin, if needed.
- Discuss wound care, if necessary.
- Teach the S/S of urinary tract infection.

HOME CARE CONSIDERATIONS

- Stress the need for medical management and self-care of the underlying condition.
- Refer the client to a dietitian for long-term nutritional support and follow-up.
- If appropriate, refer the client to social services or a psychologic counselor for stress management techniques and coping mechanisms for managing a chronic illness.

- Refer the client to the American Diabetes Association if indicated.

For more information about Hyperglycemia, see Medical-Surgical Nursing *by LeMone and Burke, p. 727.*

Hyperosmolar Nonketotic Coma (HNKC)

OVERVIEW

- HNKC is a metabolic problem characterized by significantly elevated plasma osmolarity and blood glucose levels, and altered levels of consciousness.
- It affects people with Type 2 diabetes mellitus (DM).
- The development of the condition is insidious.
- High blood glucose pulls water from body cells and fluid is lost via the urine; dehydration results.
- As water is lost, glucose and sodium increase plasma osmolarity.
- Cellular dehydration affects central nervous system (CNS) cells the most.

CAUSES

- Increased insulin resistance
- Excess carbohydrate intake
- Risk factors include:
  1. drugs such as glucocorticoids, diuretics, beta-adrenergic blockers, immunosuppressants, chlorpromazine, and diazoxide
  2. acute illness
  3. therapeutic procedures such as dialysis, hyperalimentation (oral or parenteral), surgery
  4. chronic illness such as renal or cardiac disease, hypertension, previous stroke, and alcoholism

Signs & Symptoms

- Flushed, warm, dry skin
- Extreme thirst
- Fatigue, malaise
- Nausea, vomiting; abdominal pain
- Hypotension, tachycardia
- Polyuria
- Lethargy progressing to coma; possible seizures

Diagnostics

- Serum glucose >600 mg/dL.
- Serum osmolarity >340 mOsm/L.
- Serum ketones normal.
- Serum sodiun is usually normal to slightly elevated.
- Blood urea nitrogen (BUN) and creatinine are elevated.

MEDICAL INTERVENTIONS

- HNKC is a life-threatening medical emergency.
- Treatment is immediate, and is directed toward correcting fluid and electrolyte imbalances, lowering blood glucose levels with insulin, and treating underlying conditions.

SELECTED NURSING DIAGNOSES

- Fluid Volume Deficit
- Altered Tissue Perfusion: Renal
- Knowledge Deficit

SELECTED NURSING INTERVENTIONS

- Administer IV fluids and insulin as prescribed.
- Monitor the client's response to fluids and insulin.
- Encourage fluid intake.
- Monitor fluid status through intake and output, skin turgor, vital signs, and central venous pressure. Record findings.
- Assess level of consciousness.
- Monitor blood glucose levels.
- Monitor cardiac activity.

CLIENT TEACHING

- Assess the client's knowledge of the management of diabetes.
- Provide teaching related to diet, medications, and signs and symptoms of hyperglycemia and hypoglycemia and their management.

HOME CARE CONSIDERATIONS

- Stress the need for ongoing follow-up care for management of diabetes.
- A home health care referral may be appropriate for continued teaching and monitoring of self-care activities.

For more information on Hyperosmolar Nonketotic Coma, see Medical-Surgical Nursing *by LeMone and Burke, p. 724.*

Hyperparathyroidism

OVERVIEW

- Hyperparathyroidism is defined as overactivity of the parathyroid glands with secretion of excess parathyroid hormone (PTH).
- There are three types of hyperparathyroidism:
    1. *Primary hyperparathyroidism* results from hyperplasia or an adenoma of a parathyroid gland, causing excess PTH secretion.
    2. *Secondary hyperparathyroidism* is a compensatory response to chronic hypocalcemia.
    3. *Tertiary hyperparathyroidism* is seen most often in chronic renal failure, and results from parathyroid gland hyperplasia and loss of response to serum calcium levels.
- Excess PTH affects the kidneys and bones, resulting in:
    1. increased resorption of calcium and excretion of phosphorus by the kidneys

2. increased bicarbonate excretion and decreased acid excretion by the kidneys
3. increased calcium and phosphorus release from the bones
4. soft-tissue deposits of calcium and renal stone formation

CAUSES

- Primary hyperparathyroidism is caused by intrinsic pathology of the parathyroid glands:
  1. single benign adenoma (about 80% of cases)
  2. multiple gland hyperplasia (about 15% of cases)
  3. multiple benign adenoma (about 4% of cases)
  4. carcinoma (less than 1% of cases)

H

Signs & Symptoms

Most patients are asymptomatic. When present, S/S are as follows:

- Renal: polyuria, polydipsia, renal calculi
- Musculoskeletal: backache, arthralgia, deformity, pathologic fracture, muscle weakness, atrophy
- Central nervous system (CNS): paresthesias, depression, psychosis, coma
- GI tract: nausea, anorexia, constipation, epigastric pain, peptic ulcers
- Cardiovascular: dysrhythmias, hypertension
- Metabolic: acidosis, weight loss
- Skin: subcutaneous calcification with necrosis

Diagnostics

- Serum calcium is increased in primary and tertiary hyperparathyroidism and decreased in the secondary form.
- Serum phosphorus is decreased in primary hyperparathyroidism and increased in the secondary form.
- Serum PTH is increased.
- Alkaline phosphatase is increased.
- X-rays reveal diffuse demineralization.

MEDICAL INTERVENTIONS

- Saline fluids are administered intravenously.
- Diuretics are administered to increase renal excretion of calcium.
- Oral or IV phosphates and IV calcitonin, which reduce calcium levels more rapidly, may be appropriate.
- The treatment of primary hyperparathyroidism is surgical removal of the parathyroid gland(s) affected by hyperplasia or adenoma.

SELECTED NURSING DIAGNOSES

- Risk for Injury
- Risk for Fluid Volume Excess
- Impaired Physical Mobility
- Pain
- Risk for Altered Urinary Elimination

SELECTED NURSING INTERVENTIONS

- Monitor intake and output carefully.
- Monitor serum calcium levels.
- Monitor changes in blood pressure, heart rate, and mental status, and assess for signs of heart failure.
- Administer pharmacologic agents as prescribed.
- The postoperative care for a client having parathyroid surgery includes:
  1. monitoring vital signs and serum calcium frequently.
  2. checking neck dressing front and back for excessive drainage and bleeding.
  3. assessing for respiratory distress caused by hemorrhage or tissue swelling. Keep an emergency tracheostomy tray, oxygen, and suction equipment at bedside.
  4. monitoring for signs of hypocalcemia, such as tingling and twitching of the face, and for Trousseau's and Chvostek's signs.
  5. administering calcium and vitamin D as prescribed.

CLIENT TEACHING

- Teach the client the signs of hypercalcemia and hypocalcemia.
- Preoperatively, review neck positioning and movement to prevent stress on suture line and to diminish pain.
- Teach wound care.

HOME CARE CONSIDERATIONS

- Stress the need for long-term follow-up medical care.
- Assess the client's living situation for safety if significant bone demineralization has occurred.
- The client suffering from impaired physical mobility may require a referral to a home health nurse.

For more information on Hyperparathyroidism, see Medical-Surgical Nursing *by LeMone and Burke, p. 700.*

Hypersensitivity

OVERVIEW

- Hypersensitivity is an altered immune response to an antigen that harms the client.
- Four different mechanisms may cause hypersensitivity disorders:
  1. Type I (IgE-mediated hypersensitivity)
  2. Type II (cytotoxic hypersensitivity)
  3. Type III (immune complex–mediated hypersensitivity)
  4. Type IV (delayed hypersensitivity)
- *Common hypersensitivity* reactions, such as allergic asthma, allergic rhinitis, allergic conjunctivitis, hives, and anaphylactic shock, are typical of Type I, or IgE-mediated, hypersensitivity. This entails a local or systemic response to a previously encountered antigen to which IgE has been formed and

attached to mast cells. When the antigen is reintroduced, it binds to IgE on the mast cells, which then release histamine and other chemical mediators, complement, acetylcholine, kinins, and chemotactic factors. Anaphylaxis is an acute systemic Type I response that occurs in highly sensitive persons following exposure to the antigen, usually by injection. The release of histamine and other mediators causes vasodilation and increased capillary permeability, smooth muscle contraction, and bronchial constriction, which can in turn lead to impaired tissue perfusion and hypotension, a condition known as *anaphylactic shock.*

- *Cytotoxic hypersensitivity* occurs when antibody attaches to antigens on body cells. This binding leads to phagocytosis, killer-cell activity, or complement-mediated lysis of the cell.
- *Immune-complex–mediated hypersensitivity* results when antigen, antibody, and complement proteins interact to form huge complexes that are deposited in tissues. Polymorphonuclear (PMN) leukocytes are attracted to the area, congregate, and cause local damage.
- *Delayed (cell-mediated) hypersensitivity* responses are antibody-independent responses of T lymphocytes. Antigen stimulates T cells to secrete lymphokines which then induce inflammation and attract macrophages that release additional inflammatory mediators.

CAUSES

Type I

- Allergens: pollen, dust, molds, dander, insect venom
- Foods: eggs, seafood, nuts, grains, beans, chocolate, sulfite additives
- Antibiotics: penicillin, cephalosporins, sulfonamides, amphotericin B, nitrofurantoin
- Salicylates: acetylsalicylic acid (aspirin)
- Local anesthetics: lidocaine, xylocaine
- Hormones: exogenous insulin, parathyroid hormone, vasopressin
- Enzymes: chymotrypsin, trypsin, penicillinase
- Diagnostic agents: sodium dehydrocholate, sulfobromophthalein

- Venoms: bee, yellow jacket, wasp, hornet, ant
- Vaccines/serums: antilymphocyte globulin

Type II

- Foreign tissue or cells, e.g., transfusion reaction
- Drug reaction, e.g., chlorpromazine
- Endogenous antigens leading to autoimmune disorders such as Goodpasture's syndrome, Hashimoto's thyroiditis, and autoimmune hemolytic anemia

Type III

- Drugs such as penicillin and sulfonamides
- Streptococcal infection
- Inhaled antigens such as dust from moldy hay or pigeon feces
- Systemic lupus erythematosus (SLE)

Type IV

- Contact dermatitis (e.g., poison ivy)
- Tuberculin reaction
- Foreign tissue grafts such as bone marrow or organ transplants

Signs & Symptoms

Type I

- Localized responses:
    1. asthma
    2. allergic rhinitis (runny nose; itchy, watery eyes)
    3. conjunctivitis
    4. diarrhea or vomiting
    5. atopic dermatitis
- Generalized responses:
    1. urticaria (hives)
    2. sense of foreboding or uneasiness, lightheadedness
    3. itching palms and scalp
    4. swelling of eyelids, lips, tongue, hands, feet, and genitals
    5. laryngeal edema, bronchial constriction with stridor, wheezing, air hunger, and cough
    6. hypotension and possible shock

Type II
- S/S relate to specific tissues involved
- For hemolytic disorders (transfusion reaction): fever, chills, dyspnea, chest pain, urticaria, rash, tachycardia/hypotension, back pain, hematuria, headache

Type III
- S/S relate to specific disorder
- Serum sickness: urticaria, rash, edema (face, neck, joints), fever
- Glomerulonephritis: decreased glomerular filtration rate (GFR), azotemia, hypertension, coffee-colored urine, oliguria/anuria
- Systemic lupus erythematosus: multiple (see SLE)
- Farmers' lung: fever, chills, malaise, cough, dyspnea

Type IV
- Contact dermatitis (e.g., poison ivy): itching, erythema, vesicular lesions
- Tuberculin reaction: induration at injection site
- Graft-versus-host disease: fever, rash, nausea, vomiting, diarrhea, bleeding disorders, coma

Diagnostics

- Diagnosis mainly depends on history and physical findings.
- White blood cell (WBC) count with differential is performed to detect possible high levels of circulating eosinophils.
- Radioallergosorbent test (RAST) may be performed to measure the amount of IgE directed toward specific allergens.
- Blood type and crossmatch are ordered prior to any anticipated infusions.
- Indirect and direct Coombs' tests are used to detect the presence of antibodies.
- Immune complex assays may be performed to detect the presence of circulating immune complexes. Complement assay also is useful in detecting immune complex disorders.
- A variety of skin tests (patch, prick, intradermal) may be used to determine the causes of hyper-

sensitivity reactions. Food allergy tests are conducted if the client is suspected of having a food allergy but the implicated food item has not been clearly identified.

MEDICAL INTERVENTIONS

- Immunotherapy, injections of an extract of the allergen(s) in gradually increasing doses, is used for allergic rhinitis, asthma, and reactions to insect venom.
- Other pharmacologic agents include antihistamines, cromolyn sodium, and glucocorticosterids. Epinephrine is used for immediate treatment of anaphylaxis.
- Insertion of an endotracheal tube or emergency tracheostomy may be required to maintain airway patency in clients with severe laryngospasm.
- Plasmapheresis, the removal of harmful components in the plasma, may be used to treat immune complex responses.

SELECTED NURSING DIAGNOSES WITH INTERVENTIONS

Ineffective Airway Clearance

- Place the client in Fowler's to high-Fowler's position.
- Administer oxygen per nasal cannula at a rate of 2 to 4 L per minute.
- Assess the client's airway by observing for respiratory rate and pattern, level of consciousness and anxiety, nasal flaring, use of accessory muscles of respiration, chest wall movement, audible stridor; palpate for respiratory excursion; auscultate lung sounds and any adventitious sounds, such as wheezes.
- Insert a nasopharyngeal or oropharyngeal airway, and arrange for immediate intubation as indicated by the client's status.
- Administer subcutaneous epinephrine 1:1000, 0.3 to 0.5 mL, as prescribed. This may be repeated in 20 to 30 minutes if necessary. Administer parenteral diphenhydramine as prescribed.
- Provide calm reassurance to the client, as anxiety can increase the respiratory rate, making breathing less effective.

Decreased Cardiac Output

- Monitor vital signs frequently, assessing for changes such as a fall in blood pressure, decreasing pulse pressure, tachycardia, and tachypnea.
- Assess skin color, temperature, capillary refill, edema, and other indicators of peripheral perfusion.
- Monitor the client's level of consciousness.
- Insert one or more large-bore IV catheters.
- Administer warmed intravenous solutions, such as lactated Ringer's or normal saline, as prescribed.
- Insert an indwelling catheter, and monitor urinary output frequently.
- Place a tourniquet above the site of an injected venom and infiltrate the site with epinephrine as prescribed.
- Once airway and breathing are established, place the client flat with the legs elevated.
- As the client's status begins to improve, assess for shortness of breath and crackles in the lungs.

High Risk for Injury

The risk for adverse immunologic response and injury to the client is particularly significant during a blood transfusion, which is a transplant of living tissue.

- Obtain and record a thorough history of previous blood transfusions and any reactions experienced, no matter how mild.
- Check for the presence of a signed informed consent to administer blood or blood products.
- Using two licensed health care professionals, double-check the type, Rh factor, cross match, and expiration date for all blood and blood components received from the blood bank with the client's data.
- Administer blood within 30 minutes of its delivery from the blood bank.
- Take and record vital signs within 15 minutes prior to initiating the blood transfusion.
- Infuse blood into a site separate from any other IV infusion. Use at least an 18-gauge catheter for the infusion.
- Administer 50 mL of blood during the first 15 minutes of the transfusion.
- Assess the client during transfusion for complaints of back or chest pain, an increase in the tempera-

ture of more than 1.8 F, chills, tachycardia, tachypnea, wheezing, hypotension, hives, rashes, or cyanosis.
- Stop the blood transfusion immediately if a reaction occurs, no matter how mild. Keep the IV line open with normal saline. Notify the physician and the blood bank.
- If a reaction is suspected, send the blood and administration set to the laboratory along with a freshly drawn blood sample and urine sample from the client.
- If no adverse reaction occurs, administer the transfusion within a 4-hour period.

CLIENT TEACHING

- Assist the client to identify possible allergens that prompt a hypersensitivity response. Discuss strategies to avoid these allergens if possible. Clients with food allergies should meet with a dietitian.
- Teach the client about the use of prescription and nonprescription antihistamines and decongestants for symptom relief.
- For clients anticipating surgery, discuss the advantages of autologous blood transfusion and "banking" their own blood prior to surgery.

HOME CARE CONSIDERATIONS

- Encourage the client who experiences an anaphylactic reaction to wear a MedicAlert bracelet or necklace at all times identifying the substance(s) that provoke the response.
- Encourage the client to carry an anaphylaxis kit, and teach the client and significant others how to inject the medication and use the inhaler.
- Teach clients who have undergone an organ transplant to be alert for and to promptly report signs and symptoms of rejection.

For more information on Hypersensitivity, see Medical-Surgical Nursing *by LeMone and Burke, p. 270.*

Hypertension (HTN)

OVERVIEW

- Hypertension is defined as sustained elevation in the mean arterial blood pressure.
- Elevations in the systolic blood pressure result from an increased cardiac output or decreased compliance of the aorta.
- Elevations in the diastolic blood pressure result from an increase in total peripheral vascular resistance.
- Hypertension can be primary (essential), or secondary to pathologic conditions.
- *Malignant hypertension* is a rapidly progressive form that may result in hypertensive crisis, an acute and life-threatening increase of diastolic blood pressure to greater than 120 mm Hg.
- Hypertension is the most common cardiovascular disorder; it is especially common in African Americans.
- Hypertension usually manifests in middle age.
- If untreated, complications include accelerated atherosclerosis; heart failure; cerebral vascular accident (CVA), and renal damage or failure.

CAUSES

Essential (Primary) Hypertension

- The mechanisms related to essential hypertension are poorly understood, and may involve multiple pathways such as:
  1. increased vasoconstrictor substances
  2. decreased vasodilator substances
  3. altered sensitivity to vasoactive substances
  4. altered sensitivity to electrolytes
  5. changes in the autonomic nervous system control of vascular smooth muscle tone
- Risk factors include:
  1. family history
  2. African American race
  3. high-sodium, low-calcium, high-fat diet
  4. tobacco use/alcohol abuse
  5. sedentary lifestyle

6. central obesity with increased waist-to-hip ratio
7. oral contraceptive use
8. stress
9. aging

Secondary Hypertension

- Renal disease
- Cushing's syndrome
- Conn's syndrome (primary hyperaldosteronism)
- Pheochromocytoma
- Hyperthyroidism
- Coarctation of the aorta
- Neurologic disease

Signs & Symptoms

- Stage 1: systolic 140–159, diastolic 90–99
- Stage 2: systolic 160–179, diastolic 100–109
- Stage 3: systolic ≥ 180, diastolic ≥ 110
- The client is usually symptom-free until complications develop.

Diagnostics

- Urinalysis, CBC, blood chemistry including electrolytes, BUN and creatinine, glucose, and cholesterol.
- EKG and chest x-ray are performed to rule out cardiac disease as cause or effect.
- Creatinine clearance, 24-hour urine for protein, and TSH.

MEDICAL INTERVENTIONS

- Hypertension treatment is based on the stage of the disease and risk factors for long-term consequences of elevated blood pressure.
- Lifestyle modifications are recommended for all persons with hypertension, including weight loss; limited alcohol intake; aerobic exercise for 30 to 45 minutes most days of the week; low-sodium, low-saturated fat, and low-cholesterol diet with adequate potassium; smoking cessation; stress management.
- Current pharmacologic treatment of hypertension includes use of one or more of the following

categories of drugs: diuretics, beta-adrenergic blockers, centrally acting sympatholytics, vasodilators, angiotensin-converting enzyme inhibitors, and calcium-channel blockers.

SELECTED NURSING DIAGNOSES WITH INTERVENTIONS

Noncompliance

- Assess the client's knowledge of and compliance with the prescribed medical regimen.
- Stress the importance of maintaining lifestyle changes and taking medication as prescribed to prevent long-term consequences of hypertension. Hypertension has few manifestations. Treatment controls the disease but does not cure it. Noncompliance with the prescribed regimen is common.

Fluid Volume Excess

- Carefully monitor intake and output daily and routinely throughout the shift.
- Monitor laboratory values.
- Assess for signs of fluid retention, such as dependent or sacral edema and/or ascites.
- Weigh client daily before breakfast.
- Collaborate with dietary services to provide information for the client on reducing sodium intake.
- Teach clients the importance of adhering to treatment plans such as dietary restrictions and medication schedules.

Altered Nutrition: More than Body Requirements

- Assess for causative or contributing factors for excess weight.
- Collaborate with dietary services to provide information about low-fat diets.
- Mutually determine with the client a realistic target weight and have the client weigh in regularly.
- Explore the feasibility of referring the client to an approved weight-loss program.

Altered Health Maintenance

- Assist the client and significant others in identifying unhealthy behaviors that contribute to altered health.
- Assist clients in developing a realistic health maintenance plan.

- Help clients identify strengths and weaknesses in maintaining health.

CLIENT TEACHING

- Stress the importance of adhering to dietary restrictions, limiting alcohol, avoiding smoking and second-hand smoke, and exercising regularly.
- Teach stress reduction methods such as meditation, relaxation, and deep breathing.
- Encourage frequent follow-up visits.
- Review self-monitoring of blood pressure and suggest the client keep a daily log.

HOME CARE CONSIDERATIONS

- Tell the client to report any side effects of medications to the physician. Instruct the client not to discontinue taking the medication unless instructed to do so by the physician.
- A referral to a smoking cessation program, weight-loss program, or cardiovascular fitness program may be appropriate.

For more information on Hypertension, see Medical-Surgical Nursing *by LeMone and Burke, p. 1198.*

Hyperthyroidism (Thyrotoxicosis)

OVERVIEW

- Hyperthyroidism is an endocrine derangement due to excess thyroid hormones, T_3 and T_4, that produces an increased basal metabolic rate (BMR).
- Increased thyroid hormone (TH) levels increase protein, carbohydrate, and fat metabolism in most body tissues and heighten sympathetic nervous system response to stimulation.
- Heart rate and stroke volume increase.

- The hypermetabolic effects of excess TH result in caloric and nutritional deficiencies.
- A product of the hypermetabolic state is an increase in heat production, mainly by skeletal muscles.
- The most common cause of hyperthyroidism is *Grave's disease.*
- *Thyroid storm* is an acute and profound rise in thyroid hormones that is life-threatening.

CAUSES

- *Grave's disease:* an autoimmune disorder in which antibodies [thyroid-stimulating immunoglobulin (TSI)] form that act at the thyroid-stimulating hormone (TSH) receptor, stimulating it; normal feedback regulation is lost.
- *Toxic nodular goiter:* small discrete, independently functioning nodules within the thyroid gland secrete TH.
- *Toxic carcinoma:* a rare cause of hyperthyroidism.
- *Secondary hyperthyroidism:* caused by excess TSH secretion from the pituitary gland.
- *Iatrogenic hyperthyroidism:* the result of excess exogenous thyroid medication given for hypothyroidism; may be unintentional or intentional (factitious).

Signs & Symptoms

Hyperthyroidism
- Hyperpyrexia/sweating/heat intolerance
- Nervousness/tremors/irritability
- Increased appetite with weight loss
- Tachycardia/palpitations/dysrhythmias
- Hypertension/bounding pulse
- Warm, flushed skin/thickened skin
- Friable nails/onycholysis
- Muscle fatigue/weakness
- Cardiomegaly/high-output heart failure

Grave's Disease
- S/S hyperthyroidism, severe
- Goiter: smooth, symmetric
- Exophthalmos

Diagnostics

- T_3/T_4 levels are elevated.
- Radioactive iodine (RAI) uptake test (thyroid scan) reveals increased ^{131}I uptake.
- Increased BMR.
- TSH level is decreased with primary types of hyperthyroidism; increased with hyperpituitarism.
- TSI autoantibodies are positive.

MEDICAL INTERVENTIONS

- Hyperthyroidism is treated pharmacologically by administering antithyroid medications that reduce thyroid hormone production.
- Radioactive iodine damages or destroys thyroid tissue so that it produces less thyroid hormone.
- A subtotal thyroidectomy is performed on clients with breathing or swallowing problems caused by an enlarged thyroid. A total thyroidectomy is indicated to treat cancer of the thyroid; the client then requires lifelong hormone replacement.

SELECTED NURSING DIAGNOSES WITH INTERVENTIONS

Risk for Decreased Cardiac Output (if CHF)

- Monitor blood pressure, pulse rate and rhythm, respiratory rate, and breath sounds. Assess for peripheral edema, jugular vein distention, and increased activity intolerance.
- Provide an environment that is cool and as free of distraction as possible. Decrease stress by explaining interventions and teaching relaxation procedures.
- Balance activity with rest periods.

Sensory-Perceptual Alterations: Visual

- Monitor visual acuity, photophobia, integrity of the cornea, and lid closure if exophthalmos.
- Teach the client measures for protecting the eye from injury and maintaining visual acuity.

Risk for Altered Nutrition: Less than Body Requirements

- Weigh the client daily at the same time, and record the results.

- Provide a diet high in carbohydrates and protein.
- Monitor nutritional status through laboratory data.

Body Image Disturbance

- Encourage the client to verbalize feelings about self and to ask questions about the illness and treatment.
- Provide reliable information and clarify misconceptions.
- Encourage significant others to ask questions about changes they have noticed. Explain the effects of the illness on the client's physical and emotional status.

CLIENT TEACHING

- Teach the client taking oral medications the need for lifelong treatment. Also review medication regimen, effects, and side effects.
- Teach the necessity to consume a diet high in carbohydrates and protein, including between-meal snacks. Caloric intake may need to be increased to 4000 kcal per day if weight loss exceeds 10% to 20% for height and frame.
- Review the signs and symptoms of hyper- and hypothyroidism.
- Discuss the risks and benefits of surgery versus radioactive iodine therapy.

HOME CARE CONSIDERATIONS

- Tell the postoperative client to inspect the wound for redness, tenderness, swelling, and drainage, and to report temperature elevation, sore throat, or other symptoms of infection.
- Stress the importance of follow-up visits with the physician.
- Arrange for a dietary consultation.
- Depending on the age of the client and the support systems available, referral to a home health agency may be necessary.

For more information on Hyperthyroidism, see Medical-Surgical Nursing *by LeMone and Burke, p. 684.*

Hypervolemia

OVERVIEW

- Hypervolemia is an increased volume of extracellular fluid (ECF), especially the intravascular volume.
- It may be caused by excess infusion or retention of water, or sodium and water, or of fluid shifting from the intracellular fluid (ICF) compartment into the vascular compartment.
- It can lead to pulmonary edema and heart failure.

CAUSES

- Iatrogenic: excess infusion of IV fluids
- Retention of water: syndrome of inappropriate antidiuretic hormone (ADH) secretion (SIADH)
- Retention of sodium and water via renin-angiotensin-aldosterone system:
  1. chronic renal underperfusion: heart failure (HF), cirrhosis
  2. aldosteroma (Conn's syndrome)
  3. renal failure: acute or chronic
  4. glucocorticoid administration
- Fluid shift:
  1. excess hypertonic solutions: dextran, mannitol, albumin, saline
  2. burns: fluid remobilization following treatment

Signs & Symptoms

- Dyspnea/orthopnea/shortness of breath (SOB)
- Rales/rhonchi/wheezes
- Increased heart rate and blood pressure
- Bounding pulse/distended neck veins
- Increased central venous pressure (CVP)
- Increased pulmonary capillary wedge pressure (PCWP)
- Increased mean arterial pressure (MAP)
- Gallop rhythm
- Edema/weight gain
- Moist skin
- Ascites

H

Diagnostics

- Blood urea nitrogen (BUN) and hematocrit (HCT) may be decreased due to hemodilution.
- If pulmonary edema is present, arterial blood gases (ABGs) reveal decreased PaO_2, decreased $PaCO_2$, and increased pH.
- Serum sodium/osmolarity are decreased if hypervolemia is due to water retention or excess sodium infusion.
- Urine sodium is increased if kidneys are excreting excess sodium.
- Chest x-ray may show pulmonary edema.

MEDICAL INTERVENTIONS

- Treat primary underlying disorder.
- General treatment includes fluid restriction, diuretics, and dialysis if renal function is impaired.

SELECTED NURSING DIAGNOSES

- Fluid Volume Excess
- Risk for Ineffective Breathing Pattern

SELECTED NURSING INTERVENTIONS

- Administer drug therapy such as diuretics as prescribed and monitor effects and side effects.
- Restrict fluid intake and sodium intake. Measure intake and output carefully.
- Weigh client daily at the same time of day.
- Assess for pulmonary edema and depression of vital organ function.

CLIENT TEACHING

- Teach the client about fluid and sodium restrictions.
- Teach the signs and symptoms of imbalances for which the client is at risk, and to report symptoms to primary care provider.
- Review medication regimen, effects, and side effects.

HOME CARE CONSIDERATIONS

- A referral to a dietitian or home health services may be appropriate.

For more information on Hypervolemia, see Medical-Surgical Nursing *by LeMone and Burke, p. 112.*

Hypoglycemia

OVERVIEW

- Hypoglycemia is defined as a blood glucose level of less than 60 mg/dL.
- The brain normally uses glucose as its major fuel; if blood glucose remains low, serious and permanent damage to neurons may occur.
- Damage to neurons may affect cognitive (memory, learning) or motor function.
- A prolonged state of severe hypoglycemia may be fatal.

CAUSES

Diabetics

- Excess insulin (insulin reaction/shock)
- Excess oral hypoglycemic agent
- Insufficient food for the dose of insulin or hypoglycemic agent that has been taken
- Vomiting
- Excessive exercise

Other

- Endogenous insulin secreted out of phase
- Dumping syndrome: status post gastrectomy
- Drug ingestion (pentamidine)
- Pancreatic tumor
- Hepatitis
- Renal disease
- Idiopathic

Signs & Symptoms

- Headache
- Hunger
- Tachycardia
- Skin changes: diaphoresis (cold sweat), pallor
- Motor changes: weakness, tremors, ataxia, "drunk" appearance, slurred speech, hemiplegia
- Behavior changes: irritability, apprehension, combativeness, confusion
- Coma

Diagnostics

- Plasma glucose <60 mg/dL.
- Dextrostix/Chemstrips may show color change indicative of glucose <45 mg/dL.
- Plasma insulin levels may define degree of hypoglycemic episode.
- Five-hour glucose tolerance test: is used to define phase of insulin secretion.

MEDICAL INTERVENTIONS

- Treat primary underlying disorder (e.g., administer IV glucose to diabetic clients).
- For pancreatic tumors, surgical resection or treatment with diazocide and octreatide may be necessary.

SELECTED NURSING DIAGNOSES

- Altered Nutrition: Less than Body Requirements
- Risk for Altered Thought Processes
- Ineffective Management of Therapeutic Regimen: Individual

SELECTED NURSING INTERVENTIONS

- Observe for signs of hypoglycemia: change in mental status, diaphoresis, cool, clammy skin.
- Provide quiet, darkened environment conducive to rest.
- Provide a source of glucose: orange juice, candy, glucagon, 50% glucose.
- Provide small, frequent meals.
- Monitor blood glucose levels carefully.

CLIENT TEACHING

- Teach the client the signs and symptoms of hyper- and hypoglycemia.
- Teach self-management of medications, insulin, diet, and exercise and the correlations between these factors.
- Review with the client self-monitoring of blood glucose.

HOME CARE CONSIDERATIONS

- Referral to a dietitian for long-term nutritional support and follow-up may be appropriate.
- The client may require referral to social services or a psychological counselor for coping mechanisms for managing a chronic illness.
- Provide information on obtaining a MedicAlert bracelet or necklace.
- Provide the client with information about the American Diabetes Association, if appropriate.

H

For more information on Hypoglycemia, see Medical-Surgical Nursing *by LeMone and Burke,* *p. 727.*

Hypoparathyroidism

OVERVIEW

- Hypoparathyroidism is a deficit of parathyroid hormone (PTH) that results in impaired renal tubular regulation of calcium and phosphate and produces hypocalcemia.
- Hypocalcemia may induce neuromuscular symptoms such as paresthesias, or result in life-threatening tetany.

CAUSES

- Damage to or removal of parathyroid glands during thyroidectomy
- Congenital lack of parathyroid gland development
- Radiation to the neck
- Ischemia
- Hypercalcemia
- Hypomagnesemia

Signs & Symptoms

- Neuromuscular irritability/increased deep tendon reflexes
- Tetany/carpopedal spasms/abdominal pain
- Cardiac dysrhythmias
- Dysphagia
- Positive Chvostek's sign, Trousseau's sign
- Seizures
- Psychoses
- Dry skin/hair/alopecia
- Brittle/ridged nails
- Weak tooth enamel/dental caries

Diagnostics

- PTH level is reduced.
- Serum calcium level is reduced.
- Serum phosphorus level is increased.
- EKG shows increased Q-T interval and ST segment.

MEDICAL INTERVENTIONS

- Intravenous calcium is given immediately to reduce tetany.
- Long-term therapy includes supplemental calcium, increased dietary calcium, and vitamin D therapy.

SELECTED NURSING DIAGNOSES

- Risk for Injury
- Pain
- Anxiety

SELECTED NURSING INTERVENTIONS

- Assess for tetany, muscle cramping, carpopedal spasms, mental changes, Chvostek's sign, and Trousseau's sign.
- Institute seizure precautions.
- Administer medications as prescribed.
- Encourage dietary intake of foods high in calcium and low in phosphorus.

CLIENT TEACHING

- Stress to the client that dietary modifications and other aspects of care must be maintained permanently to prevent recurrence.

HOME CARE CONSIDERATIONS

- Encourage the client to wear a MedicAlert bracelet or necklace.
- Referral to a home health nurse may be appropriate.

For more information on Hypoparathyroidism, see Medical-Surgical Nursing *by LeMone and Burke,* p. 701.

Hypothyroidism

OVERVIEW

- Hypothyroidism is a deficit of the thyroid hormones, T_3/T_4 that reduces the basal metabolic rate (BMR) and heat production, affecting all body systems.
- Primary and secondary forms exist.
  1. Primary (more common) form may be due to congenital defect, treatment of hyperthyroidism, surgery, thyroiditis, or iodine deficiency.
  2. Secondary form may result from pituitary TSH deficiency or peripheral resistance to thyroid hormones.

- Hashimoto's thyroiditis (chronic autoimmune thyroiditis) is the most common form of primary hypothyroidism, in which antibodies develop that destroy thyroid tissue.
- The incidence of hypothyroidism is higher in women and increases after age 50.
- Myxedema is a serious lack of thyroid hormones that produces multiple symptoms.
- Myxedema coma is a life-threatening condition secondary to a profound reduction of thyroid hormones.
- Other complications of untreated hypothyroidism include adrenal insufficiency and cardiovascular disorders.

CAUSES

- Hashimoto's thyroiditis is due to autoimmune destruction of thyroid follicular cells
- Infection
- Thyroidectomy for the treatment of hyperthyroidism/neoplasms
- Radiation therapy for the treatment of hyperthyroidism/neoplasms
- Antithyroid medication for the treatment of hyperthyroidism
- Reduced thyroid-stimulating hormone (TSH) from the pituitary gland
- Reduced thyroid-releasing hormone (TRH) from the hypothalamus
- Iodine deficiency (necessary for TH synthesis and secretion)

Signs & Symptoms

Hypothyroidism/Myxedema

- Reduced temperature, cool skin, cold intolerance
- Slow pulse, ventilation rate
- Nonpitting generalized edema, puffy face, periorbital edema, enlarged tongue
- Anorexia with weight gain and constipation
- Dry, loose skin; thick, brittle nails; dry, coarse hair; loss of lateral eyebrows
- Forgetfulness, mental dullness, emotional instability

Hashimoto's Thyroiditis

- S/S of hypothyroidism/myxedema
- Goiter: diffuse, tender

Myxedema Coma

- Progressive reduction in level of consciousness to coma
- Hypothermia
- Bradycardia, hypoventilation, hypotension
- Hypoglycemia
- Hyponatremia

Diagnostics

- T_3/T_4 levels are decreased.
- TSH is increased if due to primary thyroid malfunction; decreased, if due to pituitary malfunction.
- Decreased BMR

MEDICAL INTERVENTIONS

- Hypothyroidism is treated with pharmacologic preparations that replace thyroid hormone.
- If the client has a goiter large enough to cause respiratory difficulties or dysphagia, a subtotal thyroidectomy may be performed.

SELECTED NURSING DIAGNOSES WITH INTERVENTIONS

Decreased Cardiac Output

- Assess blood pressure, rate and rhythm of apical and peripheral pulses, respiratory rate, and breath sounds.
- Maintain the environment to avoid chilling; increase room temperature, use additional bed covers, avoid drafts.
- Alternate activity with rest periods. Ask the client to report any breathing difficulties, chest pain, heart palpitations, or dizziness.

H

Constipation

- Encourage the client to maintain a liquid intake of up to 2000 mL per day. If kilocalorie intake is restricted, ensure that liquids have no kilocalories or are low in kilocalories.
- Discuss with client ways to maintain a high-fiber diet.
- Encourage activity as tolerated.

Risk for Altered Skin Integrity

- Monitor skin surfaces for redness or lesions, especially if the client's activity is greatly reduced.
- Provide measures to promote optimal circulation, such as turning, repositioning, and using pillows, pads, or cushions.
- Teach and implement a schedule of range-of-motion exercises.
- Use alcohol-free skin oils and lotions, and use gentle motions when washing and drying skin.

CLIENT TEACHING

- Teach the client the importance of maintaining a high-fiber diet.
- Discuss self-care for skin integrity, such as assessing any lesions, using warm (not hot) water when cleansing skin, taking showers rather than baths, and so on.
- Review medication regimen, including effects and side effects, and the contraindications of thyroid medications with many over-the-counter medications.
- Stress the need for lifelong monitoring and care.

HOME CARE CONSIDERATIONS

- Provide the client with information on obtaining a MedicAlert bracelet or necklace.
- The older adult may need referrals to social services or home health services, especially if home support is not available.

For more information on Hypothyroidism, see Medical-Surgical Nursing *by LeMone and Burke,* *p. 694.*

Hypovolemia

OVERVIEW

- Hypovolemia is a reduction in the extracellular fluid (ECF) volume, especially the intravascular volume.
- It may be due to excess fluid loss, insufficient fluid ingestion, or fluid shifts from the ECF compartments to a "third space."
- Depending on the type of fluid lost, there may be accompanying osmolar, acid-base, or electrolyte imbalances.
- When plasma volume loss is severe, hypovolemic shock can result.
- With shock, the sympathetic nervous system (SNS) attempts to compensate and maintain cardiac output by increasing heart rate and contractile (inotropic) state, and also peripheral vascular resistance.
- Endocrine compensation includes:
  1. increased antidiuretic hormone (ADH; vasopressin), which causes thirst, enhances water reabsorption, and constricts blood vessels
  2. increased aldosterone, which causes increased sodium and H_2O reabsorption
- Prolonged hypovolemic shock may produce acute renal failure.

CAUSES

- Insufficient fluid ingestion may result from:
  1. unavailability of fluids
  2. insufficient IV therapy
  3. immobility
  4. coma
- Fluids may be lost via:
  1. diuresis: usually hypotonic fluid losses; may be of renal, endocrine, or osmotic etiology
  2. hemorrhage: isotonic loss of red blood cells, fluid, plasma proteins, and all electrolytes

3. vomiting/GI suctioning: hydrogen ions lost; may produce metabolic alkalosis
4. diarrhea: bicarbonate lost; may produce metabolic acidosis
5. diaphoresis: hypotonic fluid loss
6. excess ventilatory rate: hypotonic fluid loss
- Third spacing may result from:
  1. burns
  2. peritonitis
  3. GI obstruction
  4. ascites

Signs & Symptoms

- Weight loss will parallel fluid loss

Mild Hypovolemia
- Weakness/fatigue
- Lightheadedness
- Anorexia

Moderate Hypovolemia
- Tachycardia
- Orthostatic hypotension
- Oliguria

Severe Hypovolemia
- Rapid, thready pulse
- Supine hypotension
- Cold, clammy skin
- Confusion leading to stupor leading to coma
- Oliguria leading to anuria

Diagnostics

- Blood urea nitrogen (BUN) may be increased owing to hemoconcentration, decreased renal perfusion or function.
- Hematocrit (HCT) may be increased owing to hemoconcentration.
- Serum electrolyte changes are related to type of fluid lost.
- Serum osmolarity is increased secondary to dehydration.

- Carbon dioxide (CO_2) (HCO_3-) may be increased with alkalosis; decreased with acidosis.
- Arterial blood gases (ABGs) will show metabolic acidosis if due to lower GI losses, shock, or diabetic ketoacidosis (DKA); will show alkalosis if due to upper GI losses or diuresis.
- Urine specific gravity is increased owing to renal compensation to concentrate urine.

MEDICAL INTERVENTIONS

- Treat primary underlying disorder (e.g., replace fluids and transfuse blood with hemorrhage).
- Hyponatremic hypovolemia is treated with isotonic saline or lactated Ringer's solution.
- Hypernatremic hypovolemia is treated with isotonic saline initially, followed by hypotonic saline.

H

SELECTED NURSING DIAGNOSES

- Ineffective Breathing Pattern
- Altered Tissue Perfusion
- Decreased Cardiac Output
- Fluid Volume Imbalance

SELECTED NURSING INTERVENTIONS

- Ensure a patent airway.
- Assess cause of hypovolemia.
- Cover obvious wounds with clean cloth or dressing.
- As prescribed, insert an IV line and infuse lactated Ringer's solution or normal saline until blood products become available.
- Administer oxygen as needed.
- Apply MAST trousers if needed.
- Elevate the client's feet, keeping the head flat or elevated to 30°.
- Monitor vital and neurologic signs.
- Prepare the client for surgery as necessary to treat underlying cause.
- Monitor central venous pressure, pulmonary artery pressure, and pulmonary wedge pressure, if possible.

CLIENT TEACHING

- Teaching would depend on the cause of hypovolemia and is aimed at preventing future episodes.
- Teach proper diuretic therapy, fluid and electrolyte requirements, and early S/S of dehydration.

HOME CARE CONSIDERATIONS

- Hypovolemia should be totally corrected by discharge.
- For clients with chronic disease that may result in future episodes of hypovolemia, long-term follow-up is expected and preparations for continuity of care should be instituted.

For more information on Hypovolemia, see Medical-Surgical Nursing *by LeMone and Burke, p. 169.*

Increased Intracranial Pressure

OVERVIEW

- Increased intracranial pressure (ICP) is a rise in pressure within the closed cranial space of >20 mm Hg (normal is 3–15 mm Hg) or 270 mm H_2O (normal is 40–200 mm H_2O), as measured by cerebrospinal fluid (CSF) tap.
- The cranium is a closed vault with a constant volume and pressure; increased volume for any reason results in increased pressure.
- When pressure within the cranium rises above normal, it exerts a damaging force on central nervous system (CNS) neurons and their blood vessels.
- Increased intercranial pressure (ICP) of great magnitude and/or duration is a life-threatening condition.
- Initially, pressure will force more CSF into the spinal canal or arachnoid veins.
- This will be followed by reduced cranial perfusion, causing brain hypoxia, ischemia, and finally necrosis.
- To compensate for reduced blood flow, the CNS cardioregulatory center sends out a massive excitatory response (Cushing's reaction), which raises blood pressure to extremely high levels.
- If the pressure is unrelieved, there will eventually be herniation of the brain stem through the foramen magnum, which is fatal.

CAUSES

- Bleeding/hemorrhage: intracranial, subarachnoid, subdural, epidural
- Hematoma formation
- Neoplasms: benign or malignant
- Abscess/cyst formation
- Edema formation: infection, trauma, surgery
- Obstruction of CSF flow: hydrocephalus

Signs & Symptoms

- Change in level of consciousness (LOC): drowsiness to coma (use Glasgow coma scale)
- Headache
- Vomiting
- Restlessness, irritability, combativeness
- Eye changes: unequal/sluggish pupillary responses, diplopia
- Motor changes: hemiparesis, ataxia, slurred speech
- Decorticate or decerebrate posture
- Aphasia
- Cardiovascular S/S: bradycardia; hypertension with increased pulse pressure; dysrhythmias
- Respiratory changes: altered rate, depth, pattern; labored effort
- Seizures

Diagnostics

- Skull x-ray can show fracture and/or tissue shifting.
- Cerebral angiogram may reveal abnormal vascular anatomy.
- CT scan may show ischemia/necrosis or subdural, epidural, or intracranial hematomas.

MEDICAL INTERVENTIONS

- Osmotic diuretics and mannitol are commonly used to reduce ICP and are the mainstays of pharmacologic treatment.
- Other pharmacologic agents include barbiturates to induce coma, and anticonvulsants to manage seizure activity.
- Clients with increased ICP may undergo various intracranial surgical procedures to treat the underlying cause.
- ICP monitoring facilitates continual assessment of ICP, and is more precise than reliance on clinical manifestations.

SELECTED NURSING DIAGNOSES WITH INTERVENTIONS

Altered Tissue Perfusion: Cerebral

- Assess for and report any of the indicators of increasing ICP every 1 to 2 hours and as necessary. Assessment areas include level of consciousness, behavior, motor/sensory functions, pupillary size and reaction to light, and vital signs.
- For the client on a ventilator, maintain patency of the airway, pre-oxygenate and hyperventilate the client with 100% oxygen before suctioning, limit suctioning to 10 seconds, and suction gently.
- Monitor arterial blood gases.
- Elevate the head of the bed 30° to 45°. Maintain the alignment of the head and neck to avoid hyperextension or exaggerated neck flexion. Avoid the prone position. Avoid extreme hip flexion.
- Maintain the head and neck in the neutral plane.
- Assess for bladder distention and bowel constipation. Administer stool softeners and use the Credé technique to empty the bladder. Evaluate the pros and cons of catheterization if the bladder remains distended.
- Assist the client to move up in bed. Avoid the use of a footboard or restraints.
- Plan nursing care so that activities are not clustered together. Avoid turning the client, getting the client on the bedpan, or suctioning within the same time period. Provide rest periods between procedures.
- Provide a quiet, calm environment. Caution visitors to refrain from unpleasant conversations or those that may be emotionally stimulating to the client.
- Maintain fluid limitations if prescribed.

Risk for Infection

- Keep dressings over the ICP catheter dry, and change dressings on a prescribed basis.
- Monitor the insertion site for leaking CSF, drainage, or infection. Monitor for physical signs of infection, including changes in vital signs, chills, increased white blood cell count, and positive cultures of drainage.

- Use strict aseptic technique when in contact with the device, and check drainage system for loose connections.

CLIENT TEACHING

If the client is able to understand and follow instructions:

- Teach the client about the disease process, treatment, and rehabilitation.
- Teach the client to avoid coughing, blowing the nose, straining to have a bowel movement, pushing against the bed rails, or performing isometric exercises.
- Advise the client to maintain head and neck alignment when resting in bed.
- Advise frequent rest periods.
- Encourage significant others to avoid conversations that may be upsetting to the client.

HOME CARE CONSIDERATIONS

- Referral to a home health nursing service may be appropriate.
- Referral for the client and significant others to counseling or pastoral services may be helpful.

For more information on Increased Intracranial Pressure, see Medical-Surgical Nursing *by LeMone and Burke, p. 1709.*

Influenza

OVERVIEW

- Influenza is a highly contagious infection of the respiratory tract caused by a continuously mutating virus.
- "Flu season" is late autumn to late spring.
- It may develop into a pneumonia.

- It can occur in isolated cases, but more frequently occurs in epidemics or pandemics.
- The severity depends on age and health status, with the very young, very old, and chronically ill being most at risk.
- New strains of influenza virus develop at fairly regular intervals and are usually named for the geographic location in which they first arise.
- Effective vaccines are developed based on the strains of viruses from the previous year.

CAUSES

- Myxovirus influenzae: Type A, Type B, Type C
- Airborne droplet transmission

Signs & Symptoms

- Rapid onset of chills
- Fever: 101F to 104F (38.3C–40C)
- Headache
- Malaise
- Myalgia
- Nonproductive cough
- Cervical adenopathy
- S/S of upper respiratory tract infection: sore throat, hoarseness, rhinitis, rhinorrhea
- May develop S/S of lower respiratory infection (see Pneumonia)

Diagnostics

- Viral cultures of nose and throat.
- Serum antibody titers are increased.
- White blood cell count may be done to rule out complications such as pneumonia; it commonly is decreased in influenza and increased in bacterial infections.

MEDICAL INTERVENTIONS

- Yearly immunization with influenza vaccine is the single most important measure to prevent or minimize manifestation of influenza.
- Amantadine may be used for prophylaxis in persons who have not been vaccinated but have been exposed to the virus.

- Analgesics such as aspirin and acetaminophen provide symptomatic relief of fever and muscle aches.
- Antibiotics are not indicated unless secondary bacterial infection occurs.

SELECTED NURSING DIAGNOSES WITH INTERVENTIONS

Ineffective Breathing Pattern

- Monitor respiratory rate and pattern for changes from baseline.
- Monitor for changes in pulse rate.
- Pace activities to provide for periods of rest.
- Elevate the head of the bed.

Ineffective Airway Clearance

- Monitor the effectiveness of the client's cough and ability to remove airway secretions.
- Maintain adequate hydration. Assess mucous membranes and skin turgor for evidence of dehydration.
- Increase the humidity of inspired air with a bedside humidifier.
- Teach the client how to cough effectively.
- Administer analgesic medications as prescribed.

Sleep Pattern Disturbance

- Assess the client's sleep patterns using subjective and objective information.
- Place the client in a semi-Fowler's or Fowler's position for sleep.
- Provide antipyretic and analgesic medications at bedtime or shortly before.
- If necessary, request a cough suppressant medication for nighttime use.

CLIENT TEACHING

- Stress the importance of yearly influenza vaccination for clients in high-risk groups and their significant others.
- Teach clients how the disease is spread, including measures for reducing the risk of contracting influenza, such as avoiding crowds and persons who are ill.
- Encourage appropriate self-care, including hygiene measures such as hand washing and covering

mouth when coughing, importance of adequate rest, and use of nonprescription medications.

HOME CARE CONSIDERATIONS

- Teach clients about the possible complications of influenza and their manifestations. Tell them to report complications promptly to the physician.

For more information on Influenza, see Medical-Surgical Nursing *by LeMone and Burke, p. 1345.*

Inguinal Hernia

OVERVIEW

- An inguinal hernia ia a prolapse of the small or large intestine into the inguinal canal and possibly the scrotum.
- It is the most common type of hernia; it may be reducible, incarcerated, or strangulated.
- The contents of a reducible hernia can be returned manually to the abdominal cavity through the inguinal canal.
- The contents of an incarcerated hernia are trapped and do not reduce back through the canal. Incarceration may be due to a narrow neck or opening to the hernia or to adhesions that have formed.
- In a strangulated hernia, the blood supply to the contents in the hernia is compromised, owing to twisting or edema. Necrosis and obstruction result.

CAUSES

- Weakness of the abdominal muscles due to congenital malformation, trauma, or aging
- Increased intra-abdominal pressure due to lifting, pregnancy, coughing, straining, or obesity

Signs & Symptoms

- Lump in inguinal area upon sitting or standing that disappears when recumbent
- Pain in groin area; steady but decreases with hernia reduction
- Severe pain indicates strangulation

Diagnostics

- The diagnosis is made primarily by a physical examination.
- X-ray may show bowel obstruction.
- White blood cell count may be elevated if there is bowel obstruction.

MEDICAL INTERVENTIONS

- Herniorrhaphy—surgical repair of a hernia—usually involves suturing or using wire mesh over the defect that allowed the herniation of abdominal contents.
- If incarceration has occurred or strangulation is suspected, the abdomen is explored at the time of surgery and any infarcted bowel resected.
- Heavy lifting and heavy manual labor are restricted for 3 weeks after surgery.

SELECTED NURSING DIAGNOSIS WITH INTERVENTIONS

Risk for Altered Tissue Perfusion: Gastrointestinal

- Assess the client's comfort level, taking particular note of any acute increase in abdominal, groin, perineal, or scrotal pain, which may indicate bowel ischemia due to strangulation.
- Assess bowel sounds and abdominal distention at least every 8 hours.
- Notify the physician if the hernia becomes painful or tender, as this may indicate incarceration and increased risk for strangulation. If signs of obstruction or strangulation occur, notify the physician and place the client in a supine position with the hips elevated and the knees slightly bent. Keep the client NPO and begin preparations for surgery.

CLIENT TEACHING

- Reassure clients that surgical intervention is generally without complications, and carries a lower risk than not repairing the hernia.
- Reinforce postoperative teaching about pain management and activity restrictions following surgery.
- Teach the client wound care and how to identify signs of infection.

HOME CARE CONSIDERATIONS

- Schedule an appointment for the client to return to the surgeon for follow-up after discharge.

For more information on Inguinal Hernia, see Medical-Surgical Nursing *by LeMone and Burke, p. 861.*

I

Intestinal Obstruction

OVERVIEW

- An intestinal obstruction is a partial or complete blockage of the lumen of any structure within the GI tract; usually the small or large bowel.
- Small bowel obstruction (SBO) accounts for about 90% of all obstructions and is the most serious type.
- With complete obstruction bowel absorption ceases but secretion continues, which dilates the bowel wall.
- Bacterial growth is thus enhanced and toxins may be produced and absorbed.
- A complete blockage is a life-threatening condition owing to loss of plasma fluid into the obstructed area with resultant shock.
- Obstructions may be mechanical, vascular, or neurologic in nature.

CAUSES

Mechanical

- Adhesions/strictures
- Atresias
- Neoplasms
- Intussusception
- Volvulus

Vascular

- Thrombosis
- Embolus

Neurologic

- Paralytic ileus
- Neurologic conditions

Other

- Toxins
- Electrolyte disorders

Signs & Symptoms

- Pain: colicky
- Nausea/vomiting: vomiting feces is common
- Abdomen: distended; tender, especially on rebound
- Constipation: absolute with complete obstruction
- Bowel sounds: may be borborygmus and/or rushes (early mechanical); may be absent

Diagnostics

- X-rays may show excess gas and fluid in bowel.
- Electrolytes are reduced owing to vomiting.
- White blood cell count is slightly elevated, especially with strangulation, necrosis, or peritonitis.
- Amylase may be increased if the pancreas is inflamed.

MEDICAL INTERVENTIONS

- Ninety percent of partial small bowel obstructions are successfully treated with gastrointestinal decompression using a nasogastric or long intestinal tube.

- Surgical intervention is required for complete mechanical obstructions as well as for strangulated or incarcerate obstructions of the small intestine.

SELECTED NURSING DIAGNOSES WITH INTERVENTIONS

Fluid Volume Imbalance

- Monitor vital signs, pulmonary artery pressures, cardiac output, and central venous pressure hourly.
- Measure urinary output hourly and nasogastric suction volume every 2 to 4 hours.
- Maintain IV fluids and blood volume replacement as prescribed. The amount of fluid administered is calculated to meet the client's current fluid needs and to replace existing and current losses.
- Measure abdominal girth every 4 to 8 hours. Mark the area to be measured on the client's abdomen.
- Notify the physician of changes in the client's status.

Altered Tissue Perfusion: Gastrointestinal

- Monitor blood pressure, rate and rhythm of pulse, and respiratory rate every hour.
- Assess skin color, temperature, and capillary refill.
- Monitor intake and output hourly. Notify the physician if output falls to less than 30 mL per hour.
- Measure the client's temperature at least every 4 hours.
- Assess the client's pain frequently.
- Administer nothing by mouth until peristalsis is restored.

Ineffective Breathing Pattern

- Assess the client's respiratory rate, pattern, and lung sounds at least every 2 to 4 hours.
- Monitor arterial blood gas results for indications of respiratory alkalosis or acidosis.
- Elevate the head of the bed.
- Provide a pillow or folded bath blanket for the client to use in splinting the abdomen while coughing postoperatively.
- Maintain the patency of nasogastric or intestinal suction.
- Assist the client to use incentive spirometry or other assistive devices.
- Contact respiratory therapy as indicated.
- Provide good oral care at least every 4 hours.

CLIENT TEACHING

- Prior to surgery, teach the client postoperative pain-relief measures and how to cough, move, and breathe more comfortably with the incision.
- If a temporary colostomy has been created, teach the client and significant others about its care. Discuss planned reanastomoses.
- For the client with recurrent obstructions, discuss their cause, early identification of symptoms, and possible preventive measures.
- Teach health-promotion activities, such as increasing intake of dietary fiber and fluids, and exercising daily.

HOME CARE CONSIDERATIONS

- Provide instruction regarding wound care.
- Discuss activity level after discharge, return to work, and any other restrictions.
- Clients with a colostomy may require continuing care for a period of time.

For more information on Intestinal Obstruction, see Medical-Surgical Nursing *by LeMone and Burke, p. 864.*

Irritable Bowel Syndrome (Spastic Colon)

OVERVIEW

- Irritable bowel syndrome is a chronic disorder of the bowel producing diarrhea alternating with constipation and accompanied by abdominal cramps.
- Small bowel motility is often increased in clients with predominant diarrhea, and decreased in those with constipation. Large bowel pressures also may be altered with changes in the frequency and strength of contractions. Hypersecretion of colonic mucus is a common feature of the syndrome.

CAUSES

- Usually associated with psychologic stress
- May be associated with:
  1. diverticulitis
  2. ingestion: food allergy; irritants; lactose intolerance

Signs & Symptoms

- Pain: lower abdomen; relieved by passing gas and/or defecation
- Diarrhea: usually daytime; alternating with constipation
- Stool changes: varying size; varying shape; excess mucus
- Possible: dyspepsia, distention

Diagnostics

- Sigmoidoscopy/colonoscopy reveals a normal appearance of the bowel with increased mucus, marked spasm, and possible hyperermia (increased redness), but no suspicious lesions.
- Barium enema may demonstrate increased motility of the GI tract.
- Complete blood count (CBC) and erythrocyte sedimentation rate (ESR) are performed to assess for possible anemia or infectious/inflammatory processes.
- Stool sample is obtained to rule out bacteria, parasites, and bleeding.

MEDICAL INTERVENTIONS

- An anticholinergic drug may be prescribed to inhibit bowel motility. In clients with diarrhea, loperamide or diphenoxylate may be given before meals.
- If chronic anxiety is identified as a probable precipitating factor, an antianxiety medication may be prescribed on a short-term basis. As depression is commonly associated with irritable bowel syndrome, an antidepressant may be prescribed.
- Dietary management measures include limiting intake of milk and milk products; gas-forming foods such as cabbage, bananas, and nuts; foods

containing fructose; alcohol; and caffeinated drinks. Many clients benefit from additional dietary fiber.

SELECTED NURSING DIAGNOSES

- Constipation
- Diarrhea
- Anxiety
- Ineffective Individual Coping

SELECTED NURSING INTERVENTIONS

- Assist the client to identify and reduce or eliminate factors that lead to symptoms.
- Encourage regular exercise to promote bowel elimination and to reduce stress.

CLIENT TEACHING

- Tell the client that any prescribed medications are generally considered temporary measures. Encourage long-term management through dietary changes, exercise, and stress reduction.
- Teach stress- and anxiety-reduction techniques, such as meditation, visualization, "time out," and progressive relaxation.
- Emphasize the need for routine follow-up appointments. Stress the importance of notifying the physician if the disease manifestations change.

HOME CARE CONSIDERATIONS

- Refer the client to a dietitian for nutritional support.
- Refer the client to a counselor or other mental health professional for assistance in dealing with psychologic factors.

For more information on Irritable Bowel Syndrome, see Medical-Surgical Nursing *by LeMone and Burke, p. 787.*

Kaposi's Sarcoma

OVERVIEW

- Kaposi's sarcoma (KS) is a malignant neoplasm of blood vessels.
- It is most often associated with AIDS; non–AIDS-related cases are seen but are rare.
- It is most frequently seen in cohorts of AIDS patients with risk factors of male homosexuality and partners of bisexual males. An unknown infectious cofactor is believed to exist and be the reason for the high incidence in these groups.
- The percentage of AIDS patients who develop KS has been declining owing to the reduced percentage of male homosexuals and increased number of cases in other risk groups.
- Histologically, there is an overgrowth of endothelial cells and spindle-shaped cells that cause narrowing of vascular lumens and increase the number of blood vessels. Red blood cells spill into the tissue spaces and hemolyze; the hemosiderin produced is ingested by numerous phagocytes.
- Macroscopically, lesions of KS appear as tiny (1 mm) red to purple macules that may develop into large raised plaques or nodules.
- While the skin is the most common site of formation, lesions can form anywhere including mucous membranes and visceral organs; the GI tract, lungs, and lymph nodes are most common.
- KS is locally destructive and rarely invasive or metastatic.

CAUSES

- Acts like a neoplasm, but may be a viral infection of blood vessels cells; cytomegalovirus (CMV) and herpes viruses have been proposed.
- Closely associated with HIV/AIDS, especially in homosexual males.

K

Signs & Symptoms

Skin (Most Common Site of Lesions)

- Early, small red to purple macules; painless, non-itchy
- Progression to larger plaques/nodules; may be edematous or ulcerate, becoming painful

Mucous Membranes

- Lesions similar to those on skin; frequently bleed

Lymphatics

- Swollen lymph nodes
- Edema

Gastrointestinal

- Mucosal bleeding may result in hemorrhage, anemia, and/or obstruction
- Gallbladder involvement may result in biliary obstruction/jaundice

Pulmonary

- Shortness of breath secondary to pulmonary effusion

Other

- Any organ system can be affected and produce organ-specific S/S

Diagnostics

- Biopsy of lesions is diagnostic.
- Chest x-ray may show pulmonary effusion.

MEDICAL INTERVENTIONS

- Radiation therapy.
- Chemotherapy (systemic or intralesional).
- Laser or cryotherapy.

SELECTED NURSING DIAGNOSES

- Impaired Skin Integrity
- Self-Esteem Disturbance
- Pain

- Fear
- Anticipatory Grieving

SELECTED NURSING INTERVENTIONS

- Assess and monitor progression of lesions. Document size, location, distribution, and so on. Monitor lesions for signs of infection or impaired healing.
- Institute measures to relieve pressure, such as air or water mattress, egg-crate mattress, or sheepskin pads. Turn the client at least every 2 hours, or more frequently if necessary.
- Keep skin clean and dry using mild, nondrying soaps or oils for cleansing. Avoid the use of heat or occlusive dressings.
- Prepare client as appropriate for chemotherapy or radiation treatments.
- Administer prescribed analgesics for pain.
- Assist client in identifying ways of dressing to cover KS lesions.
- Encourage the client to express feelings about his or her appearance.

CLIENT TEACHING

- Teach the client the importance of standard precautions, skin care, and wound care if applicable.
- As appropriate, provide the client and significant others with information about HIV infection and its effects. Discuss safe sex practices. Discuss the risks and benefits of sexual intercourse with latex condoms and spermicidal lubricant. Encourage the client and significant others to discuss fears and concerns with each other.
- Talk to the client about measures to maintain optimal health, including diet, rest, exercise, and stress reduction. Teach the client the importance of washing the hands and avoiding people with infectious diseases. As appropriate, encourage the client to stop smoking and eliminate the use of alcohol and illicit drugs.

K

HOME CARE CONSIDERATIONS

- Emphasize the importance of long-term follow-up care with the primary physician.
- Refer the client and significant others to local support groups for persons, partners, and families and friends of persons with HIV.
- Provide addresses and phone numbers for local and national information resources and hotlines.

For more information on Kaposi's Sarcoma, see Medical-Surgical Nursing *by LeMone and Burke,* *p. 604.*

Legionnaire's Disease (Legionella)

OVERVIEW

- Legionnaire's disease is a pneumonia caused by *Legionella pneumophila*, a gram-negative, aerobic bacillus.
- It was named for an epidemic at an American Legion convention in 1976. Other species of *Legionella* have since been identified; many also cause pneumonia.
- The organism is present everywhere in the environment, especially in and around warm, standing water.
- Infection usually results when the organism has been concentrated as in air conditioner filters, stagnant heating/cooling systems, hot tubs, and nebulizers.
- Cases may be isolated or can occur in epidemics.
- The diagnosis of Legionella may be missed as the organism requires special culture media.
- The overall mortality rate is 15%, but in immunocompromised patients the rate is much higher (untreated, 80%; treated, 25%).

CAUSES

- Respiratory inoculation with *Legionella pneumophila*

Signs & Symptoms

- Abrupt onset.
- Prodrome: headache, malaise/weakness, myalgia
- Fever and chills follow above one day later
- Cough is at first nonproductive; later, small amounts of purulent secretions or hemoptysis may be present
- Pleuritic pain and dyspnea may mimic pulmonary embolism
- Gastrointestinal S/S include nausea, vomiting, diarrhea, and abdominal pain

L

- Neurologic S/S include altered level of consciousness, hallucinations, delirium, seizures, and coma
- Complications include empyema/lung abscess, disseminated intravascular coagulation, hypotension/shock, renal failure, and thrombocytopenic purpura

Diagnostics

- White blood cell (WBC) count increased to >20,000/μL; differential reveals a shift to the left.
- Sputum Gram stain and culture and sensitivity tests are used to identify the causative organism.
- Arterial blood gases (ABGs) are measured to determine blood oxygen and carbon dioxide levels.
- X-ray shows infiltrates and effusions.
- Direct fluorescent antibody (DFA) specimen staining is positive.
- Serum indirect fluorescent antibody (IFA) can detect antibody formed against *Legionella*.

MEDICAL INTERVENTIONS

- Fiberoptic bronchoscopy may be done to obtain a sputum specimen or remove secretions from the bronchial tree.
- A macrolide antibiotic such as erythromycin is typically prescribed.
- Bronchodilators are used when bronchospasm is present. Mucolytic agents and expectorants also may be prescribed.
- Oxygen therapy is indicated if the client is tachypneic or if blood gas measurements reveal hypoxemia.

SELECTED NURSING DIAGNOSES

- Ineffective Airway Clearance
- Impaired Gas Exchange
- Pain
- Fatigue
- Activity Intolerance

SELECTED NURSING INTERVENTIONS

- Assess the client's respiratory status, including vital signs, breath sounds, and skin color, at least every 4 hours.

- Assess cough and sputum.
- Monitor ABG measurements and pulse oximetry readings.
- Position the client in Fowler's position, and assist the client to cough, deep breathe, and use assistive devices. Encourage use of incentive spirometry.
- Encourage a fluid intake of at least 2500 to 3000 mL per day. Monitor intake and output.
- Administer medications as prescribed and monitor for their effects.
- Administer oxygen therapy as prescribed.
- Encourage the client to avoid climbing stairs or participating in any activity that may increase dyspnea and fatigue.
- Encourage frequent rest periods.

CLIENT AND FAMILY TEACHING

- Teach the client about the disease process, treatments, medication regiment, and the need for rest.
- Teach the client to avoid upper respiratory tract infections and viruses by avoiding crowds, people with colds or flu, and respiratory irritants such as smoke.
- The course and symptoms of the disease can be long-lasting.

HOME CARE CONSIDERATIONS

- Stress the importance of notifying the physician if chills, fever, persistent cough, dyspnea, hemoptysis, chest pain, or fatigue recur or fail to resolve.
- Encourage an annual influenza vaccine and a pneumococcal vaccine.
- Provide clients who smoke with a referral to a smoking cessation program.
- Provide the client with the name and address of the local chapter of the American Lung Association.

For more information on Legionnaire's Disease, see Medical-Surgical Nursing *by LeMone and Burke,* p. 1393.

Leukemia

Acute Lymphocytic Leukemia (ALL)
Acute Myelocytic Leukemia (AML)
Chronic Lymphocytic Leukemia (CLL)
Chronic Myelocytic Leukemia (CML)

OVERVIEW

- Leukemias are malignant neoplasms of white blood cell (WBC) precursors within the bone marrow that disseminate into the general circulation and organs.
- They are classified by the predominant type of abnormal cells involved as *lymphocytic* or *myelocytic* and also by the maturity of the leukemic cells.
- Acute forms of leukemia are associated with very immature bone marrow cells called *blast cells;* the course is rapidly fatal.
  1. ALL is the result of a proliferation of immature lymphocyte precursors (B cell or T cell); it usually affects children less than 15 years of age. The 5-year survival rate in children with aggressive chemotherapy is 60%; in adults, the prognosis is poor.
  2. AML is the result of a proliferation of immature myeloid cell lines. It accounts for 20% of all leukemias, and is usually seen in adults between 15 and 40 years of age. About 20% of clients achieve 5-year disease-free survival.
- Chronic leukemias result from more differentiated cells; the course is much slower.
  1. CLL is the result of a proliferation of small mature lymphocytes. It accounts for 25% of all leukemias; the male to female ratio is 2:1. It usually occurs in adults older than 50 years; the prognosis is 2 to 10 years survival.
  2. CML is the result of proliferation of mature granulocytes. It accounts for 15% to 20% of all leukemias. It is associated with the Philadelphia chromosome (translocation of long arm of No. 22 to No.9), and usually affects adults between

25 and 60 years of age. The prognosis is poor—death usually follows a "blast crisis" resembling acute leukemia.

- All types of leukemia display an increased proliferation of WBCs at the expense of red blood cells (RBCs), thrombocytes, and platelets.

CAUSES

- The cause of leukemia is presently unknown
- Both genetic and environmental factors are considered important

Genetic Factors

- Identical twins show a high concordance rate for leukemia within the first year of life
- Families with an incidence of leukemia greater than the general population have been identified
- Acute leukemias have a higher incidence in persons with genetic diseases such as Down, Fanconi, and Klinefelter's syndromes

Environmental Factors

- Ionizing radiation increases risk for myeloid types
- Chemicals (aromatic hydrocarbons, alkylating agents) increase risk for AML
- Human T-cell leukemia virus (HTLV-1) is associated with adult T-cell leukemia (ATL)
- Epstein-Barr virus (EBV) is associated with a type of ALL

Signs & Symptoms

- Pallor
- Fatigue
- Fever
- Increased incidence of infection, e.g., herpes zoster
- Abnormal bleeding (gingival, epistaxis, petechiae/ecchymosis)
- Hyperuricemia
- Weight loss
- Lymphadenopathy
- Hepatomegaly/splenomegaly

L

Diagnostics

- RBC count, hemoglobin (Hg) and hematocrit (HCT) are all reduced.
- WBC count is usually >50,000/μL.
- Bone-marrow aspiration shows leukemic cell lines; distinguishes type.
- Uric acid is elevated.
- Prothrombin time/partial thromboplastin time may be increased.

MEDICAL INTERVENTIONS

- Systemic chemotherapy is used to eradicate leukemic cells and produce remission.
- Radiation therapy may be used to damage the DNA in the leukemic cells.
- Bone marrow transplantation may be used in conjunction with chemotherapy or radiation.
- Colony stimulating factors may be used to reduce the depth and length of postchemotherapy nadirs.

SELECTED NURSING DIAGNOSES WITH INTERVENTIONS

Risk for Infection

- Institute measures to prevent exposure to known or potential sources of infection:
  1. If prescribed, maintain protective isolation.
  2. Ensure that all people who are in contact with the client maintain meticulous hand washing.
  3. Provide careful and thorough hygiene daily.
  4. Restrict visitors with colds, flu, or infections.
  5. Provide oral hygiene after every meal.
  6. Avoid invasive procedures that may provide a portal of entry for infection.
  7. Monitor for manifestations of infection.
- Monitor vital signs and oxygenation every 4 hours. Assess for temperature spikes with chilling, tachypnea, tachycardia, restlessness, change in Pao_2, and hypotension.
- Monitor decreasing levels of neutrophils to detect risk of infection.
- Explain the reasons for precautions and restrictions,

and explain that these measures are usually temporary.

Altered Nutrition: Less Than Body Requirements

- Evaluate weight over time to determine degree of malnutrition. A weight that is 10% to 20% below ideal for height and weight indicates malnutrition.
- Provide interventions to eliminate causative or contributing factors to inadequate food and fluid intake:
  1. Perform oral hygiene before and after meals. Use a soft toothbrush or sponge as necessary.
  2. Use a solution of hydrogen peroxide and water to swish out the mouth. Use an equal amount of hydrogen peroxide, or less, to water.
  3. Provide liquids with different tastes and textures.
  4. Increase liquid intake with meals.
  5. Avoid intake of milk and milk products, which makes mucus more tenacious.
  6. Have the client assume a sitting position when eating.
  7. Ensure that the environment is clean and odor-free.
  8. Provide medications for pain or nausea 30 minutes before meals, if prescribed.
  9. Provide rest periods before meals.
  10. Offer small, frequent meals six times per day.
  11. Use commercial supplements, such as Ensure.
  12. Avoid painful or unpleasant procedures immediately before or after meals.
- Increase food tolerance by suggesting that the client:
  1. Eat dry foods when arising.
  2. Eat salty foods, if permitted.
  3. Avoid very sweet, rich, or greasy foods.
  4. Eat small amounts of food more frequently.

Risk for Injury: Bleeding

- Assess all body systems for manifestations of bleeding once every shift.
- Monitor vital signs as well as platelet counts every 4 hours.
- Avoid the following invasive procedures, if possible:
  1. use of rectal suppositories or taking of rectal temperature

L

2. use of vaginal douches, suppositories, or tampons
3. urinary catheterizations
4. parenteral injections

- Diagnostic procedures such as biopsy or lumbar puncture should not be done if the platelet count is <50,000 μL.
- Apply pressure to puncture sites for 3 to 5 minutes; apply pressure to arterial blood gas sites for 15 to 20 minutes.
- Use soft toothbrushes or sponges for oral hygiene.
- Administer corticosteroids and other medications as ordered.
- Administer platelet transfusions for acute, life-threatening bleeding, as prescribed.
- Teach the client to avoid the following:

1. picking crusts from the nose
2. blowing the nose forcefully
3. straining to have a bowel movement
4. forceful coughing or sneezing

Anticipatory Grieving

- Assess the client's and significant others' previous experiences with loss.
- Use therapeutic communication skills to allow open discussion of losses as well as permission to grieve.
- Identify agencies that may help in resolving grief, and make referrals as indicated. Consider self-help groups, cancer support groups, widow-to-widow groups, single-parent groups, and bereavement groups.

CLIENT TEACHING

- Explain the pathophysiology of the illness, the function of bone marrow, and the potential complications of the condition.
- Discuss chemotherapy, radiation, and/or bone marrow transplantation. Discuss pain control, including nonpharmacologic measures, and provide teaching as appropriate.

HOME CARE CONSIDERATIONS

- Encourage meticulous personal hygiene, including daily showering or bathing, brushing with a soft-bristle toothbrush, and inspection of the skin and mucous membranes for bleeding.

- Encourage the client to balance activity with rest.
- Teach the client to take measures to avoid infection, such as avoiding people who are ill, eating fruits and vegetables cooked, not raw, avoiding immunizations, using an electric razor rather than razor blades, and so on.
- Encourage the client to report any signs of infection or injury to the physician immediately.
- Promote nutrition by encouraging the client to eat several small meals a day, increase fiber in the diet, drink several glasses of water each day, and report any continued weight loss to the physician. A referral to a dietitian may be appropriate.
- Provide referrals to the American Cancer Society, hospice services, and support groups as appropriate.

For more information on Leukemia, see Medical-Surgical Nursing *by LeMone and Burke, p. 1305.*

Lyme Disease

OVERVIEW

- Lyme disease is a systemic inflammatory disorder caused by *Borrelia burgdorferi,* a spirochete bacterium transmitted primarily by deer or mice ticks.
- It manifests as a skin rash, arthritis, and neurologic symptoms. The inflammatory joint changes closely resemble those of rheumatoid arthritis.
- It is common along the Atlantic coastal states, Midwest (Minnesota, Wisconsin), and Pacific coastal states (California, Oregon); also present in other parts of the world.
- There are three stages of infection:
    1. *Stage 1*—occurs when the spirochete enters and infects the skin at the puncture site.
    2. *Stage 2*—begins when the organism infects the blood.

3. *Stage 3*—occurs when the organism spreads via the blood to the central nervous system (CNS), joints, and possibly the heart, colonizing these tissues.

CAUSES

- Infection, via tick bite, with the spirochete *Borrelia burgdorferi*

Signs & Symptoms

Stage 1 (Local Infection)
- Rash:
    1. initially forms at bite site as a small red macule
    2. red macule expands to a red ring surrounding a central area ("bull's eye" lesion)
    3. central area usually remains clear, but may turn red or blue, ulcerate, or become necrotic
    4. lesions are usually painless

Stage 2 (Disseminated Infection)
- After several days, skin lesions similar to above form in a disseminated pattern
- Fever/chills
- Malaise/fatigue is usually profound
- Headache is severe
- Stiff neck is mild compared with meningitis
- Myalgia—migratory
- Arthralgia—migratory
- Less common S/S include conjunctivitis/iritis, hepatitis, splenomegaly, sore throat, cough, meningitis, cranial neuritis, carditis, cardiomyopathy, first-degree heart block

Stage 3 (Persistent Infection)
- Recurrent attacks of arthritis of large or small joints
- Chronic skin lesions
- Chronic neurologic impairment

Diagnostics

- ELISA will be positive for *B. burgdorferi* antibodies approximately 4 weeks after the initial lesion.

MEDICAL INTERVENTIONS

- Pharmacologic intervention includes antibiotics and aspirin or other NSAIDs for symptom relief.
- The joint may be splinted.

SELECTED NURSING DIAGNOSES

- Activity Intolerance
- Pain
- Fatigue

SELECTED NURSING INTERVENTIONS

Vary according to stage of disease and symptoms.

- Administer prescribed antibiotics and aspirin or other NSAIDs. Emphasize the importance of complying with the prescribed antibiotic regimen for the full course of treatment. Tell the client that NSAIDs should be taken on a regular schedule rather than as needed for pain.
- Administer analgesics as prescribed.
- Teach the client to recognize symptoms of Lyme disease, including neurologic and cardiac symptoms, and to notify the physician if these occur.
- Provide opportunities for adequate rest until client's energy returns. Reassure client that fatigue is temporary.

CLIENT TEACHING

- Teach clients how to avoid contact with the tick that spreads Lyme disease and what to do if a tick bite occurs:
  1. Avoid tick-infested areas, including tall grasses and dense brush. Wear protective clothing and use an insect repellant.
  2. After being outdoors, inspect skin and clothing for ticks. Remove any ticks immediately with tweezers and wash the area thoroughly with soap and water. Apply an antiseptic.

HOME CARE CONSIDERATIONS

- Tell the client to notify the physician if a "bull's eye" rash ever develops around a tick bite.

For more information on Lyme Disease, see Medical-Surgical Nursing *by LeMone and Burke, p. 1668.*

Lymphoma, Non-Hodgkin's

OVERVIEW

- Lymphomas are malignant neoplastic diseases of lymphoid tissues (B or T lymphocytes, histiocytes). Two general categories are described: Hodgkin's lymphoma (or Hodgkin's disease) and non-Hodgkin's lymphoma (NHL). Hodgkin's lymphoma is discussed separately. (See Hodgkin's Disease.)
- NHLs are a diverse group of lymphomas classified according to cell type (T or B), size, growth pattern, and tumor grade.
- Specific NHLs may be due to the presence of low-, intermediate-, or high-grade malignant cells.
- They are usually seen in lymph nodes initially; then in spleen, thymus, gastrointestinal tract; secondary lesions occur in bone marrow.
- The incidence of NHL is about 40,000 per year in the United States.
- The prognosis is highly related to type and stage of disease.

CAUSES

- Unknown
- Associated with previous viral infection: Burkitt's lymphoma, Epstein-Barr virus (EBV), human T-cell lymphoma virus (HTLV-1)
- Risk factors include immunosuppression and autoimmune disease

Signs & Symptoms

- Painless lymphadenopathy (regional or general)
- Enlarged tonsils/adenoids
- Splenomegaly
- Gastrointestinal bleeding or obstruction
- Fever
- Pallor and fatigue
- Itching

Diagnostics

- Biopsy of lymph nodes or other tumors shows pathologic cell types and tissue structures.
- Complete blood count (CBC) may show mild to severe anemia.
- Serum uric acid is elevated.
- Serum calcium is elevated if bone marrow is affected.
- X-rays of chest and bone may show degree of metastasis.
- Scans of the liver and spleen may show degree of metastasis.
- Lymphangiogram may show degree of metastasis.
- Computed tomography (CT) scan may show degree of metastasis.

MEDICAL INTERVENTIONS

- The goal of therapy in non-Hodgkin's lymphoma is to control the disease in the area where it is evidenced; many lymphomas are highly responsive to radiation and have a high remission rate. In many cases, radiation therapy is used in conjunction with chemotherapy.
- Chemotherapy is the primary treatment for disseminated non-Hodgkin's lymphoma.
- A therapeutic splenectomy may be performed in clients with non-Hodgkin's lymphoma.

SELECTED NURSING DIAGNOSES WITH INTERVENTIONS

Altered Protection

- Assess the onset, sites, precipitating factors, and methods of relieving pruritis.

- Provide and teach the client and significant others interventions to enhance comfort and relieve itching: use cool water and a mild soap to bathe; blot (rather than rub) skin dry; apply plain cornstarch or nonperfumed lotion or powder to the skin unless contraindicated; use light-weight blankets and clothing; maintain adequate humidity and a cool room temperature; wash bedding and clothes in mild detergent and put them through the second rinse cycle.

Nausea

- Assess factors that precipitate nausea and/or vomiting, the frequency and type of vomiting, and relief measures used by the client.
- Use prescribed antiemetics before chemotherapy is started.
- Provide teaching to prevent or relieve nausea and vomiting:
    1. Eat soda crackers and suck on hard candy.
    2. Eat cold or room-temperature foods.
    3. Eat soft, bland foods.
    4. Avoid unpleasant odors and get fresh air.
    5. Do not eat immediately before chemotherapy.
    6. Use distraction or progressive muscle relaxation.
    7. Do not eat for several hours if vomiting occurs. Resume oral intake with clear liquids or ice, and progress to bland foods.

Fatigue

- Assess the client's subjective experience of malaise and fatigue.
- Allow the client to verbalize feelings regarding the impact of the disease and of the fatigue on lifestyle.
- Encourage enjoyable but quiet activities, such as reading, listening to music, or doing puzzles.
- Assist the client to establish priorities, and include rest periods or naps when scheduling daily activities.
- Help the client determine how to delegate some responsibilities to other family members.
- Assist the client in the use of energy-saving equipment.
- Encourage a diet high in carbohydrates and fluids.

Altered Nutrition: Less than Body Requirements

- Provide small feedings of high-kilocalorie, high-protein foods and fluids.

- Assist the client with oral care, general hygiene, and environmental control of temperature, appearance, and odors.
- Identify and provide foods the client prefers.
- Place the client in a sitting position during and immediately after meals.

CLIENT TEACHING

- Teach the client about the disease process, treatment options, and prognosis.
- Teach the client the strategies for self-care described in the previous section, including skin care, rest, nutrition, and so on.

HOME CARE CONSIDERATIONS

- Emphasize the importance of maintaining medical follow-up care.
- Encourage the client to contact a support group, local chapter of the American Cancer Society, Leukemia Society of America, or other community service for information, financial assistance, and counseling.

L

For more information on Lymphoma, Non-Hodgkins, see Medical-Surgical Nursing *by LeMone and Burke, p. 1318.*

Magnesium Imbalance

Hypermagnesemia
Hypomagnesemia

OVERVIEW

- Most magnesium (Mg^{++}) is contained in bone; 1% is present in the extracellular fluid; it is the second most abundant ion in the intracellular fluid.
- Physiologically, magnesium mainly acts in the intracellular fluid as a cofactor in many enzymatic reactions, including sodium/potassium pump (Na^+/K^+-ATPase).
- The concentration of magnesium is regulated by gastrointestinal absorption and renal excretion rate, both of which depend on vitamin D.
- The normal serum magnesium level is 1.5 to 2.5 mEq/L.
- When serum concentrations fall outside the normal range, cell membranes in excitable tissues such as nerve and muscle become unstable.

Hypermagnesemia

- Reduces acetylcholine release at neuromuscular junction, resulting in weakness.
- Other excitable cells such as neurons have reduced function, resulting in a general slowing of nerve function and conduction and reduced level of consciousness; vascular smooth muscle is relaxed.

Hypomagnesemia

- Makes excitable cells fire more easily, and speeds conduction.
- Increases acetylcholine release at neuromuscular junction, may produce tetany.
- Associated with low calcium and potassium levels.

CAUSES

Hypermagnesemia
(Serum Magnesium >2.5 mEq/L)

- Renal failure: decreased excretion
- Excess use of antacids/laxatives that contain magnesium: Maalox; milk of magnesia; magnesium sulfate (for toxemia of pregnancy)
- Dehydration, severe
- Hypoadrenalism: Addison's disease; adrenal trauma; adrenalectomy

Hypomagnesemia
(Serum Magnesium <1.5 mEq/L)

- Hyperaldosteronism (Conn's syndrome): dilutional
- Chronic malnutrition, malabsorption, alcoholism
- Hyperalimentation (with insufficient magnesium)
- Excess ingestion of antacids containing phosphate: prevents magnesium absorption
- Prolonged gastrointestinal fluid losses: nasogastric suctioning; diarrhea/steatorrhea
- Gastrointestinal mucosal damage/necrosis
- Medications:
    1. diuretics (furosemide, thiazides, osmotics)
    2. antibiotics (aminoglycosides)
    3. antifungals (amphotericin B)
    4. chemotherapeutics (cisplatin)
    5. glucocorticosteroids
    6. cyclosporine
    7. digitalis

Signs & Symptoms

Hypermagnesemia
- Hypotension/bradycardia
- EKG changes: prolonged P-R & Q-T intervals; wide QRS complex; elevated T wave
- Dysrhythmias: premature ventricular contractions (PVCs) heart block
- Somnolence, lethargy, coma
- Muscle weakness, reduced deep tendon reflexes
- Respiratory muscle paresis/paralysis

M

- Nausea, vomiting
- Diaphoresis

Hypomagnesemia

- Cardiac dysrhythmias: PVCs, atrial fibrillation (AF); ventricular fibrillation (V Fib), fatal
- Tremors, increased deep tendon reflexes
- Tetany:
  1. carpopedal spasms
  2. laryngospasm
  3. positive Chvostek's sign
  4. positive Trousseau's sign
- Convulsions
- Agitation, confusion, psychoses, depression
- Anorexia, nausea/vomiting, abdominal distention
- Tachycardia, hypertension possible

Diagnostics

- Serum magnesium will show deviations from normal values.
- EKG changes:
  1. *hypermagnesemia*—prolonged Q-T interval, heart block.
  2. *hypomagnesemia*—prolonged Q-T interval, wide QRS complex, low or inverted T wave, and depressed ST segment.

MEDICAL INTERVENTIONS

Hypermagnesemia

- The usual treatment includes discontinuation of all medications that contain magnesium and administration of loop diuretics.
- If cardiac symptoms occur, administration of calcium may be prescribed.
- Reducing intake of foods high in magnesium (meat, nuts, legumes, fish, vegetables, and whole-grain products) may prevent hypermagnesemia.

Hypomagnesemia

- The usual treatment of includes increasing the intake of foods high in magnesium (meat, nuts,

legumes, fish, vegetables, and whole-grain products).
- It also may include discontinuing drugs that cause excessive excretion of magnesium, such as loop diuretics, aminoglycosides, and drugs containing phosphorus.
- If severe, hypomagnesemia may be treated with IV magnesium sulfate. It may be necessary to administer drugs to increase the serum calcium concentration.

SELECTED NURSING DIAGNOSES

Hypermagnesemia
- Decreased Cardiac Output
- Risk for Impaired Gas Exchange
- Risk for Injury
- Risk for Altered Health Maintenance

Hypomagnesemia
- Altered Nutrition: Less than Body Requirements
- Knowledge Deficit
- Risk for Injury
- Decreased Cardiac Output

SELECTED NURSING INTERVENTIONS

Hypermagnesemia
- Monitor serum magnesium levels every 6 hours.
- Administer loop diuretics as prescribed.
- Monitor the client's cardiovascular and respiratory status.
- Avoid use of magnesium-containing medications (e.g., Maalox, Mylanta, milk of magnesia).
- Monitor vital signs and level of consciousness every hour.
- Encourage fluid intake.
- Administer IV calcium gluconate as prescribed.
- Observe client for flushing of skin and diaphoresis.

Hypomagnesemia
- Monitor serum magnesium levels.
- Assess the client for manifestations of neuromuscular excitability, such as muscle twitching,

M

tremors, grimaces, paresthesias, leg cramps, and hyperactive reflexes.

- Monitor the client for changes in GI function, such as nausea, vomiting, anorexia, diarrhea, and abdominal distention.
- Monitor the client for changes in cardiovascular function, such as premature atrial and ventricular beats and tachycardias; changes in the EKG, such as broad, flat, or inverted T waves, depressed ST segments, and prolonged Q-T intervals. In clients receiving digitalis, monitor for digitalis toxicity.
- Monitor laboratory results for electrolyte imbalances, particularly hypokalemia.

CLIENT TEACHING

- Teaching for the client with hypermagnesemia focuses on instructions to avoid magnesium-containing medications, including antacids, mineral supplements, cathartics, and enemas. Also provide the client with a list of foods rich in magnesium, which should be restricted.
- Teach the client experiencing mild hypomagnesemia to increase dietary intake of foods high in magnesium, and provide information about magnesium supplements.

HOME CARE CONSIDERATIONS

- If alcoholism has precipitated a magnesium deficit, a referral to Alcoholics Anonymous may be appropriate.

For more information, see the following pages in Medical-Surgical Nursing *by LeMone and Burke:*
Hypermagnesemia, p. 141
Hypomagnesemia, p. 138

Melanoma

OVERVIEW

- Melanoma is a malignant neoplasm of melanocytes, the pigment-producing cells.
- It usually affects the skin, but can also occur in the eye.
- It is generally a highly malignant lesion, although different growth patterns exist.
- The *superficial spreading type* consists of radial and shallow growth; it is a flat lesion; areas of growth restricted to the epidermis and papillary dermis.
- The *nodular type* usually begins superficially; it has a vertical growth pattern; and involves the dermis and deeper tissues.
- Metastasis is via regional lymph nodes; hematologic spread to all organs is possible.
- The usual sites involved are areas of sun exposure, but melanoma can occur on the palms, soles of feet, groin, subungual areas, or in the eye.

CAUSES

The cause is unknown; however, risk factors include:

- European American race, fair skin
- Excess sun exposure in childhood
- Positive family history
- Nevi (congenital giant, dysplastic, changing)
- Age 30 to 60 years

Signs & Symptoms

- Change in the appearance of a pre-existing skin lesion or mole
- Rapid growth of a new pigmented skin lesion with irregular borders
- Appearance of new pigmented lesion on palm, sole, or under fingernail
- Itchiness, tenderness, redness
- Ulceration, crusting, or bleeding

M

Diagnostics

- Biopsy will determine the type and stage of invasion.
- Liver function tests and computed tomography (CT) scan of the liver may be done to determine whether the tumor has metastasized to the liver.
- A chest x-ray, bone scan, and CT or magnetic resonance imaging (MRI) scan of the brain may be conducted to assess for metastasis to these organs.
- Biopsy of tissue from lymph nodes or other skin lesions is done to identify metastases.

MEDICAL INTERVENTIONS

- Surgical excision is the preferred treatment for malignant melanoma.
- Elective lymph node dissection in the treatment of localized malignant melanoma is controversial.
- Chemotherapy is used to treat metastatic melanoma or as an adjunct to other therapies.
- The use of immunotherapeutic agents such as interferons, interleukins, monoclonal antibodies, and others, is under investigation.
- Radiation frequently is used for palliation of symptoms resulting from metastasis.

SELECTED NURSING DIAGNOSES WITH INTERVENTIONS

Impaired Skin Integrity

- Monitor the client every 4 hours for manifestations of infection: fever, tachycardia, malaise, and incisional erythema, swelling, pain, or drainage that increases or becomes purulent.
- Keep the incision line clean and dry by changing dressings as necessary.
- Follow principles of medical and surgical asepsis when caring for the client's incision. Teach the importance of careful hand washing. Maintain universal precautions if drainage is present.
- Encourage and maintain adequate kilocalorie and protein intake in the diet. Suggest a consultation with the dietitian if the client does not want to eat.

Death Anxiety

- Provide an environment that encourages the client to identify and express feelings, concerns, and goals.
- Explore the client's perceptions and modify or clarify them if necessary by providing information and correcting misconceptions.
- Encourage the client to identify support systems and sources of strength and coping in the past.
- Encourage the client to participate actively in self-care as well as in mutual decision making and goal setting.
- Encourage the client to focus not only on the present but also on the future: Review past occasions for hope, discuss the client's personal meaning of hope, establish and evaluate short-term goals with the client and significant others, and encourage them to express hope for the future.

Anxiety

- Provide reassurance and comfort by setting aside time to sit quietly with the client, speaking slowly and calmly, conveying empathic understanding, and avoiding making demands or expecting the client to make decisions.
- Decrease sensory stimuli by using short, simple sentences, focusing on the here and now, and providing concise information.
- Provide interventions that decrease anxiety levels and increase coping:
  1. Provide accurate information about the illness, treatment, and prognosis.
  2. Encourage discussion of expected physical changes and coping strategies.
  3. Include significant others in teaching sessions.
  4. Provide the client with strategies for participating in the recovery process.

CLIENT TEACHING

- Teach the client techniques for avoiding sun exposure, such as wearing sunscreen of at least 15 SPF, wearing protective clothing and sunglasses, and avoiding tanning booths.
- Teach the client to conduct monthly skin self-examinations, and suggest that significant others check hard-to-see areas such as the back of the neck.

M

- Teach wound care and stress the importance of contacting the physician immediately if the client notices signs of infection.
- The client who has had a lymph node dissection is given instruction in protecting the extremity from bleeding, trauma, and infection. Describe the manifestations and side effects of chemotherapy and radiation and provide information on how to decrease nausea and vomiting, anorexia, and fatigue, and how to care for irradiated skin areas.

HOME CARE CONSIDERATIONS

- Provide the client with a brochure explaining the various types of skin cancer, treatment, and prevention, and showing photographs of cancerous lesions.
- Encourage clients to continue regular medical checkups every 3 months for 2 years following the initial diagnosis and treatment.
- A referral to a local cancer support group or psychologist may be helpful.

For more information on Melanoma, see Medical-Surgical Nursing *by LeMone and Burke, p. 611.*

Ménière's Disease

OVERVIEW

- Ménière's disease, also known as endolymphatic hydrops, is a recurrent disorder of the vestibular apparatus in the ear, producing the triad of severe vertigo, tinnitus, and sensorineural hearing loss.
- An accumulation of endolymph within the vestibular apparatus, owing to an increased rate of production or a decreased rate of reabsorption, destroys vestibular and cochlear hair cells.
- Attacks occur in a paroxysmal pattern.

- Repeated attacks may result in permanent sensorineural deafness and tinnitus.
- It is usually an ailment of adults, ages 50 to 60 most common, but can strike any age.

CAUSES

- Idiopathic
- May be brought about by impairment of autonomic control of labyrinthine circulation, or damage to the inner ear from severe otitis media or a head injury

Signs & Symptoms

- Vertigo, severe and usually disabling
- Sensorineural hearing loss
- Tinnitus
- Accompanying S/S may include:
  1. nystagmus
  2. ataxia/falling: toward the affected side
  3. nausea/vomiting
  4. diaphoresis

Diagnostics

- Audiometric studies show reduced hearing with loss of sound discrimination and recruitment.

MEDICAL INTERVENTIONS

- Antivertigo/antiemetic medications are prescribed to reduce the whirling sensation and nausea. An oral diuretic may help maintain lower labyrinthine pressure between attacks.
- A low-sodium diet, and in severe cases a salt-free neutral ash diet, may be prescribed. Alcohol, caffeine, and smoking are also prohibited.
- Surgical endolymphatic decompression and shunting relieves excess pressure in the labyrinth and relieves vertigo in about 70% of clients. Destruction of a portion of the acoustic nerve is an alternative to shunting procedures. A labyrinthectomy is used only when hearing loss is nearly complete and vertigo is persistent.

M

SELECTED NURSING DIAGNOSES WITH INTERVENTIONS

Risk for Trauma

- Assess the client for manifestations of vertigo, nystagmus, nausea and vomiting, and hearing loss.
- Place the client experiencing an acute attack of vertigo on bed rest with the side rails elevated and the call light readily accessible. Instruct the client not to get up without assistance.
- Teach the client to avoid sudden head movements or position changes.
- Administer prescribed medications, including antiemetics, diuretics, and sedatives.
- Instruct the client who senses an impending attack to respond by taking the prescribed medication and lying down in a quiet, darkened room.
- If an attack occurs while the client is driving, advise the client to pull to the side of the road and wait for the symptoms to subside.
- Discuss the importance of wearing a MedicAlert bracelet or necklace.
- Discuss the effect of unilateral hearing loss on the client's ability to identify the direction from which sounds come.

Altered Nutrition: Less than Body Requirements

- Assess the client's food and fluid intake and output.
- Obtain additional anthropometric assessment data, such as the client's height, weight, and skinfold measurements, as indicated.
- Administer antiemetic medications at the onset of an acute attack of vertigo.
- Provide fluids but do not feed the client during an acute attack unless the client requests food.
- Arrange for a dietary consultation for teaching about any prescribed dietary restrictions.
- Encourage the client on a low-sodium diet to read carefully labels of prepared foods.
- Discuss the use of seasonings such as lemon juice, pepper, and herbs to enhance the flavor of foods prepared without salt.

CLIENT TEACHING

- Teach the client about the disease process, causes, treatment options, medication regimen, methods to reduce the frequency of attacks, and prognosis.
- Teach the client safety measures, such as slowly turning the body rather than just the head to change position. Teach the client to sit or lie down immediately with the onset of vertigo. The client should not ambulate alone unless in a safe environment.
- Tell the client that surgical intervention may result in permanent hearing loss in the affected ear. Teach alternative communication strategies for the client to use postoperatively.

HOME CARE CONSIDERATIONS

- Provide a referral to a dietitian as indicated to assist the client with implementing a low-salt or salt-free ash diet.
- Support groups for the hearing impaired may provide the client with information and emotional support.

M

For more information on Ménière's Disease, see Medical-Surgical Nursing *by LeMone and Burke, p. 1938.*

Meningitis

Bacterial
Viral
Fungal

OVERVIEW

- Meningitis is an inflammation of the meninges of the central nervous system (CNS) usually due to infectious agents.

- Bacterial meningitis is the most common type, but meningitis can also be due to viruses, fungi, or chemical irritation.
- It usually involves all three meningeal layers (pia, arachnoid, and dura).
- The most common pathway for meningeal infection is via sepsis secondary to infections such as pneumonia, sinusitis, mastoiditis, otitis, pharyngitis, or osteomyelitis. Primary infections may occur with head trauma such as compound, especially basilar, skull fracture or following surgery or lumbar puncture.
- Organisms multiply rapidly, especially within arachnoid space, and are spread readily via the cerebral spinal fluid (CSF) to all areas of the brain and spinal cord. Bacteria and their exudate accumulate and may result in increased intracranial pressure (ICP).
- About 25,000 cases occur each year, most commonly in children.

CAUSES

Bacterial (Acute Pyogenic)

- *Haemophilus influenzae:* most common organism; usually in infants and children
- *Streptococcus pneumoniae:* usually in very young or very old
- *Neisseria meningitidis:* second most common organism; usually in children, adolescents, and young adults; causes meningococcal (epidemic) meningitis
- *Escherichia coli:* usually in infants

Viral (Aseptic)

- Childhood disease viruses: mumps, measles, chickenpox
- ECHO virus
- Arbovirus (epidemic): usually with encephalitis
- Coxsackie virus
- Epstein-Barr virus (EBV)
- Herpes simplex virus (HSV), Type I or II
- Cytomegalovirus (CMV)
- Varicella zoster virus (VZV)
- Polio virus

- Rabies virus: if untreated is 100% fatal
- Human immunodeficiency virus (HIV)

Fungal
- Usually seen only in immunocompromised patients
- *Cryptococcus*
- *Candida albicans*
- *Aspergillus*

Signs & Symptoms

Infection
- Fever, chills, malaise

General
- Irritability; photophobia; seizures; petechiae, purpura, ecchymosis (meningococcus); rash; deafness and joint pain (*H. influenzae*); increased deep tendon reflexes

Meningeal Irritation
- Stiff neck/back, positive Brudzinski's sign, positive Kernig's sign

Increased ICP/Herniation
- Headache
- Decreased level of consciousness; decreasing Glasgow coma scale, coma
- Projectile vomiting
- Pupils: decreased response, inequality, dilation
- Vital sign changes: increased blood pressure, increased pulse pressure, decreased heart rate, irregular respiratory pattern

Diagnostics

- Lumbar puncture for CSF culture and sensitivity (C&S):
  1. *Bacterial:* increased pressure; cloudy fluid; white cell count up to 90,000 polymorphonuclear leukocyte (PMNs)/μL; elevated protein; decreased glucose; C&S positive for specific organism.

2. *Viral:* clear fluid; normal glucose; increased pressure; increased lymphocytes; negative bacterial C&S; positive or negative viral culture.

- Cultures of blood, nose and throat mucous membranes, or urine may locate primary infection site.
- X-rays of the chest, for pneumonia; of the head, for sinusitis, or cranial osteomyelitis.
- Computerized tomography (CT) scan to rule out abscess, hematoma, hemorrhage, or tumor.

MEDICAL INTERVENTIONS

- A broad-spectrum antibiotic usually is prescribed until the results of the culture and Gram stain are available, at which time a specific antibiotic is prescribed as appropriate.
- Anticonvulsant medications may be prescribed to prevent seizure activity, and antipyretics and nonopiate analgesics may be given for symptom relief.
- An Ommaya reservoir may be surgically implanted into a lateral ventricle of the brain to enhance CSF absorption of antibiotics.

SELECTED NURSING DIAGNOSES WITH INTERVENTIONS

Altered Protection

- Assess neurologic status on a regular basis.
- Assess vital signs, including temperature, on a regular basis.
- Assess for and report decreasing levels of consciousness. Assess levels of orientation, memory, attention span, and response to overall stimuli.
- Assess for and report manifestations of seizure activity and institute seizure precautions.
- Assess for and report manifestations of cranial nerve damage; monitor extraocular movements, facial movement, dizziness, ability to hear, double vision, drooping upper eyelids, and pupillary changes.
- Assess for and report manifestations of increased ICP: decreased pulse, increased blood pressure, widening pulse pressure, respiratory changes, and vomiting.

- Administer prescribed medications and maintain prescribed fluid restrictions.

Risk for Fluid Volume Imbalance

- Assess for presence or worsening of fluid volume deficit:
  1. Measure and compare intake and output every 2 to 4 hours.
  2. Monitor daily body weights.
  3. Monitor skin turgor and tongue turgor.
  4. Monitor condition of mucous membranes.
  5. Monitor concentration of urine.
  6. Monitor blood urea nitrogen: creatinine ratio.
  7. Monitor body temperature at least every 4 hours.
- When administering fluids, either orally or parenterally, consider other illnesses that are occurring concurrently.

CLIENT TEACHING

- Teach the client and significant others about the disease process, treatment, and ways to prevent future occurrences and spread of the disease to others.
- Teach the names, dosages, and purposes of all prescribed medications, and stress the importance of taking all medication until completely gone.

HOME CARE CONSIDERATIONS

- Teach the client and significant others to report any signs or symptoms of ear infection, sore throat, or upper respiratory tract infection.

For more information on Meningitis, see Medical-Surgical Nursing *by LeMone and Burke, p. 1743.*

Mononucleosis

OVERVIEW

- Mononucleosis is an acute infection of B lymphocytes, most commonly with the herpes virus or Epstein-Barr virus (EBV).
- EBV is thought to spread via saliva, as with kissing.
- Infection spreads from oral mucosa to pharynx and lymphatic vessels, nodes, and spleen to enter B lymphocytes. The lymph nodes and spleen enlarge.
- It occurs in young adults (15 to 30 years old) primarily; most adults test positive.
- Symptoms last an average of 2 weeks but fatigue may linger for months.
- EBV is associated with Burkitt's lymphoma and nasopharyngeal carcinoma.

CAUSES

- Most commonly caused by the Epstein-Barr virus.

Signs & Symptoms

- Fever, diaphoresis, chills, malaise
- Sore throat
- Lymphadenopathy
- Left-upper-quadrant tenderness
- Fatigue, often profound
- Headache
- Myalgia, generalized
- Rash, red papular
- Anorexia

Diagnostics

- White blood cell count shows elevated lymphocytes; atypical lymphocytes.
- Monospot is positive.
- Liver enzymes show an abnormal profile.

MEDICAL INTERVENTIONS

- Treatment includes analgesics and, in severe cases of pharyngotonsillitis, corticosteroids to reduce

inflammation. Penicillin-type antibiotics are not used.
- Bed rest is an essential component of treatment.

SELECTED NURSING DIAGNOSES
- Fatigue
- Pain
- Activity Intolerance
- Risk for Altered Role Performance

SELECTED NURSING INTERVENTIONS
- Assess the client's physical limitations and toleration of activities of daily living (ADLs). Assess the client's sleep pattern and number of sleep hours per 24-hour period. Assess the client's dietary intake to ensure adequate nutrition for healing.
- Assess the client's need for assistance in caring for self or family. Develop a plan of care with the client that identifies coping mechanisms and personal strengths and acknowledges limitations.
- Encourage frequent rest periods and activity restrictions to diminish fatigue. Discuss strategies for increasing rest time, prioritizing daily tasks, and relinquishing tasks when fatigued.
- Administer analgesics as prescribed, and corticosteroids if prescribed for pharyngotonsillitis.

CLIENT TEACHING
- Teach the client about the disease process, treatment, and strategies to avoid relapse. Tell the client that symptoms normally last 2 to 3 weeks, but some degree of lethargy and debility may remain for several months.

HOME CARE CONSIDERATIONS
- A referral to social or community services may be appropriate to assist the client with self-care and care of family in the initial stages of the disease.

For more information on Mononucleosis, see Medical-Surgical Nursing *by LeMone and Burke, p. 1302.*

Multiple Myeloma

OVERVIEW

- Multiple myeloma is a primary malignancy of plasma cells, which are mature, Ig (immunoglobulin, antibody) secreting B lymphocytes.
- It most often arises in bone marrow where a single abnormal clone of plasma cells
  1. proliferates,
  2. secretes abnormal Ig,
  3. crowds out normal cells, and
  4. forms destructive bone lesions.
- Typically it initially involves the bone and marrow of vertebrae, ribs, pelvis, femur, and skull, but may affect any bone.
- Plasma cells, which usually constitute about 5% of marrow cells, increase to 30% to 90%; most are immature and malignant.
- Later, disease spreads to any organ, the most common being lymph nodes, spleen, and liver.
- It is responsible for about 15% of all white blood cell disorders.
- The incidence rises with age; it is rare before age 40, and peaks at about 65 years of age.

CAUSES

- Unknown
- Possibly related to genetic predisposition, inflammatory stimuli, oncogenic virus, and/or chronic antigenic challenge with mutation
- Risk factors include older age; male sex; African ancestry

Signs & Symptoms

- Bone pain: back, ribs, legs; increased with movement
- Pathologic fracture/loss of height
- Hypercalcemia: weakness, lethargy, constipation, polyuria
- Raynaud's phenomenon, carpal tunnel syndrome

- Joint swelling and pain
- Fever and malaise
- Weight loss
- S/S of anemia: fatigue, pallor, tachycardia
- S/S of abnormal bleeding: petechiae, purpura, ecchymosis, epistaxis
- S/S of spinal nerve-root compression: weakness, sciatica, incontinence, impotence
- S/S of recurrent infection
- S/S of renal insufficiency or failure

Diagnostics

- Complete blood count (CBC) shows moderate to severe anemia and neutropenia, but increased lymphocytes.
- Erythrocyte sedimentation rate (ESR) is elevated.
- Serum protein electrophoresis shows abnormal IgG or IgA.
- Urine studies may detect Bence Jones protein and/or hypercalciuria.
- X-rays early in the disease show osteopenia; later, they show specific, round osteolytic lesions.
- Bone marrow aspiration identifies an abnormal number of immature plasma cells.

M

MEDICAL INTERVENTIONS

- There is no cure for multiple myeloma and treatment is primarily palliative. Chemotherapy, radiation therapy, and pharmacology are used to decrease tumor size and lessen bone pain.
- Pain is controlled with analgesics and infections are controlled with antibiotics.
- Blood transfusions are used to treat anemia.

SELECTED NURSING DIAGNOSES WITH INTERVENTIONS

Chronic Pain
- Assess pain, including onset, duration, precipitating factors, and effective measures of relief.
- Determine which position allows greatest comfort, and help the client assume this position.
- Support the client with pillows.
- Allow for uninterrupted rest periods.

- Teach the client to use nonpharmacologic methods of pain control, including relaxation or guided imagery.
- Teach the client how to take prescribed analgesics. Involve significant others as needed to ensure that the client's pain is relieved.
- Report unrelieved pain to the physician.

Impaired Bed Mobility

- Gently hold the client's extremities when repositioning.
- Provide a change of position every 2 hours, or more frequently if needed.
- Provide a trapeze to assist in repositioning.

Risk for Injury

Place needed items close at hand for the client.
- Provide safety measures to prevent falls from the bed: Place the bed in a low position, use side rails, and place the call bell within reach.
- Provide safety measures to prevent injury when the client is ambulatory: Ensure that the pathway is clear, remove scatter rugs, and provide adequate lighting, a nonslippery floor, and nonskid soles on shoes.

Risk for Infection

- Ensure that all persons coming in contact with the client wash hands meticulously.
- Restrict visitors with colds, flu, or other infections.
- Provide careful and thorough hygiene care daily.
- Provide a high-protein, high-vitamin diet.
- Provide oral hygiene after every meal.
- Use strict aseptic technique for invasive procedures.
- Assess vital signs every 4 hours. Report abnormal findings to the physician.
- Monitor levels of neutrophils to detect any increasing risk of infection.
- Institute protective isolation if the neutrophil count drops below 500/μL.
- Restrict fresh flowers and plants from the client's room, as insects may harbor microorganisms that could cause infection.
- Restrict raw fruits and vegetables, and ensure that fruits and vegetables are washed well prior to cooking.

CLIENT TEACHING

- Teach the client about the disease process, palliative treatments, medication administration, and prognosis.
- Teach the client and significant others the signs and symptoms that signify complications and the need to seek medical help, including pathologic fractures and infections.

HOME CARE CONSIDERATIONS

- As the client's status deteriorates, the client and significant others may wish to consider hospice care.
- A referral to pastoral services, cancer support groups, or a psychologic counselor may be appropriate for the client and significant others to facilitate grief work.

For more information on Multiple Myeloma, see Medical-Surgical Nursing *by LeMone and Burke, p. 1303.*

M

Multiple Sclerosis

OVERVIEW

- Multiple sclerosis (MS) is a disease characterized by inflammatory demyelination and gliosis (scarring) of the central nervous system (CNS).
- Myelin is a fatty substance made by CNS oligodendrocytes that insulates axons and speeds conduction of action potentials.
- In MS, myelin is lost in scattered patches of the CNS; rapid transmission of impulses is impaired, producing progressive motor, sensory, and visual neurologic deficits.
- Although symptoms are generally progressive, the disease's course is marked with periods of remission and exacerbation; with remission, remyelination can occur and symptoms improve.

- Once myelin is lost permanently it is replaced by sclerotic plaques (scar tissue); conduction is permanently impaired.
- The course of MS is very individualized: in some clients the course is rapidly fulminating, although most have slowly progressive forms of the disease with long periods of remission.
- The disease is usually diagnosed in young adults between the ages of 20 and 40.
- MS eventually leads to severe neurologic disability.

CAUSES

- Unknown, but slow-acting viral agents combined with altered immune responses are being investigated.
- Episodes may be triggered by fever, pregnancy, extreme physical exertion, and exhaustion.
- Risk factors include:
  1. family history
  2. age 20 to 40
  3. cool to cold environments; uncommon in tropics
  4. recent viral infection

Signs & Symptoms

Motor

- Paresis, fatigue
- Paralysis, spastic type (upper-motor-neuron lesion)
- Tremor
- Ataxia
- Eyes: diplopia (eye muscles); nystagmus (cerebrum/brain stem)
- Head: slurred speech; dysphagia
- S/S of Bell's palsy
- Incontinence: urinary and/or fecal

Sensory

- Reduced general senses: touch, vibration, temperature, pain
- Special senses: *eyes*—diplopia, clouding, blurring, scotoma, loss of acuity, with eye pain due to

optic neuritis; *vestibular*—loss of proprioception, vertigo
- Paresthesias: numbness, tingling, "pins and needles" sensation
- Hypesthesia
- Trigeminal neuralgia

Emotional
- Euphoria
- Irritability/hyperexcitability
- Apathy/depression
- Uncontrollable laughter or crying

Cognitive
- Memory loss
- Poor judgment
- Inappropriate responses

Diagnostics

- Cerebrospinal fluid analysis shows increased mononuclear cells and IgG and positive myelin basic protein (MBP).
- Computed tomography (CT) scan shows ventricular enlargement.
- Magnetic resonance imaging (MRI) can show size and distribution of plaques.

M

MEDICAL INTERVENTIONS

- Interferon beta-1B is being used for ambulatory clients with relapsing-remitting MS. It appears to decrease the number of exacerbations.
- Medications used during an exacerbation include a combination of adrenocorticotropic hormone (ACTH) and glucocorticoids to decrease inflammation and suppress the immune system.
- Some clinicians report success at inducing remission with plasmapheresis in combination with ACTH therapy.
- Physical and rehabilitative therapies are individualized to the client's level of functioning.

SELECTED NURSING DIAGNOSES WITH INTERVENTIONS

Fatigue

- Encourage the client to discuss fatigue. Assess degree of fatigue and identify contributing factors.
- Arrange daily activities to include rest periods.
- Help the client set priorities.
- Encourage the client to perform tasks in the morning hours when he or she has more energy.
- Advise the client to avoid temperature extremes, such as hot showers or exposure to cold.
- Refer the client to professional services such as stress management groups, physical therapists.

Self-Care Deficit

- Fully assess the extent of the client's self-care deficit.
- Help the client to maintain as much independence in activities as possible.
- Assist with daily hygiene needs; modify toothbrush, comb, and so on, as indicated. Provide adaptive devices as needed. Maintain privacy.
- Assist the client with feeding needs. Teach the client how to use assistive devices.
- Teach routine inspection of skin.
- Teach interventions related to altered bowel and bladder function.

CLIENT TEACHING

In addition to the teaching discussed above:

- Teach the client about the disease process and how to reduce the risk of exacerbations. Stress the importance of avoiding respiratory and urinary tract infections. If appropriate, tell the client that pregnancy may exacerbate the condition.
- Review treatment options and their side effects.
- Ascertain that the client or significant others have taken steps to make the home environment safe, such as removing scatter rugs and using handrails in the shower.
- Discuss the importance of long-term follow-up care.

HOME CARE CONSIDERATIONS

- Tell the client how to obtain assistive devices.
- If the client is unable to prepare meals, refer the client to Meals-on-Wheels.
- Refer the client to the local chapter of the Multiple Sclerosis Society.

For more information on Multiple Sclerosis, see Medical-Surgical Nursing *by LeMone and Burke, p. 1827.*

Muscular Dystrophy

OVERVIEW

- Muscular dystrophy (MD) is a group of genetic muscle diseases with a variety of genetic inheritance patterns that result in progressive symmetrical skeletal muscle wasting.
- Duchenne's MD, the most common variant, is usually a sex-linked recessive hereditary disorder but may occur as a spontaneous mutation.
- The disease occurs in about 1 in 3500 live births.
- The affected gene codes for dystrophin, a specific cytoskeletal protein in skeletal and cardiac muscles.
- Skeletal and cardiac muscles show patchy necrosis; muscle is replaced by fibrous or fatty tissue.
- Symptoms are evident by early childhood (3–4 years).

CAUSES

- The disease is hereditary in two thirds of cases; the defective gene is present in both parents, while in one third of cases, MD is thought to be due to spontaneous mutation in the maternal gamete.

Signs & Symptoms

- Weakness is evident by age 3 and is symmetric; early on, it involves pelvic and shoulder girdles;

later in the course of the disease, it involves all muscles.

- Delayed walking, waddling gait, frequent falls
- Muscle pain
- Muscle wasting/pseudohypertrophy
- Cardiac S/S: tachycardia; dysrhythmias
- Total disability by age 10 to 15 years, including contracture deformity, lordosis, scoliosis, and obesity

Diagnostics

- Muscle biopsy shows increased muscle fat and fibrosis.
- Electromyography shows deficiency of electric activity.
- Serum enzymes show increased creatine kinase (CK) and increased lactate dehydrogenase (LDH).
- Serum shows increased creatinine levels.
- Urine shows increased 24-hour creatinine excretion.

MEDICAL INTERVENTIONS

- Therapy is usually supportive and rehabilitative, involving physical and occupational therapy.

SELECTED NURSING DIAGNOSES

- Impaired Wheelchair Mobility
- Self-Care Deficit
- Risk for Impaired Skin Integrity
- Ineffective Individual Coping
- Risk for Altered Development

SELECTED NURSING INTERVENTIONS

- Assess for complications of immobility. Provide active and passive range-of-motion exercises, foot support, and adequate nutrition and hydration.
- Teach the client to turn, cough, deep breathe, and use the incentive spirometer. Encourage independence as much as possible.
- Assess the client's skin frequently. Provide pressure relief for both bed and wheelchair, and keep the client's skin clean and dry. Change the client's position every 2 hours.

- Encourage the client and significant others to verbalize their feelings about this progressive, often fatal, disease. Refer them to psychological, spiritual, or religious counseling as appropriate.
- Assess the client and significant others' coping strategies for long-term needs.

CLIENT TEACHING

- Teach the client and significant others about the disease process, supportive therapies, and prognosis. Listen actively to their questions and concerns and provide accurate information.
- Teach basic care strategies to the client and caregivers. Involve the client in decision making as much as possible. Provide positive reinforcement for independent activities such as self-care, eating, and asking questions.

HOME CARE CONSIDERATIONS

- Refer the client and significant others to the local chapter of the Muscular Dystrophy Association for resources and support.

M

For more information on Muscular Dystrophy, see Medical-Surgical Nursing *by LeMone and Burke, p. 1569.*

Myasthenia Gravis

OVERVIEW

- Myasthenia gravis (MG) is a chronic disease that causes progressive weakness and easy fatigability of skeletal muscles.
- The axons of motor neurons divide as they enter skeletal muscle. The transmission of nerve impulses to the muscle occurs when acetylcholine (ACh) is released from the axonal endings, crosses the synaptic cleft, attaches to receptors on the muscle

fibers, and stimulates the muscle. In MG, antibodies destroy or block receptor sites, resulting in a decrease in the number of ACh receptors. There are also structural changes that result in diminished ACh uptake. The net result is a decrease in the muscle's ability to contract despite a sufficient amount of ACh.

- Muscles supplied by cranial nerves are particularly susceptible, but MG may occur in any skeletal muscle.
- There is a bimodal age distribution: *early onset,* ages 20 to 30 with women affected more often than men; *late onset,* after age 50 with men affected more often than women.
- The course is unpredictable, with remissions and exacerbations.

CAUSES

- Autoimmune: destruction of ACh receptors on skeletal muscle cell membrane of myoneural junction; most common form
- Genetic types exist, but are rare
- MG is associated with:
  1. other autoimmune disorders
  2. thymomas
  3. small (oat) cell carcinoma of lung

Signs & Symptoms

- Skeletal muscle weakness
- Easy fatigability of skeletal muscles, especially following repetitive movements
- S/S of eye muscles are usually the first to be detected: ptosis, diplopia, incomplete closure
- Cranial muscles: reduced facial expression, difficult vocalization, difficulty chewing and swallowing
- Respiratory muscles: respiratory distress or failure, which can be life threatening

Diagnostics

- Electromyographic (EMG) studies show fatigue following repeated muscle stimulation.

- Tensilon test: IV injection of edrophonium chloride (Tensilon), a short-acting anticholinesterase, brings dramatic improvement of muscle function within 30 to 60 seconds and lasts about 5 minutes.
- Anti-ACh receptor antibody serum levels are increaed in about 80% of clients.

MEDICAL INTERVENTIONS

- Anticholinesterases are used to promote ACh concentration at receptor sites.
- Immunosuppression with glucocorticoids improves muscle strength.
- Approximately 75% of clients with MG have dysplasia of the thymus gland; therefore, thymectomy is often performed within the first 2 years of diagnosis.
- Plasmapheresis may be used in conjunction with other therapies.

SELECTED NURSING DIAGNOSES WITH INTERVENTIONS

M

Ineffective Airway Clearance

- Assist the client with turning, deep breathing, and coughing at least every 2 hours. Teach proper coughing techniques. Use an incentive spirometer every 2 hours while the client is awake.
- Position the client in semi-Fowler's position.
- Maintain the client's hydration status and monitor for dehydration. Use a humidifier as needed.
- Assess lung sounds, rate and character of respirations, and pulse oximetry readings at least every four hours.

Impaired Swallowing

- Assess the client's ability to manage safely various consistencies of foods.
- Have the client eat slowly, using small bites of food. Schedule mealtimes during periods when the client is adequately rested.
- If necessary, give cues while the client is eating; for example, "Chew your food thoroughly; now swallow."
- Teach caregivers the Heimlich maneuver and how to suction.

CLIENT TEACHING

- Teach the client about the disease process, treatment options, and prognosis.
- Teach about medication side effects and scheduling, and instruct the client to avoid nonprescription drugs without first consulting the physician.
- Teach methods to avoid fatigue and undue stress. Teach strategies for avoiding upper respiratory tract infections. Stress the importance of avoiding extreme heat or cold.
- Discuss family planning as appropriate, since pregnancy can exacerbate symptoms, and medications used to control MG can cross the placenta.

HOME CARE CONSIDERATIONS

- A referral to a physical or occupational therapist, and/or social services may be appropriate.
- Provide information on local MG support groups.
- Refer significant others to local CPR certification classes.

For more information on Myasthenia Gravis, see Medical-Surgical Nursing *by LeMone and Burke,* p. 1853.

Myocardial Infarction

OVERVIEW

- Myocardial infarction (MI) is the death of functional myocytes due to ischemia.
- MI usually presents as an acute event brought on by a sudden reduction of coronary perfusion secondary to final closure of the atheromatous vessel, most often due to thrombosis.
- The amount of myocardial damage depends on the location, size, and degree of occlusion; number of collateral vessels present; and oxygen demand at the time of the infarction.

- An inner necrotic area is surrounded by an ischemic zone, which is salvageable; eventually the area of necrosis is replaced by scar tissue.
- MI is one of the most common disorders in Western civilizations.
- Approximately 1.5 million MIs occur in the United States each year.

CAUSES

- Any condition that creates a myocardial oxygen demand greater than supply
- Atherosclerosis is the most common cause, but genetic types of coronary blockage exist
- Dissecting aneurysm
- Anemia
- Hypercoagulability syndromes
- Coronary embolus
- Connective tissue disease
- Poisoning: carbon monoxide; cyanide; cocaine
- Risk factors include:
  1. male gender or postmenopausal status in females
  2. age greater than 45
  3. high fat/calorie/cholesterol diet
  4. obesity
  5. diabetes mellitus
  6. hypertension
  7. sedentary lifestyle
  8. smoking
  9. genetic forms of atherosclerosis

M

Signs & Symptoms

- Pain: visceral; substernal chest; severe; crushing; radiating to left arm and possibly jaw, neck, abdomen, back; not improved by rest or nitroglycerin
- Shortness of breath/dyspnea
- Diaphoresis, cool, clammy extremities, pallor
- Indigestion, nausea, vomiting
- Fatigue
- Anxiety
- Sudden collapse without any of the above signs and symptoms is also possible

Diagnostics

- EKG may show a variety of abnormalities, depending on the area of myocardial damage; dysrhythmias seen are:
  1. premature ventricular contractions
  2. ventricular tachycardia
  3. ventricular fibrillation
  4. sinus tachycardia or bradycardia
  5. heart block
- Echocardiogram shows wall motion changes.
- Cardiac catheterization shows reduced coronary perfusion and amount of wall damage.
- Serial serum enzymes: creatine phosphokinase-MB isoenzyme rises within 8 to 24 hours and returns to normal by 48 to 72 hours; troponin T and troponin I are more specific and remain elevated for 5–7 days.

MEDICAL INTERVENTIONS

- Drug therapy can help reduce oxygen demand and increase oxygen supply. Thrombolytic agents, analgesics, and antidysrhythmic agents are among the principal classes of drugs used.
- Thrombolytic therapy may be followed by immediate percutaneous transluminal coronary angioplasty (PTCA). Or cardiac catheterization and PTCA may be performed 5 to 10 days after the MI.
- For clients with large MIs and evidence of pump failure, invasive devices may be used to take over the function of the heart temporarily, allowing the injured myocardium to heal. The intra-aortic balloon pump is a widely used device to augment cardiac output. Ventricular assist devices are indicated for clients requiring more artificial support than can be provided by the intra-aortic balloon pump alone.
- Cardiac rehabilitation, a planned program of activity and exercises, psychologic support, and client education are appropriate for all clients with MI.

SELECTED NURSING DIAGNOSES
WITH INTERVENTIONS

Pain

- Assess the client for verbal and nonverbal signs of pain. Document characteristics of the pain and the client's rating on a scale of 0 to 10. Accept verbal reports of pain. If the client exhibits nonverbal indicators of pain, confirm the meaning of these with the client.
- Assess and document vital signs.
- Administer oxygen at 2 to 5 mL/minute per nasal cannula.
- Provide for physical and psychologic rest. Provide information and emotional support.
- Titrate IV nitroglycerin as prescribed to relieve chest pain, maintaining the systolic blood pressure at above 100 mm Hg.
- Administer 2 to 4 mg of morphine by IV push for chest pain unrelieved by nitroglycerin.
- Administer other medications as prescribed.

Altered Tissue Perfusion

- Assess and document vital signs. Report increases in heart rate and changes in heart rhythm, blood pressure, and respiratory rate.
- Assess the client for changes in level of consciousness; decreased urine output; moist, cool, pale, mottled, or cyanotic skin; dusky or cyanotic mucous membranes and nail beds; diminished to absent peripheral pulses; delayed capillary refill.
- Auscultate heart and breath sounds. Note the presence of abnormal heart sounds or adventitious sounds in the lungs.
- Monitor the client's EKG rhythm continuously. Obtain a 12-lead EKG to assess the client's complaints of chest pain. Report marked changes to the physician.
- Monitor oxygen saturation levels with pulse oximetry. Administer oxygen as prescribed. Obtain and assess arterial blood gases as indicated.
- Administer antidysrhythmic medications as needed.
- Obtain serial creatine kinase and isoenzymes as prescribed.

M

- Anticipate the need to insert invasive hemodynamic monitoring catheters.
- Administer medications to improve cardiac output and tissue perfusion as prescribed.
- Continuously monitor the client's response to these interventions.

Fear

- Identify the client's level of fear. Note both verbal and nonverbal signs of fear.
- Acknowledge the client's perception of the situation and allow the client to verbalize concerns.
- Encourage the client to ask questions, and provide consistent, factual answers. Repeat information as needed.
- Recognize opportunities for client independence. Encourage self-care. Allow the client to make decisions regarding the plan of care.
- Administer antianxiety or hypnotic medications as prescribed.
- Teach the client nonpharmacologic methods of stress reduction such as relaxation methods, mental imagery, and breathing exercises.

CLIENT TEACHING

- Teach the client about the disease process; treatments, including medications, dosage, effects, and side effects; and risk factor modifications that may be required.
- For the client who has had PTCA, advise a return to moderate activities in 1 to 2 weeks, per the physician's recommendation. Tell the client to avoid heavy lifting. If there is bleeding from the insertion site, the client or caregiver should apply manual pressure. Tell the client to call the physician if bleeding is extensive or lasts for more than 15 minutes.

HOME CARE CONSIDERATIONS

- Emphasize the importance of complying with the medical regimen and keeping follow-up appointments. Provide the client with telephone numbers and addresses of resource personnel who are available to respond to questions and concerns after discharge.

- Provide information about community resources, such as the local chapter of the American Heart Association.
- Encourage significant others to learn CPR in the event of an emergency, and provide information on community agencies that offer CPR classes.

For more information on Myocardial Infarction, see Medical-Surgical Nursing *by LeMone and Burke,* p. 1100.

Myocarditis

OVERVIEW

- Myocarditis is an inflammation of cardiac myocytes that can result in necrosis and degeneration of the myocardium; the endocardium may be affected.
- Focal or scattered patterns of inflammation are possible.
- It can be acute or chronic.
- It affects all age groups.

CAUSES

- Often the etiology is unknown: types include giant cell myocarditis and Fiddler's myocarditis
- May be associated with sarcoidosis
- Infectious:
  1. Viral (most common): coxsackie A and B, ECHO, poliovirus, influenza A and B, rubeola, rubella
  2. Bacterial: diphtheria, gonococcus, pneumococcus, staphylococcus, tetanus, tuberculosis, typhoid fever
- Parasitic:
  1. Trypanosoma cruzi: Chagas' disease; common in South America
  2. Toxoplasmosis
  3. Trichinosis

M

- Also can be caused by acute rheumatic fever or can accompany other autoimmune diseases such as systemic lupus erythematosus
- May be caused by toxins such as lead, chronic heavy alcohol ingestion, and drugs such as lithium and cocaine
- Other causes include heat stroke, radiation, and transplant rejection

Signs & Symptoms

- May be entirely asymptomatic
- Usually vague and nonspecific
- Fever, malaise
- Fatigue
- Dyspnea
- Chest pain: mild, continuous
- Palpitations
- S/S of congestive heart failure

Diagnostics

- Cardiac serum enzymes show elevated creatine phosphokinase, isoenzyme 2 (CPK_2), and lactate dehydrogenase (LDH).
- White blood cell count is elevated.
- Erythrocyte sedimentation rate is elevated.
- Antistreptolysin titers are elevated.
- EKG reveals ST segment and T wave disturbances; prolonged P-R interval; supraventricular dysrhythmias.
- Endomyocardial biopsy shows characteristic inflammatory lesions.

MEDICAL INTERVENTIONS

- Corticosteroid drugs may be prescribed to reduce inflammation.
- Strenuous exercise and labor is prohibited until the EKG is normal.

SELECTED NURSING DIAGNOSES

- Risk for Decreased Cardiac Ouput
- Activity Intolerance
- Risk for Altered Role Performance
- Pain

SELECTED NURSING INTERVENTIONS

- Administer medications as prescribed.
- Encourage bed rest and activity restriction until fever and cardiac symptoms subside.
- Discuss with the client and significant others the change in the client's role performance, their questions, and concerns. Assess the need for home care, social services, or other community assistance to provide for client's and significant others' immediate needs.
- Assess the client's level of pain. Administer pain medications as prescribed.

CLIENT TEACHING

- Teach the client about the disease process; treatment, including medication regimen; strategies for preventing reccurrences; and prognosis.
- Teach the client and significant others the manifestations of streptococcal pharyngitis and stress the importance of reporting these symptoms to the physician immediately for antibiotic therapy.

HOME CARE CONSIDERATIONS

- Explain to the client that prophylactic antibiotic therapy is necessary for the rest of the client's life in the event of streptococcal infection.
- A referral to social or community services may be appropriate for the client experiencing altered role performance due to activity restrictions.

M

For more information on Myocarditis, see Medical-Surgical Nursing *by LeMone and Burke, p. 1162.*

Occupational Lung Disease

Pneumoconiosis
Hypersensitivity Pneumonitis

OVERVIEW

- *Pneumoconiosis* is a chronic fibrotic lung disease that is caused by exposure to inorganic dusts, mainly as a result of heavy exposure at work. The most common types include asbestosis, silicosis, and coal miner's pneumoconiosis.
- *Hypersensitivity pneumonitis* is an allergic pulmonary disease caused by exposure to inhaled organic dusts and gases. Some common types include byssinosis, bagassosis, and farmer's lung.
- Dusts are deposited within alveoli and ingested by pulmonary macrophages, which then secrete fibroblast-stimulating factor. This results in fibrosis of lung parenchyma.
- Fibrotic lung tissues are stiff and difficult to inflate, producing a restrictive type of lung disease. The breathing pattern is rapid and shallow.
- They occur in occupations such as asbestos workers, miners, sandblasters, stonecutters, and farmers.
- The incidence increases with exposure and, therefore, age.

CAUSES

Pneumoconiosis

- Asbestosis is caused by exposure to asbestos, as in insulators: electricians, plumbers, construction workers, and their wives (laundry exposure) are at risk
- Coal miner's pneumoconiosis is caused by exposure to coal dust
- Silicosis is caused by exposure to silica; mining, stonecutting, sandblasting, and quarrying increase the risk
- Other inorganic dusts implicated include talc, beryllium, iron, graphite, cadmium, cement, and antimony

Hypersensitivity Pneumonitis

- Byssinosis results from exposure to cotton dust
- Bagassosis results from exposure to moldy cane sugar
- Farmer's lung results from exposure to molds or fungi on grain, hay, or straw

Signs & Symptoms

- Respiratory insufficiency
- Respiratory pattern is rapid and shallow; keeps work of breathing minimal
- Progressive dyspnea
- Chronic cough
- S/S of congestive right heart failure, including peripheral edema, ascites, jugular vein distention, hepatomegaly, abdominal distress, and increased central venous pressure

Diagnostics

- Chest x-ray can show the type and extent of damage.
- Pulmonary function test can define the type of respiratory disease (restrictive versus obstructive) as well as monitor disease progress; restrictive-type disease will show reduced lung volumes and capacities and a reduced FEV_1.
- Sputum for cytology and culture can be used to rule out neoplasia and infection.

MEDICAL INTERVENTIONS

- There is no specific therapy available.
- Anti-inflammatory drugs such as corticosteroids may be used to reduce the inflammatory process.
- Further exposure to the offending agent must be avoided.

SELECTED NURSING DIAGNOSES

- Ineffective Breathing Pattern
- Activity Intolerance
- Caregiver Role Strain
- Ineffective Family Coping
- Anticipatory Grieving
- Situational Low Self-Esteem

O

SELECTED NURSING INTERVENTIONS

- Teach controlled cough techniques. Explain the need to avoid respiratory irritants (dust, fumes).
- Instruct clients on breathing retraining techniques (e.g., pursed lip and diaphragmatic breathing).
- Instruct client on energy conservation measures.
- Institute progressive range-of-motion (ROM) exercises as tolerated. Encourage rest periods between treatments.
- Encourage client and significant others to verbalize their fears and concerns. Listen and answer questions in a nonjudgmental manner.
- Provide support and reassurance—focus on positive ways of handling stress.
- Provide realistic hope by focusing on short-term goals.

CLIENT TEACHING

- Preventive teaching includes information about occupational lung diseases and methods to reduce their risk. Teach workers measures to reduce dust in their areas and the use of personal protective devices such as masks.
- Teach affected clients to avoid exposure to cigarette smoke, environmental pollutants, and other respiratory irritants. The client should also avoid further exposure to the offending agent.
- Recommend immunizations for influenza and pneumococcal pneumonia.
- Recommend that clients with silicosis receive yearly tuberculin testing.
- Teach the client about pulmonary hygiene measures such as maintaining good fluid intake, coughing, and deep-breathing exercises.
- If the client requires oxygen therapy, teach its use and care of equipment.
- Teach the client about the use and effects of any prescribed or recommended over-the-counter medications.

HOME CARE CONSIDERATIONS

- Referral to a smoking cessation program may be appropriate.

- The client may obtain further information and support from the local chapter of the American Lung Association.

For more information, see the following pages in Medical-Surgical Nursing *by LeMone and Burke:*
Pneumoconiosis, *p. 1449*
Hypersensitivity Pneumonitis, *p. 1449*

Osteoarthritis (Degenerative Joint Disease)

OVERVIEW

- Osteoarthritis (OA) is a degenerative disorder of articular cartilage with accompanying remodeling of bone in the joint.
- Early in the disease, proteoglycans and collagen are lost from the cartilage as a result of enzymatic degradation. Surface ulcerations occur, and fissures develop in deeper layers of cartilage.
- Later, large areas of articular cartilage are lost and underlying bone is exposed. Cysts can develop, and cartilage-coated outgrowths called *osteophytes* occur. As these enlarge, small pieces may break off, leading to mild synovitis.
- OA involves the major weight-bearing joints (vertebrae, hips, knees) most often; it is also seen in the distal and proximal interphalangeal joints of the hands.
- The incidence of OA increases with age.
- OA is the most common form of arthritis.
- Primary and secondary forms have been described.

CAUSES

- *Primary:* genetic and/or metabolic factors
- *Secondary:* trauma, sepsis, obesity, pre-existing congenital deformity, frostbite

Signs & Symptoms

- Onset is usually insidious
- Joint stiffness/pain: deep; aching; worse in morning and with exercise and weather changes
- Crepitus: grating type, with motion
- Decreased range of motion (ROM)
- Joint spurs/deformity: Heberden's and Bouchard's nodes in finger; enlargement of large joints

Diagnostics

- X-ray of joint shows joint-space narrowing, bone cysts, osteophytes, subchondral sclerosis, and absence of the gross inflammation typical of rheumatoid arthritis.
- Erythrocyte sedimentation rate is normal.

MEDICAL INTERVENTIONS

- Analgesics typically are used to manage the pain of OA. Corticosteroids may be injected into the joint space for relief of severe pain. However, this procedure can hasten the rate of cartilage breakdown if performed more frequently than every 4 to 6 months.
- Surgery may be indicated for chronic pain and loss of joint function. Arthroscopy may be employed for clients with OA of the knee. Osteotomy, an incision into or transection of the bone, may be performed to realign an affected joint. Arthroplasty reconstructs or replaces a joint.

SELECTED NURSING DIAGNOSES WITH INTERVENTIONS

Chronic Pain

- Assess the client's level of pain, including intensity, location, quality, and aggravating and relieving factors.
- Administer prescribed analgesic or anti-inflammatory medication as needed.
- Encourage rest of painful joints.
- Apply heat to painful joints using the shower, a tub or sitz bath, warm packs, hot wax baths, heated gloves, or diathermy.

- Emphasize the importance of proper posture and good body mechanics of walking, sitting, lifting, and moving.
- Encourage the overweight client to reduce.
- Teach the client to use splints or other devices on affected joints as needed.
- Encourage the client to use nonpharmacologic pain-relief measures such as progressive relaxation, meditation, visualization, and distraction.

Impaired Physical Mobility

- Assess the ROM of affected joints.
- Perform a functional mobility assessment, evaluating the client's gait, ability to sit and rise from a chair, step into or out of a tub or shower, and negotiate stairs.
- Teach the client active and passive ROM exercises, as well as isometric, progressive resistance, and low-impact aerobic exercises.
- Provide analgesics or other pain-relief measures prior to exercise or ambulation.
- Teach the client the importance of proper posture and good body mechanics when moving. Encourage the client to avoid heavy lifting.
- Encourage the client to plan periods of rest during the day.
- Teach the client how to use ambulatory aids such as a cane or a walker as prescribed.
- Assess the client's home for hazards to safe mobility, such as scatter rugs. Encourage use of devices such as hand rails and grab bars.

Bathing/Hygiene Self-Care Deficit

- Perform a functional assessment of the upper and lower extremities.
- Assess the client's home to determine the need for assistive devices.
- Assist the client to obtain assistive devices.

CLIENT TEACHING

- Teach the client about the disease process and its chronic degenerative nature, treatments, including medication regimen, and ways to slow joint destruction, as discussed above.

- For the client who has undergone a total joint replacement, teach proper use and weight-bearing of the affected limb. Teach the proper use of splints, braces, and so on, and of assistive devices such as walkers or canes.
- Discuss possible complications, including signs of infection or dislocation, and instruct the client to notify the physician promptly if these occur.

HOME CARE CONSIDERATIONS

- Provide referrals to physical or occupational therapy, or other community agencies as indicated.
- The obese client may benefit from a referral to a weight-reduction program.

For more information on Osteoarthritis (Degenerative Joint Disease), see Medical-Surgical Nursing *by* LeMone and Burke, p. 1618.

Osteomalacia (Rickets)

OVERVIEW

- Osteomalacia is a metabolic disorder of bone characterized by reduced ossification of bone protein matrix (osteoid); soft, weak bone results.
- It is usually secondary to a deficiency of vitamin D, which is necessary for precipitation of hydroxyapatite (calcium phosphate crystals).
- In children the condition is called *rickets*. It results in skeletal deformity, especially bowed legs.
- It usually affects weight-bearing bones: pelvis, spine, legs.
- It is more common later in life, and affects women more than men.

CAUSES

- Lack of vitamin D activity from:
  1. inadequate ingestion

2. inadequate sunlight exposure
3. altered metabolism, as in renal disease, or hereditary disorders
- Phosphate depletion, as in renal tubular disorders
- Malabsorption, as in small bowel disease
- Hypoparathyroidism
- Drugs: anticonvulsants, tranquilizers, sedatives, muscle relaxants

Signs & Symptoms

- Skeletal deformity: scoliosis, kyphosis, bowed legs
- Bone pain
- Muscle cramps
- Pathologic fracture, usually of the hip

Diagnostics

- Serum calcium is reduced in severe cases.
- X-rays demonstrate the effects of generalized bone demineralization.
- Bone biopsy is definitive.

MEDICAL INTERVENTIONS

- Therapy typically includes vitamin D supplementation. Calcium and phosphorus supplements also may be prescribed.
- Ultraviolet irradiation may be an adjunct therapy.

SELECTED NURSING DIAGNOSES WITH INTERVENTIONS

Altered Nutrition: Less than Body Requirements

- Review with the client the dietary sources of calcium, phosphorus, and vitamin D.
- Provide consultation with appropriate specialists, especially the dietitian and gastroenterologist.
- Teach clients about foods fortified with vitamin D.

Risk for Injury

- Evaluate the home setting of clients with a high risk of fractures.
- Teach the client safety measures and ways to acquire safety aids for the home.
- Consult with a physical therapist regarding the use of ambulatory or gait devices.

Impaired Physical Mobility

- Instruct the client to space activities to conserve energy.
- Instruct the client to use ambulatory or gait devices.

CLIENT TEACHING

- Teach the client about the disease process, treatments, and expected outcomes. Discuss foods high in vitamin D and calcium, including dairy products. Encourage clients to perform appropriate exercise on a regular basis.
- Encourage clients, especially homebound and institutionalized clients, to get daily brief exposure to the sun, even in winter.
- Teach clients taking large doses of vitamin D about the potentially toxic effect of hypercalcemia.
- Instruct older adults to monitor their intake of fat while taking vitamin D.

HOME CARE CONSIDERATIONS

- Stress the importance of follow-up visits with the physician.
- A referral to a home health nurse may be appropriate.

For more information on Osteomalacia (Rickets), see Medical-Surgical Nursing *by LeMone and Burke, p. 1536.*

Osteomyelitis

OVERVIEW

- Osteomyelitis is an acute or chronic bacterial infection of bone.
- Bacteria can inoculate the bone directly from compound fractures, penetrating injuries, or surgery; or

secondarily from hematogenous spread of bacteria or extension of local soft-tissue infection.

- It usually remains localized, but may spread within marrow to the cortex and periosteum.
- Acute osteomyelitis is the more common form; the chronic form is rare.
- A client with osteomyelitis requires immediate treatment because microorganisms in the microscopic channels of the bone multiply unimpeded. Also, the infection stimulates osteoclastic activity and the resorption weakens the bone.

CAUSES

- Inoculation of bone with virulent bacteria
- *Staphylococcus aureus* is the most common organism. Others include: *Escherichia coli, Pseudomonas, Klebsiella, Neisseria gonorrhea, Haemophilus influenzae, Streptococcus (A, B, G), Mycobacterium tuberculosis, Proteus,* or *Salmonella*
- Population particularly at risk are elderly, malnourished, and immunocompromised patients, or those who have diabetes mellitus, sickle cell disease, chronic obstructive pulmonary disease, or a recent history of open trauma, biopsy, surgery (especially implant), or sepsis

Signs & Symptoms

Local

- Pain in local infection site
- Redness in skin over infection site
- Decreased range of motion (ROM) in nearest joints

Systemic

- Fever/malaise, usually sudden onset
- Nausea
- Tachycardia

Diagnostics

- Differential white blood cell (WBC) count is elevated.
- Blood cultures frequently are positive.
- Erythrocyte sedimentation rate is elevated.

high-protein diet; vitamin D and/or calcium deficiency; estrogen (postmenopausal females) or androgen (aging males) deficiency; history of high caffeine or alcohol intake or smoking

Secondary

- Surgical menopause (bilateral oophorectomy) or castration (bilateral orchiectomy)
- Endocrine disorders: hyperparathyroidism, primary or secondary to renal disease; Cushing's syndrome/disease; hyperthyroidism; hypogonadism
- Metastatic disease: multiple myeloma
- Osteogenesis imperfecta
- Connective tissue disease
- Drugs: glucocorticosteroids; heparin; anticonvulsants; antacids (phosphate binders); isoniazid
- Immobilization
- Alcoholism
- Malnutrition, scurvy

Signs & Symptoms

- May be asymptomatic until fracture occurs
- Pain, usually in the back
- Loss of height/deformity: kyphoscoliosis secondary to multiple vertebral crush fractures
- Pathologic fracture after minimal stress to bone; usually the hip

Diagnostics

- X-ray will show fracture if present; it is not diagnostic for the disease.
- Single or dual photon absorptiometry can measure bone density.
- Bone biopsy is diagnostic, but invasive.

MEDICAL INTERVENTIONS

- Hormonal replacement in postmenopausal women may be used to preserve existing bone mass.
- Other pharmacologic agents include calcium supplements and calcitonin to increase bone formation and decrease resorption. Sodium fluoride enhances trabecular bone mass, but its use remains controversial.

SELECTED NURSING DIAGNOSES WITH INTERVENTIONS

Impaired Physical Mobility

- Teach clients who are able to participate in weight-bearing exercises to perform exercises at least three times a week for a sustained period of 30 to 40 minutes.
- Encourage older adults to use assistive devices to maintain independence in activities of daily living.
- Teach older clients about safety and fall precautions.
- Evaluate and closely monitor the cleint's medications.

Altered Nutrition: Less than Body Requirements

- Teach adolescents, pregnant or lactating women, and adults through the mid-thirties to eat foods high in calcium, to maintain a daily intake of 1200–1500 mg.
- Encourage postmenopausal women to maintain a calcium intake of 1500 mg daily, either through diet or a calcium supplement.
- Collaborate with the dietitian to help the client understand which foods and liquids prevent the absorption of calcium.
- Provide current information regarding the absorption of supplemental calcium.
- Teach clients taking calcium supplements the importance of taking the medication at the proper time and the side effects that may occur.

CLIENT TEACHING

- Teach clients the disease process, and how to limit the severity by diet, activity, supplements, and estrogen replacement therapy as appropriate.
- Discuss the effects of smoking, and encourage the client not to smoke.
- Encourage clients to limit caffeine intake and to avoid diuretics.
- Encourage clients to limit alcohol intake.
- Encourage moderate exposure to sunlight.
- Discuss home safety measures such as tub mats, shower rails, no scatter rugs, use of a walker, and so on.

HOME CARE CONSIDERATIONS

- A dietary consult may be appropriate for this client.
- Provide the name and address of a local osteo-porosis support group.

For more information on Osteoporosis, see Medical-Surgical Nursing *by LeMone and Burke, p. 1527.*

Otitis

Otitis Externa (Swimmer's Ear)
Otitis Media

OVERVIEW

- Otitis is an inflammation of the ear, most often due to infection

Otitis Externa

- Otitis externa affects the skin in the external auditory canal and is usually an acute infection, most common in the summer; a chronic type may indicate underlying systemic disease.

Otitis Media

- Otitis media is an inflammation of the middle ear that can be acute (suppurative) or chronic (serous). Both types are associated with upper respiratory infection and auditory tube dysfunction.
  1. Acute (suppurative) otitis media occurs when edema of the auditory tube impairs drainage of the middle ear, causing mucus and serous fluid to accumulate. This fluid is an excellent environment for the growth of bacteria. This growth and the resultant migration of white blood cells (WBCs) cause pus formation, increasing pressure sufficiently to rupture the tympanic membrane.

2. Chronic (serous) otitis media occurs when the auditory tube is obstructed for a prolonged period, preventing air from entering the middle ear. The resulting negative pressure causes sterile serous fluid to move from the capillaries into the space.

CAUSES

Otitis Externa

- Bacteria: *Proteus vulgaris; Streptococcus; Staphylococcus aureus*
- Fungi: *Aspergillus niger; Candida albicans*
- Skin diseases: psoriasis, seborrhea, hypersensitivity reaction
- Risk factors: working in dirty, dusty conditions; swimming in contaminated water; plugging ears (earphones); inserting object into ear

Otitis Media

- Suppurative: associated with upper respiratory tract infection, that ascends the auditory tube; organisms usually *Pneumococcus, Haemophilus influenzae, beta-hemolytic streptococci, Staphylococcus,* gram-negative organisms
- Serous: inadequately treated acute otitis media, viral infection, allergy, barotrauma

Signs & Symptoms

Otitis Externa

- Bacterial: fever, ear canal pain, local swelling/lymphadenopathy, foul discharge, hearing loss
- Fungal: may be asymptomatic; black/gray tissue growth in canal; red tissue if removed

Otitis Media

- Acute suppurative:
  1. pain, deep and throbbing
  2. fever, low to high
  3. nausea, vomiting, dizziness
  4. hearing loss, mild conductive
  5. bulging, red tympanic membrane on examination; distorted ear anatomy

O

- Acute serous
  1. severe hearing loss
  2. full feeling in ear
  3. abnormal sounds with jaw movement (crackling, popping, echo)
  4. clear fluid behind tympanic membrane on examination

Diagnostics

Otitis Externa

- Culture and sensitivity will identify specific organism.
- Otoscopic examination will show structural manifestations.

Otitis Media

- Otoscopic examination will show structural manifestations.
- Complete blood count (CBC) may show elevated white blood cells indicative of acute bacterial infection.
- Impedance audiometry will show reduced compliance.

MEDICAL INTERVENTIONS

- Systemic antibiotics and analgesics are the drugs of choice. Oral and nasal decongestants also may be prescribed.
- Surgical myringotomy or tympanocentesis may be performed if the tympanic membrane continues to bulge after antibiotic therapy is complete. Antibiotic eardrops may be prescribed postoperatively.

SELECTED NURSING DIAGNOSES WITH INTERVENTIONS

Pain

- Assess the client's pain for severity, quality, and location.
- Instruct the client to use mild analgesics such as aspirin or acetaminophen every 4 hours as needed to relieve pain and fever.

- Advise the client to apply heat to the affected side unless contraindicated.
- Instruct the client to avoid air travel, rapid changes in elevation, or diving until the condition is completely resolved.
- Instruct the client to report promptly an abrupt relief of pain.

Impaired Tissue Integrity

- Stresss the importance of completing the full prescribed course of antibiotics.
- Discuss the desired and potential adverse effects of the prescribed antibiotic. Tell the client to report any adverse effects to the physician.
- Instruct the client who has ventilation tubes inserted to avoid swimming, diving, or submerging the head while bathing as long as the tubes are in place.
- Instruct the client to avoid air travel, rapid changes in elevation, or diving, all of which can cause bruising, hematoma, or hemorrhage.
- Encourage the client to rest, drink ample amounts of fluid, and consume a nutritious diet.

CLIENT TEACHING

In addition to the teaching listed above:

- Teach the client about the disease process, causes and prevention, treatments, and expected recovery time.
- If surgery is necessary, teach the client about the procedure and postoperative care. Provide instruction about any special postoperative precautions, such as avoiding water in the ear canals.
- Tell the client to avoid inserting foreign objects into the ear canal.

HOME CARE CONSIDERATIONS

- Encourage the client to contact the health care provider if symptoms recur or persist despite therapies.

For more information on Otitis, see Medical-Surgical Nursing *by LeMone and Burke, p. 1929.*

Ovarian Cancer

OVERVIEW

- Ovarian cancer is a malignant disease of ovarian structures.
- Most cases (90%) are carcinomas, arising from surface epithelium; germ cell or stromal types account for most of the rest of cases.
- Usually the tumors are nonsecretory.
- Ovarian cancer is the second most common gynecologic cancer, but the most lethal; it is the leading cause of reproductive cancer death in women.
- The incidence increases with age but may occur at any time, including childhood and pregnancy.
- Ovarian cancer spreads rapidly by seeding of intraperitoneal membranes and/or organs.
- It is usually found in advanced stages because it is asymptomatic in early stages.

CAUSES

- Unknown
- Risk factors: family history; primiparous status; previous ovarian, breast, or visceral cancer; upper socioeconomic status
- More common in European American women than African American women

Signs & Symptoms

- Often lacking until the development of ascites or metastatic complications
- Lower abdominal pain
- Urinary S/S: retention, frequency
- Gastrointestinal S/S: dyspepsia, constipation, bloating, full feeling, distention, obstruction
- Weight loss
- Feminization/masculinization (rare)
- Dysfunctional uterine bleeding or postmenopausal bleeding; both are uncommon

Diagnostics

- Ultrasonography may reveal location and size of cancerous mass.
- Computed tomography (CT) scan may reveal areas of metastasis.
- X-rays of the chest, kidneys, and abdomen may show metastasis.
- Barium enema and intravenous pyelogram may show obstruction in bowel or kidneys.
- Peritoneal aspiration may identify atypical cells.
- Exploratory laparotomy with lymph node biopsy is used for definitive diagnosis.

MEDICAL INTERVENTIONS

- Combination chemotherapy is palliative or adjunctive only.
- Usually, total hysterectomy with bilateral salpingo-oophorectomy is performed. Second-look surgery may be done at 6-month or yearly intervals to monitor for possible tumor recurrence.
- Radiation therapy is performed for palliative purposes only.

SELECTED NURSING DIAGNOSES

- Pain
- Risk for Infection
- Death Anxiety
- Altered Family Processes
- Anticipatory Grieving
- Hopelessness

SELECTED NURSING INTERVENTIONS

- Assess level of pain, characteristics, and duration. Provide pain medications as prescribed and monitor for effects. Instruct the client in nonpharmacologic measures to reduce pain, including meditation, guided imagery, distraction, and so on.
- Postoperatively, assess the client frequently for signs of infection. Assess temperature, pulse rate, drainage, appearance of wound, and secretions. Monitor laboratory values.

O

- Encourage the client to express feelings of anxiety. Discuss coping strategies that have worked in the past. Make her a part of the decision-making process whenever feasible. Provide diversion through television, radio, games, and occupational therapies whenever possible.
- Assess interaction between client and significant others. Teach significant others as well as the client about the disease process, treatment options, and prognosis. Also teach skills required for client care.
- Provide referral to home health services, financial assistance, psychologic counseling, clergy, and social services as appropriate.
- Assess past experience of the client and her significant others with loss, existing support systems, and current grief work. Discuss the phases of the grieving process with the client and significant others. Refer them to appropriate resources, including religious or spiritual counselors, legal assistance, or financial assistance.
- Encourage active participation in cancer support groups. Arrange for visits from cancer survivors. Provide positive reinforcement for behaviors that demonstrate initiative, including self-disclosure, self-care, increased appetite, and so on.

CLIENT TEACHING

- Provide pre- and postoperative teaching for the client undergoing hysterectomy, and provide teaching to help the client cope more effectively with side effects from chemotherapy and/or radiation therapy.
- Explain the importance of planned rest periods to the client who has undergone surgery.
- Emphasize the importance of involving family members or significant others in dealing with the client's body image changes.
- Emphasize the importance of follow-up outpatient care for further treatment of cancer as necessary.

HOME CARE CONSIDERATIONS

- As noted above, referrals to home care, cancer support groups, social services, legal services, psychologic counselors, and/or spiritual counselors are appropriate for this client.
- Emphasize the importance of keeping all scheduled follow-up visits.

For more information on Ovarian Cancer, see Medical-Surgical Nursing *by LeMone and Burke, p. 2035.*

O

Pancreatic Cancer

OVERVIEW

- Pancreatic cancer is a primary malignant neoplasm of the pancreas, usually in the head of the gland.
- Most tumors are adenocarcinoma of the duct system (90%), with islet-cell tumors accounting for the rest.
- Pancreatic cancer claims the lives of 95% of those with the disease; it causes about 29,000 deaths per year in the United States. It is a leading cause of cancer death.

CAUSES

- Unknown
- Associated with mutations of the c-K-*ras* genes
- Risk factors: age (rare prior to age 20); slightly more common in males than in females, in blacks than in whites; cigarette smoking (two to three times the risk in heavy smokers); high meat/fat diet; pancreatitis; exposure to naphthalene

Signs & Symptoms

- Often has an insidious/elusive onset
- Abdominal pain: visceral; gnawing; possibly radiating to back
- Anorexia, weight loss, cachexia
- Palpable gallbladder
- S/S of gall bladder obstruction (tumors in head): jaundice; clay colored stools; dark urine
- Splenomegaly
- Glucose intolerance (infrequent)
- Gastrointestinal hemorrhage
- Migratory thrombophlebitis

Diagnostics

- Biopsy will be diagnostic for malignant cells.
- Carcinoembryonic antigen (CEA) may be positive.
- CA 19-9 tumor marker may be positive.

MEDICAL INTERVENTIONS

- The client with an early diagnosis of cancer of the head of the pancreas may have a resectable tumor. In this case, a pancreatoduodenectomy (or Whipple's procedure) is performed.
- Advanced pancreatic cancer is usually treated with palliative chemotherapy and radiation for pain and symptom relief.

SELECTED NURSING DIAGNOSES

- Pain
- Altered Nutrition: Less than Body Requirements
- Anticipatory Grieving
- Impaired Skin Integrity

SELECTED NURSING INTERVENTIONS

- Maintain the client on bed rest, in a comfortable position.
- Ask the client to rate his or her pain on a scale of 0 to 10, considering the frequency, duration, character, and intensity of the pain.
- Administer analgesics as prescribed.
- Administer chemotherapy as prescribed.
- Teach and assist the client with alternative pain-relieving techniques, such as progressive relaxation, therapeutic touch, imagery, and music.
- Encourage the client to change position every 2 hours, to cough, and to deep breathe.
- Administer total parenteral nutrition (TPN) via a central or Hickman catheter as prescribed.
- Monitor intake and output every 8 hours.
- The client's skin may itch because of bile salts excreted through the skin. Keep fingernails short to avoid injury from scratching. Apply hand mitts if necessary.
- Avoid the use of soap. Use bath oils, creams, and lotions to keep skin soft and to prevent itching.
- Use protective barriers around drainage tubes to prevent excoriation.
- Administer medications as prescribed: antiemetics, antacids, pancreatic enzymes, bile salts, and insulin.
- Ask the past experience of the client and significant others with loss. Assess support systems and current

P

grief work. Discuss phases of the grieving process with the client and significant others. Assist them to verbalize their fears and concerns, and provide referrals to appropriate resources.

CLIENT TEACHING

- Teach the client about the disease process, treatment options, and prognosis.
- Teach nonpharmacologic comfort measures such as guided imagery, distraction, meditation, and so on.
- Teach the client recovering from Whipple's procedure wound care and activity restrictions to reduce the risk for infection or injury to the incision site.

HOME CARE CONSIDERATIONS

- Refer the client and significant others to support groups such as the American Cancer Society, social services, psychologic counselors, and religious/spiritual caregivers as appropriate.
- A referral to a long-term care facility or hospice service may be appropriate.

For more information about Pancreatic Cancer, see Medical-Surgical Nursing *by LeMone and Burke, p. 550.*

Pancreatitis

Acute
Chronic

OVERVIEW

- Pancreatitis is an acute or chronic destructive inflammation of the acinar (exocrine) secretory cells.

Acute Pancreatitis

- Develops over a short time course and is potentially reversible; it is associated with the release of proteolytic enzyme; may be mild and self-limiting (edematous) or highly destructive to pancreatic tissue (necrotizing).

Chronic Pancreatitis

- A progressive, permanent destruction of pancreatic acinar cells; associated with atrophy, fibrosis, calcification, and fatty degeneration.

CAUSES

Acute

- Alcoholism (more common in men)
- Cholelithiasis (more common in women)
- Genetics: inherited lipid disorders
- Trauma, surgery
- Metabolic disorders: hypercalcemia, renal failure or transplant, hypertriglyceridemia, fatty liver of pregnancy
- Infections: viral, mycoplasma, parasitic
- Connective tissue disease: systemic lupus erythematosus; thrombotic thrombocytopenic purpura
- Ruptured peptic ulcer
- Drugs: thiazide diuretics; estrogens; salicylates, steroids, nonsteroidal anti-inflammatory drugs (NSAIDs)

Chronic

- Alcoholism
- Genetic: cystic fibrosis; hemochromatosis; deficiencies of trypsinogen or enterokinase, amylase, lipase, protease, $alpha_1$-antitrypsin
- Malnutrition
- Neoplasms: gastrinoma, pancreatic, duodenal
- Surgery: subtotal gastrectomy, vagotomy, pyloroplasty, pancreatic resection

Signs & Symptoms

Acute

- Acute attack often precipitated by heavy eating or alcohol ingestion
- Pain: visceral; mild to severe; constant; boring; epigastric; radiates to periumbilical region, back, chest, flanks, pelvic region; aggravated by lying

P

supine; relieved by sitting forward with knees on chest
- Nausea, vomiting
- Hypoactive bowel sounds, abdominal distention
- Fever
- S/S of shock: tachycardia, hypotension

Chronic
- Weight loss (owing to malabsorption)
- Steatorrhea
- S/S of diabetes mellitus (DM): polyuria, polydipsia, polyphagia
- Abdominal pain: can be absent, sporadic, or chronic

Diagnostics

- Serum/stool/urine lipase is elevated (acute).
- Serum/stool/urine amylase is elevated (acute).
- Serum calcium is low (if fat necrosis).
- Serum glucose is elevated if glucose intolerance/DM.
- White blood cell count is elevated, especially polymorphonuclear leukocytes (PMNs).
- X-rays of the chest or abdomen may identify pleural effusion or elevation of the diaphragm on the left side.
- Computed tomography (CT) scan may identify pancreatic enlargement, fluid deficits, or areas of necrosis.

MEDICAL INTERVENTIONS

- Meperidine hydrochloride may be prescribed to relax smooth muscle and decrease pain. Antibiotics may be administered to prevent or treat infection. Antacids and H_2 antagonists or proton pump inhibitors may be given to neutralize or decrease gastric secretions. Carbonic anhydrase inhibitors or antispasmodics may be administered to decrease the volume of pancreatic secretions.
- The client with severe pancreatitis is given nothing by mouth; instead, a nasogastric tube is inserted and connected to suction, and total parenteral nutrition (TPN) is initiated.

- Surgical resection of all or part of the pancreas may be performed. A cholecystectomy may be performed to remove gallstones.

SELECTED NURSING DIAGNOSES WITH INTERVENTIONS

Pain

- Administer prescribed analgesics on a regular schedule. Assess the location, radiation, duration, character, and intensity of the pain, asking the client to rate the pain on a scale of 0 to 10. Also assess nonverbal indicators of pain.
- Maintain NPO status and nasogastric tube patency as prescribed.
- Maintain client on bed rest in a calm, quiet environment.
- Provide oral and nasal care every 1 to 2 hours. Encourage the client to maintain a comfortable position, such as side-lying with knees flexed and head elevated to 45°.
- Encourage the client to relax and use guided imagery or other nonpharmacologic methods to reduce pain.
- Provide careful explanations of all procedures and care. Listen to the client's concerns and evaluation of pain relief.

Risk for Altered Nutrition: Less than Body Requirements

- Monitor nutritional parameters, including serum albumin, serum transferrin, total lymphocyte count, blood urea nitrogen (BUN), hematocrit, and hemoglobin.
- Weigh the client daily at the same time each day.
- Maintain stool chart; include frequency, color, odor, and consistency of stools.
- Assess the presence and character of bowel sounds.
- Administer prescribed IV fluids and/or TPN.
- Provide oral hygiene before and after meals. Offer small, frequent feedings.

CLIENT TEACHING

- Explain the disease process, treatments, medications, effects, side effects, prognosis, and strategies for preventing further attacks of inflammation.

- Discuss the type of foods to select to meet nutritional needs and to maintain a high-carbohydrate, low-protein, low-fat diet. Also discuss foods to avoid, including alcohol, caffeine, spicy foods, and gas-producing foods. Emphasize the need to avoid large meals and to restrict dietary fats.
- Tell the client that smoking and stress stimulate the pancreas and should be avoided.
- Since an abscess may form months after the initial attack, stress the importance of reporting symptoms of infection, including fever, pain, rapid pulse, and malaise.

HOME CARE CONSIDERATIONS

- Emphasize the importance of follow-up with the physician.
- Provide referrals to a smoking cessation program or to Alcoholics Anonymous as appropriate.
- A referral for home care may be appropriate.

For more information, see the following pages in Medical-Surgical Nursing *by LeMone and Burke:*
Acute Pancreatitis, p. 542
Chronic Pancreatitis, p. 543

Parkinson's Disease

OVERVIEW

- Parkinson's disease is an idiopathic, progressive, bilateral degeneration of the dopaminergic neurons in the basal ganglia of the brain.
- The usual balance of neurotransmitter activity in the brain is disrupted when dopamine production decreases; acetylcholine is no longer inhibited by dopamine. The failure to inhibit acetylcholine is responsible for the symptoms of the disorder.
- Secondary parkinsonism is a syndrome sometimes seen in clients taking tranquilizers or clients with

carbon monoxide or cyanide poisoning. It may also occur as a result of encephalitis. It consists of tremors, rigidity, motor dysfunction, and akinesia.

- Parkinson's disease is relatively common; it mostly begins between 45 and 65 years of age.

CAUSES

- Unknown

Signs & Symptoms

- Akinesia: loss of spontaneous movement (arm swinging, eye blinking)
- Bradykinesia: slowing of voluntary movement
- Rigidity: cogwheel type; of limb muscles
- Rhythmic "pill-rolling" movements of fingers seen mostly during rest
- Tremor of the hands typically seen at rest and disappearing during conscious motion
- Stooped posture
- Shuffling gait with difficult starting and stopping movement
- Loss of facial expression, staring
- Monotonous vocalization
- Dementia in about 25% of cases

Diagnostics

P

- There is no test that clearly differentiates Parkinson's disease from other neurological disorders. Thus, tests are commonly performed to rule out disorders that produce secondary parkinsonism.
- An electroencephalogram (EEG) may indicate slowed pattern and disorganization.

MEDICAL INTERVENTIONS

- Throughout the disease process, drugs and combinations of drugs such as anticholinergics, levodopa, and dopamine agonists may be used for symptom control. Eventually, pharmacotherapeutic agents lose their efficacy and the disease continues to progress despite treatment.

- Surgical destruction of tissue may improve symptoms in clients who do not respond to drug therapy. Autologous adrenal medullary transplant also may be performed.
- Clients frequently benefit from rehabilitation therapy.

SELECTED NURSING DIAGNOSES WITH INTERVENTIONS

Impaired Physical Mobility

- Perform range-of-motion (ROM) exercises at least twice a day, emphasizing the trunk, neck, arms, hips, and legs.
- Consult with a physical therapist to develop an individualized exercise program.
- Ambulate the client at least four times a day.
- Incorporate assistive devices such as canes, splints, or braces as indicated.

Impaired Verbal Communication

- Assess the client's current communication abilities: speech, hearing, and writing.
- Develop methods of communication appropriate to the client's coordination abilities, such as a write-on, wipe-off slate, flash cards with common phrases, pointing to objects, and so on.
- Consult with a speech pathologist to develop oral exercises and interventions that will facilitate speaking.
- Remind the client to speak more loudly, if possible.

Altered Nutrition: Less than Body Requirements

- Assess the client's nutritional status and self-feeding abilities.
- Provide foods of proper consistency as determined by the client's swallowing function.
- Weigh the client weekly, or teach the client or significant others to weigh weekly and notify the physician of significant weight loss.
- Teach eating methods to decrease tremors, such as holding a piece of bread in the hand that is not holding an eating utensil.
- Monitor the diet for foods high in bulk and for high fluid intake.

CLIENT TEACHING

In addition to the teaching described above:

- Teach the client about the disease process, treatment options including medication regimen, and prognosis.
- Teach the client measures to prevent falls, malnutrition, constipation, skin breakdown,and joint contracture.

HOME CARE CONSIDERATIONS

- Coordinate referrals for speech therapy, physical therapy, occupational therapy, psychotherapy, and social services as appropriate.
- Referral to a home health nurse for home care and a home safety check may be appropriate.
- A referral to respite care for caregiver relief may be required. Alternatively, a referral to a long-term-care facility may be necessary if significant others are absent or unable to provide the appropriate level of care.
- Provide the name and address of local support groups.

For more information on Parkinson's Disease, see Medical-Surgical Nursing *by LeMone and Burke,* p. 1838.

P

Pelvic Inflammatory Disease (PID)

OVERVIEW

- Pelvic inflammatory disease (PID) is an infection of the reproductive tract of women that is accompanied by peritonitis.
- Inflammation of each pelvic organ usually occurs: cervicitis (cervix); endometritis (uterus); salpingitis (uterine tubes); parametritis (uterine ligaments); oophoritis (ovary).

- Scarring, usually of uterine tubes, follows.
- PID is most frequently caused by ascending infections due to sexually transmitted diseases (STDs).
- Organisms can also be acquired secondarily: by instrumentation or intrauterine device (IUD); as a postpartum endometritis; following surgery, including cesarean section.
- The disorder can be acute, with overt, systemic manifestations, or subacute and go unnoticed.

CAUSES

Infection due to:
- *Neisseria gonorrhoeae*
- *Chlamydia trachomatis*
- *N. gonorrhoeae* and *C. trachomatis* account for most cases
- *Haemophilus influenzae*
- *Staphylococcus*
- *Streptococcus*
- *Escherichia coli*

Signs & Symptoms

Acute Infection

- Vaginal discharge that is copious, purulent, or mucopurulent
- Pain that is visceral, pelvic, dull/aching, diffuse, increased with cervical motion; possible right-upper-quadrant (RUQ) or pleuritic pain
- Abnormal uterine bleeding prior to, or along with, pain
- Fever is not always present

Subacute Infection

- Will lack above S/S
- Infertility is usually presenting complaint

Diagnostics

- Complete blood count (CBC) with differential reveals a markedly elevated white blood cell count.
- Gram stain of secretions may be diagnostic for causative organisms.

- Culture and sensitivity of secretions may identify causative organism.
- Ultrasound is used to rule out ectopic pregnancy.
- Laparoscopy is the most specific diagnostic tool for salpingitis.

INTERVENTIONS

- Combination antibiotic therapy with broad-spectrum antibiotics is the typical treatment for PID.
- Surgical procedures include draining of any abscess, removal of adhesions, or hysterectomy.

SELECTED NURSING DIAGNOSES WITH INTERVENTIONS

Risk for Injury

- Administer antibiotic therapy as prescribed, and monitor closely for adverse effects.
- Teach the client to recognize and report side effects of medications, as well as manifestations of ectopic pregnancy.
- Provide information about safe sex practices and family planning. Instruct client to remove diaphragm within 6 hours after use. IUDs are contraindicated. Latex condoms offer the most protection against infection.
- Teach the client to report any unusual vaginal discharge or odor to the health care provider.

Anxiety and Fear

- Provide an atmosphere conducive to unhurried expression of feelings and fears; include the partner if appropriate.
- Explain the treatment options, emphasizing those that could preserve fertility, if this is desired.
- Suggest a support group or counselor as needed.

Pain

- Assess the client's level of pain, characteristics of pain, and duration of pain. Note verbal and nonverbal indicators of pain. Administer analgesics as prescribed. Monitor for effects.
- Encourage use of sitz baths and apply heat to lower back or abdomen. Teach other nonpharmacologic

Compromised Mucosal Barrier

- Infection by *H. pylori*
- Prostaglandin E (PGE) inhibitors: aspirin, non-steroidal anti-inflammatory drugs, glucocortico-steroids
- Severe burns or shock (Curling's ulcer)
- Risk factors: alcohol ingestion, chronic gastritis, bile regurgitation, presence of *H. pylori*

Signs & Symptoms

- Pain: epigastric, gnawing/burning; increased between meals; reduced after eating or ingesting antacids
- Dyspepsia, bloating, eructations
- Nausea, vomiting (possibly blood or coffee-ground)
- Black, tarry stools (indicate bleeding)
- S/S of anemia (slow bleeds): pallor, fatigue, tachycardia
- S/S of shock (fast bleeds): pallor, tachycardia, hypotension, cool and clammy skin
- S/S of perforation: sudden, sharp pain; rigid abdomen; shallow breathing; absent bowel sounds; shock

Diagnostics

- Endoscopy can visualize lesions.
- Barium swallow can identify lesions.
- Testing for *H. pylori*

MEDICAL INTERVENTIONS

- Pharmacologic agents used in the treatment of peptic ulcer disease include antacids, which neutralize hydrochloric acid and reduce pepsin activity, H_2-receptor antagonists and proton pump inhibitors, which reduce gastric acid.
- Sucralfate and bismuth subsalicylate may be used to provide a protective coating and promote wound healing; antibiotics are used to eradicate *H. pylori*.
- Surgical procedures for clients with severe peptic ulcer disease include partial gastrectomy, total gastrectomy, pyloroplasty, and vagotomy.

SELECTED NURSING DIAGNOSES WITH INTERVENTIONS

Pain

- Assess pain, including location, type, severity, frequency and duration, and its relationship to food intake or other contributing factors.
- Administer antacids, H_2-receptor antagonists, or mucosal protective agents as prescribed. Monitor for effectiveness and side effects.
- Provide and teach adjunctive relief measures such as distraction, relaxation, and breathing exercises.

Altered Nutrition: Less than Body Requirements

- Assess the client's current diet, including pattern of food intake, eating schedule, and foods that precipitate pain or are being avoided in anticipation of pain.
- Arrange a consultation with a dietitian to identify a meal plan that minimizes PUD symptoms yet meets the nutritional needs of the client.
- Monitor for complaints of anorexia, fullness, nausea, and vomiting or symptoms of dumping syndrome. Adjust dietary intake or medication schedule as indicated.
- Assess and monitor laboratory values for indications of anemia or other specific nutritional deficits. Monitor for therapeutic and side effects of therapeutic measures such as oral iron replacement. If the client is receiving iron orally, do not administer iron and antacids at the same time: wait at least 1 to 2 hours before giving the second medication.

Fluid Volume Deficit

- Monitor and record blood pressure and apical pulse every 15 to 30 minutes until stable. Monitor cardiovascular pressure or pulmonary artery pressure as indicated. Insert a Foley catheter and monitor urinary output hourly.
- Monitor stools and gastric drainage for overt and occult blood.
- Maintain IV therapy with fluid volume and electrolyte replacement solutions; administer whole blood or packed cells as prescribed.

- Insert a nasogastric tube and maintain its position and patency; irrigate with sterile normal saline until returns are clear, if prescribed. Initially, measure and record gastric output every hour, then every 4 to 8 hours.
- Monitor laboratory data for hemoglobin and hematocrit, serum electrolytes, blood urea nitrogen, and creatinine. Report abnormal findings.
- Assess abdomen, including bowel sounds, distention, girth, and tenderness, every 4 hours and record findings.
- Maintain client on bed rest with the head of the bed elevated.

Client Teaching

- Teach the client the disease process as well as preventive and therapeutic strategies.
- Provide written and verbal instruction about the medications prescribed, dosage, effects, and side effects. Stress the importance of continuing medications even when symptoms are relieved, and of avoiding aspirin and other nonsteroidal antiinflammatory drugs.
- Provide information about the relationship between PUD and smoking, alcohol intake, and caffeine.
- Teach the client the symptoms that may indicate complications, such as increased abdominal pain or distention, vomiting, black or tarry stools, light-headedness, or fainting.

HOME CARE CONSIDERATIONS

- Refer the client to a smoking cessation or alcohol treatment program as appropriate.
- A referral for counseling, classes, or support groups for stress reduction may be appropriate.

For more information on Peptic Ulcer Disease, see Medical-Surgical Nursing *by LeMone and Burke, p. 488.*

Pericarditis

OVERVIEW

- Pericarditis is an inflammatory condition of the visceral and parietal pericardial membranes.
- Primary pericarditis is rare, and usually viral; the secondary type is most common; multiple causes exist.
- The condition may be acute (<6 weeks), subacute (6 weeks to 6 months), or chronic (>6 months); acute is most common.
- Chronic constrictive pericarditis results in scarring, thickening, and rigidity of the membranes, impairing ventricular filling and thus cardiac output.
- Chronic adhesive pericarditis results in elimination of the pericardial space and the adhesion of the parietal layer to surrounding structures in the mediastinum, increasing the resistance to outflow of cardiac output; ventricular hypertrophy results.
- Pericarditis may be dry (fibrinous) or exudative with serous, purulent, or bloody fluids.

CAUSES

- Frequently idiopathic
- Infection due to viruses; bacteria, including syphilis; tuberculosis; fungi; parasites
- Immune mediated (hypersensitivity or autoimmune): rheumatic fever, rheumatoid arthritis, scleroderma, systemic lupus erythematosus
- Chest trauma, surgery or radiation
- Neoplasia: primary or metastatic tumors
- Myocardial infarction (MI): acute or post-MI (Dressler's syndrome)
- Drugs: procainamide, hydralazine
- Uremia
- Myxedema

Signs & Symptoms

Acute

- Pain: visceral; retrosternal/left precordial chest and/or pleuritic; may radiate to back, neck,

P

shoulders or arms; severe; sharp; aggravated by inspiration, coughing, movement; relieved by sitting or leaning forward
- Friction rub: during cardiac cycle; up to three components; rubbing, grating, scratching; usually high-pitched; best heard with expiration at lower left sternal border; disappears if effusion develops
- S/S of pericardial effusion: previously present friction rub disappears; faint heart sounds; dyspnea; enlarged cardiac silhouette on x-ray
- S/S of cardiac tamponade: hypotension with increased central venous pressure (CVP); paradoxical pulse; cardiovascular collapse; death

Chronic Constrictive
- Weakness, fatigue
- Anorexia, weight loss, cachexia
- Dyspnea on exertion, orthopnea
- Jugular vein distention
- Positive Kussmaul's sign (failure of CVP to fall during inspiration)
- S/S of right congestive heart failure: ascites, congestive hepatomegaly, peripheral edema

Diagnostics

Acute
- White blood count (WBC) is normal or elevated.
- EKG changes may include diffuse ST segment elevation in all leads or decreased QRS voltage across the leads.
- Echocardiography is the most specific test; it shows effusions.
- Computed tomography (CT) or magnetic resonance imaging (MRI) may identify pericardial effusions or thickening.

Chronic
- Echocardiography can show thickening of the pericardial sac.
- Cardiac catheterization.
- Angiography.
- Biopsy.

MEDICAL INTERVENTIONS

- Nonsteroidal anti-inflammatory drugs (NSAIDs) are used to reduce inflammation and promote comfort. In severe cases, corticosteroids may be used.
- Removal of fluid from the pericardial sac, called pericardiocentesis, may be performed.
- The client with constrictive pericarditis may require a partial or total pericardiectomy: removal of part or all of the pericardium.

SELECTED NURSING DIAGNOSES WITH INTERVENTIONS

Pain

- Assess the client's complaints of chest pain using a rating scale of 0 to 10 and noting the quality and radiation of the pain. Ask the client about factors that aggravate or relieve the pain. Note nonverbal cues of pain and validate them with the client.
- Auscultate heart sounds every 4 hours.
- Administer NSAIDs on a regular basis as prescribed with food. Document effectiveness within 1 hour after administration.
- Provide supportive measures: Maintain a calm, quiet environment, and provide position changes, back rubs, heat/cold therapy, diversional activity, and emotional support.

Ineffective Breathing Pattern

- Assess and document the client's respiratory rate and effort, and auscultate breath sounds every 4 hours. Note and report the presence of adventitious sounds or areas of diminished breath sounds.
- Assess the client for depth of respirations every 2 hours. Help the client breathe deeply and use the incentive spirometer. Provide pain medication for the client at least 30 minutes before respiratory therapy treatments, as needed.
- Administer oxygen as needed.
- Elevate the head of the bed to Fowler's or high-Fowler's position. Assist the client to assume a position of comfort.

P

Risk for Decreased Cardiac Output

- Assess and document vital signs every hour during an acute inflammatory process.
- Assess heart sounds and peripheral pulses, and observe for neck vein distention and pulsus paradoxus, every hour. Notify the physician of the presence of distant, muffled heart sounds, new murmurs or extra heart sounds, decreasing quality of peripheral pulses, and distended neck veins.
- Observe and document changes in trends of hemodynamic parameters and rhythm disturbances. Notify physician of changes.
- Document and notify physician of other signs of decreased cardiac output: changes in level of consciousness; decreased urine output; cold, clammy, mottled skin; delayed capillary refill; and weak peripheral pulses.
- Ensure that at least one IV access line is established, and maintain its patency.
- If emergency pericardiocentesis and/or surgery is needed to evacuate pericardial fluid, prepare the client for the procedure, providing appropriate explanations and reassurance. Observe the client during the pericardiocentesis procedure for adverse effects.

CLIENT TEACHING

- Teach the client about the disease process; treatments, including any procedures such as pericardiocentesis; medications, activity restrictions, and so on.
- If surgery is scheduled, provide preoperative and postoperative teaching as appropriate.

HOME CARE CONSIDERATIONS

- Stress the importance of continuing anti-inflammatory medications as prescribed. Tell the client to take the medications with food to minimize gastric distress, and to monitor his or her weight at least weekly, as these drugs may cause fluid retention. Advise the client to avoid aspirin and over-the-counter preparations containing aspirin while taking other NSAIDs. Finally, encourage the client to maintain a fluid intake of at least 2500 mL per day to avoid renal toxicity.

- Teach the client specific measures to maintain activity restrictions as prescribed.
- Teach the client and significant others about manifestations that may indicate recurrence, and the importance of reporting these promptly to the physician.

For more information on Pericarditis, see Medical-Surgical Nursing *by LeMone and Burke, p. 1165.*

Peripheral Vascular Disease (PVD)

OVERVIEW

- PVD is a general term that usually refers to obliterative arterial disease of the extremities, due to the formation of atheromatous plaques.
- Atheroma formation occurs in the medium to large arteries throughout the body, including coronary and cerebral vessels, but the term PVD is generally reserved for occlusive disease in the extremities; usually the legs.
- Symptoms of PVD develop secondary to the formation of plaques within the extremities themselves (femoral, popliteal, tibial, peroneal) or due to occlusion of feeder vessels (abdominal aorta, iliac).
- Although the atherosclerotic process is slow, an acute closure can occur abruptly because of plaque changes (cracking, bleeding), embolus, vessel spasm; or thrombus formation.
- A reduced blood flow through the narrowed or blocked vessel results in ischemia of cells supplied by the vessels; prolonged ischemia may result in necrosis.

P

CAUSES

- Atherosclerosis is the most common cause; risk factors include: male gender and postmenopausal status in females; age over 45 years; high fat/calorie/cholesterol diet; obesity; diabetes mellitus; hypertension; sedentary lifestyle; smoking; genetic forms of atherosclerosis
- Embolism (acute arterial occlusion); sudden S/S
- Vasculitis
- Trauma to legs
- Buerger's disease
- Raynaud's phenomenon

Signs & Symptoms

- Intermittent claudication: severe cramping pain that accompanies exercise; subsides with rest
- Reduced or absent pulses/bruits on auscultation
- Cyanotic extremities/increased capillary filling time
- Decreased hair, smooth shiny skin, thickened nails
- Poor wound healing, leg ulcers, gangrene

Diagnostics

- Angiography will identify areas of narrowing.
- Doppler flow studies measure blood flow in arteries.
- Digital subtraction angiography allows visualization of specific areas of arteries.
- A lumbar sympathetic nerve block evaluates peripheral circulation.

MEDICAL INTERVENTIONS

- Beta-blockers and vasodilators may be prescribed to decrease pain and improve functional abilities. Analgesics also may be prescribed. Low doses of aspirin are recommended for all clients with severe peripheral vascular disease.
- Conservative measures include daily walking, weight reduction, and smoking cessation.

- Surgery may be indicated if intermittent claudication becomes worse or significantly interferes with the client's physical activities.

SELECTED NURSING DIAGNOSES WITH INTERVENTIONS

Altered Peripheral Tissue Perfusion

- Assess the extremities for peripheral pulses, pain, color, temperature, and capillary refill times at least every 4 hours or more often as needed. If pulses cannot be palpated, use an electronic ultrasound device to locate them.
- Teach the client the importance of keeping extremities in a dependent position.
- Keep extremities warm using lightweight blankets, socks, and slippers. Do not use electric heating pads or hot water bottles to warm extremities.
- Encourage the client to change position at least every hour and to avoid leg crossing.
- Provide meticulous leg and foot care daily, using mild soaps and moisturizing lotions.

Impaired Skin Integrity

- Assess the skin of the extremities at least once each shift and more often if needed. Document findings and changes with each assessment.
- Provide meticulous daily skin care, being sure to keep skin clean, dry, and supple.
- Apply a bed cradle.

CLIENT TEACHING

- Provide the client with information about the disease process and conservative strategies that will help the client to manage the condition. Teach the importance of stress reduction, smoking cessation, exercise, maintaining a healthy weight, and taking medications as prescribed.
- Teach the client and significant others about care of the legs and feet: Keep the legs and feet clean, dry, and well lubricated. Wear well-fitting shoes. Keep toenails trimmed straight across. Avoid exposure to extremes of temperature. Avoid constricting leg garments.

P

HOME CARE CONSIDERATIONS

- A referral to a weight reduction program and/or smoking cessation program may be appropriate.
- A list of support groups, public health services, and other community agencies should be provided to all clients.

For more information on Peripheral Vascular Disease, see Medical-Surgical Nursing *by LeMone and Burke, p. 1214.*

Peritonitis

OVERVIEW

- Peritonitis is an acute or chronic inflammation of the peritoneal membranes.
- Peritonitis most commonly results from a breach in the gastrointestinal wall.
- If the stomach ruptures, a caustic inflammation results from exposure to hydrochloric acid.
- When the colon ruptures, coliform bacteria invade the peritoneal space, causing infection.
- Infectious agents may also ascend the genital tract in females, to reach the peritoneal space.
- Acute peritonitis usually causes a generalized inflammation of the entire abdominal cavity; chronic peritonitis may result in a localized abscess.
- Bacterial peritonitis is the most common form.

CAUSES

- Pelvic inflammatory disease (PID)
- Ruptured viscus: stomach, duodenum, gallbladder, appendix, diverticulum
- Bowel infarct
- Peritoneal dialysis
- Penetrating abdominal trauma
- Spontaneous bacterial peritonitis (accompanies cirrhosis)

Signs & Symptoms

- Pain: visceral; epigastric or abdominal; severe; sharp; increases with movement (patients lie motionless); may be relieved by flexing knees; rigid abdomen; rebound tenderness
- Fever/malaise
- Diaphoresis
- Weakness, prostration
- Nausea, vomiting
- Hiccoughs
- Vital sign changes: tachycardia, hypotension, rapid shallow breathing
- S/S of ileus/obstruction: abdominal distention, hyperresonant abdomen, hyperactive followed by absent bowel sounds

Diagnostics

- White blood cell (WBC) count is elevated, often to >20,000/μL.
- Paracentesis is performed to extract fluid for analysis or culture and sensitivity.
- X-ray of abdomen may show abnormal presence of fluid and/or gas.

MEDICAL INTERVENTIONS

- Antibiotics are prescribed for the client with peritonitis. In addition, narcotic analgesics and possibly sedatives may be given to promote comfort and rest.
- If peritonitis is the result of a perforation, gangrenous bowel, or inflamed appendix, a laparotomy will be performed. Peritoneal lavage may be done during surgery.
- Intestinal decompression may be initiated to relieve abdominal distention, facilitate closure, and minimize postoperative respiratory problems.

SELECTED NURSING DIAGNOSES WITH INTERVENTIONS

Pain
- Assess the client's pain, including its location, severity, and type.

413

- Place the client in a Fowler's or semi-Fowler's position with the knees and feet elevated.
- Once the diagnosis has been established, administer analgesics as prescribed.
- Teach and assist the client to use alternative pain management techniques along with pharmacologic interventions.
- Frequently evaluate the client's response to analgesics.

Fluid Volume Deficit

- Monitor and record the client's intake and output carefully. Urine output is measured every 1 to 2 hours. Report output of less than 30 mL per hour to the physician. Measure GI output at least every 4 hours.
- Monitor vital signs, including blood pressure, pulse, respirations, venous pressure, cardiac output, and pulmonary artery pressures every hour or as indicated.
- Weigh the client daily at the same time of day using the same scale and consistent clothing.
- Assess the client's skin turgor, color, temperature, and mucous membranes at least every 8 hours.
- Measure or estimate fluid losses through abdominal drains and on dressings.
- Monitor laboratory values, including hemoglobin and hematocrit, urine specific gravity, serum osmolality, serum electrolytes, and blood gases. Report changes to the physician.
- Provide IV fluid and electrolyte replacement as prescribed.
- Provide good skin care and frequent oral hygiene.

Altered Protection

- Monitor the client for manifestations of infection, including increased temperature, increased pulse, redness and increased swelling around incisions and drain sites, increased or purulent drainage, and changes in the character of urine output.
- Obtain cultures of purulent drainage from any site.
- Monitor laboratory work for evidence of immune function, including WBC count and differential WBC count, serum protein, and albumin.

- Practice meticulous hand washing on entering and leaving the client's room.
- Use strict aseptic technique when performing dressing changes and wound or peritoneal irrigations.
- Maintain fluid balance and adequate nutrition through either enteral or parenteral feedings, as indicated.

Anxiety

- Assess the anxiety level of the client and significant others and their present coping skills.
- Present a calm, reassuring manner. Encourage the client and significant others to express their concerns. Listen carefully, and acknowledge their validity.
- Minimize changes in caregiver assignments.
- Explain all treatments, procedures, tests, and examinations.
- Reinforce and clarify information provided by physicians.
- Teach and assist the client to practice relaxation techniques such as meditation, visualization, and progressive relaxation.

CLIENT TEACHING

- Explain the disease process, manifestations, treatment, including medication regimen, and prognosis.
- Teach procedures for wound care, including any dressing changes or irrigations that will be required.
- Describe the signs and symptoms of further infection and other potential complications. Stress the importance of reporting these immediately to the physician.
- Discuss the need to consume a diet with adequate kilocalories and protein to meet the needs of the body for healing and optimal immune function.

HOME CARE CONSIDERATIONS

- Tell the client to avoid heavy lifting, strenuous labor, and driving a car until wound healing has occurred.
- Provide information on where to obtain necessary supplies.

P

- A referral to home health care for assessment, wound care, and further teaching may be appropriate.

For more information on Peritonitis, see Medical-Surgical Nursing *by LeMone and Burke, p. 799.*

Pheochromocytoma

OVERVIEW

- Pheochromocytomas are tumors most often arising from chromaffin cells in the adrenal medulla (90%) or in sympathetic ganglia (10%).
- Pheochromocytomas synthesize, store, and secrete catecholamines (epinephrine, norepinephrine); manifestations are due to this excess secretion.
- These tumors are benign 90% of the time and usually unilateral; most are small (<100g).
- They are not common, and are usually seen in adults.

CAUSES

- Sporadic, unknown
- Genetics: 5% are due to an autosomal dominant trait

Signs & Symptoms

- S/S usually appear in paroxysms, varying in duration and frequency
- Hypertension: often severe or malignant; unresponsive to conventional treatment; can be episodic constantly elevated
- Tachycardia or dysrhythmia or angina
- Headache
- Profuse diaphoresis
- Extreme anxiety
- Nausea or vomiting
- Pallor or flushing

- Hypotension/shock: may occur during anesthetic induction, due to down regulation (decrease) in catecholamine receptors

Diagnostics

- Magnetic resonance imaging (MRI) may localize the tumor.
- Computed tomography (CT) may localize the tumor.
- Serum and/or urine chemistries may reveal an elevation of vanillylmandelic acid; metanephrines; free catecholamines

MEDICAL INTERVENTIONS

- Surgical removal of the tumor(s) by adrenalectomy is the treatment of choice.
- Inoperable tumors may be managed with alpha- and beta-adrenergic blocking agents.

SELECTED NURSING DIAGNOSES WITH INTERVENTIONS

Pain
- Administer prescribed analgesics.
- Provide a quiet environment.

Risk for Altered Tissue Perfusion
- Remain with the patient during episodes of hypertension.
- Monitor blood pressure every 10 to 15 minutes.
- Observe the client for any neurologic or respiratory changes.
- Provide a calm, restful environment.

Risk for Altered Nutrition: Less than Body Requirements
- Assess nutritional status and food preferences.
- Assist the client in selecting daily menu (help incorporate basic food groups).
- Ask family or significant others to bring favorite foods from home, within the limits of the prescribed diet.
- Consult with a dietitian to reduce tyramine-containing foods in the diet.
- Monitor daily kilocalorie intake and client's weight.

P

Anxiety

- Explain to the client the basic concepts of the disease and potential risk factors.
- Encourage the client and significant others to ask questions and express their fears and concerns.
- Encourage the client to avoid dietary stimulants (e.g., caffeine, chocolate).
- Provide an environment conducive to rest.

CLIENT TEACHING

See Nursing Interventions.

HOME CARE CONSIDERATIONS

- Emphasize to the client the importance of ongoing outpatient care.
- Provide information on obtaining a MedicAlert® bracelet and card if necessary.
- Explain the need to avoid over-the-counter medications without first consulting a physician.

For more information on Pheochromocytoma, see Medical-Surgical Nursing *by LeMone and Burke, p. 712.*

Phosphate Imbalance

Hyperphosphatemia
Hypophosphatemia

OVERVIEW

- Elemental phosphorus exists in the body as inorganic phosphate and as part of organic molecules such as serum and cell membrane phospholipids.
- Most (85%) body phosphate is complexed with calcium in the bone; about 15% is found in the soft-tissue intracellular fluid (ICF); only 0.1% is present in the extracellular fluid (ECF).

- In serum, 20% of phosphate ions are bound to plasma proteins; 80% is filterable, either as phosphate anions (50%), or as a salt of sodium, calcium, or magnesium (50%).
- Serum phosphate concentration is regulated by a number of factors, including gastrointestinal ingestion and absorption, vitamin D activity, parathyroid hormone function, bone metabolism, nutrient metabolism, acid-base status, and renal excretion.
- Inorganic phosphate is the primary ICF anion.
- High-energy bonds formed with phosphate and nucleotides (ATP, GTP) are important as forms of currency for numerous energy-requiring metabolic reactions.
- Multiple enzyme systems are activated or inactivated via phosphorylation.
- Phosphate is a major renal buffer of hydrogen.
- Phosphate balance is intimately associated with calcium balance; the relationship is reciprocal.
- The normal serum phosphate concentration is 2.5 to 4.5 mg/dL (1.7–2.6 mEq/L).
- Hyperphosphatemia that develops acutely may reduce calcium levels and cause tetany; chronic elevations may cause metastatic calcification of soft tissues or osteodystrophy (renal).
- Hypophosphatemia can result in intracellular phosphate trapping and reduced ATP. Hypophosphatemia can cause respiratory, muscular, neurologic, leukocytic, and erythrocytic dysfunction; skeletal demineralization; metabolic acidosis (if due to decreased vitamin D); rhabdomyolysis; cardiomyopathy.

CAUSES

Hyperphosphatemia (Serum Phosphate >4.5 mg/dL [2.6 mEq/L])

- Increased absorption: phosphate cathartics; excess vitamin D intake; vitamin D–secreting disease (sarcoidosis, TB)
- ICF to ECF shifts: acute acidosis (metabolic or respiratory); insulin deficiency; drugs (clonidine)
- Decreased excretion: renal insufficiency/failure; hormone mediated (hypoparathyroidism, hyperthyroidism, hypoadrenalism, growth hor-

mone excess); drugs (biphosphonate)
- Other: excess serum protein binding (plasma cell dyscrasias); hemolysis; tumor lysis; infarcted tissue; rhabdomyolysis; parenteral (phosphate salts, phospholipids)

Hypophosphatemia (Serum Phosphate <2.5 mg/dL [1.7 mEq/L])

- Decreased absorption: nutritional deficiency (rare); vitamin D deficiency; vomiting; phosphate-binding antacids; malabsorption; diarrhea; steatorrhea
- ECF to ICF shifts: respiratory alkalosis; hormone mediated (insulin, glucocorticoids, epinephrine); nutrient induced (glucose, fructose, amino acids, lactate); neoplasia (lymphoma, leukemia); recovery from hypothermia
- Increased excretion: hormone mediated (hyperparathyroidism, hyperaldosteronism, Cushing's syndrome, SIADH); renal tubular dysfunction; licorice poisoning; diuretics
- Other: chronic alcoholism/alcohol withdrawal; severe burns; hyperalimentation; renal transplantation; exhaustive exercise, diabetic ketoacidosis; volume expansion

Signs & Symptoms

Hyperphosphatemia

- Most S/S are not due to hyperphosphatemia directly, but secondary to hypocalcemia
- Muscle weakness
- Muscle spasms, tetany, hyperreflexia
- Tachycardia
- Anorexia, nausea, vomiting
- Chronic hyperphosphatemia can cause soft-tissue calcification and necrosis

Hypophosphatemia

- Most S/S are related to deficiency of cellular ATP or erythrocyte diphosphogluceric acid
- Acute: muscle dysfunction (skeletal, cardiac, respiratory); neurologic disturbance (irritability,

paresthesia, ataxia, confusion, seizures, coma); skeletal (demineralization); infection, due to leukocyte dysfunction; metabolic acidosis, due to reduced phosphate buffer and reduced NH^{4+}

- Chronic: memory loss; lethargy; bone pain

Diagnostics

- Serum phosphate will be outside the normal range of 2.5 to 4.5 mg/dL (1.7–2.6 mEq/L).
- Parathyroid hormone level will show an elevation in hyperparathyroidism and a decrease in hypoparathyroidism.
- Blood urea nitrogen and creatinine is tested to identify renal failure as a cause of hyperparathyroidism.
- X-rays may show bone changes indicative of hypophosphatemia, or osteodystrophy.

MEDICAL INTERVENTIONS

- The treatment of hyperphosphatemia is aimed at management of the underlying hypocalcemia.
- The treatment of hypophosphatemia is aimed at eliminating drugs that cause loss of phosphate, such as antacids, osmotic diuretics, and calcium supplements, and increasing phosphates in the diet. IV phosphorus is administered only when serum phosphorus levels are less than 1 mg/dl and serious signs of hypophosphatemia are exhibited.

P

SELECTED NURSING DIAGNOSES WITH INTERVENTIONS

Impaired Walking

- Encourage the client to ask for assistance when ambulating.

Impaired Gas Exchange

- Monitor the client's respiratory rate and oxygen saturation levels.

Decreased Cardiac Output

- Monitor EKG for any changes or abnormalities.

Hyperphosphatemia

Altered Nutrition: More than Body Requirements

- Have the client avoid ingestion of milk and dairy products.
- Provide adequate hydration to enhance renal excretion of phosphorus.
- Administer phosphate-binding agents as prescribed.

Hypophosphatemia

Altered Nutrition: Less than Body Requirements

- Offer nutritional snacks, such as Ensure.
- Provide phosphorus-rich foods, such as milk and dairy products.
- Monitor serum phosphate levels frequently.

CLIENT TEACHING

- Teach the client about the disease process, including causes, treatment, and strategies to prevent recurrences.
- For the client with hyperphosphatemia, discuss the importance of avoiding phosphate enemas and over-the-counter medications containing phosphorus. Encourage the client to eliminate foods high in phosphorus from the diet, and supply a list of these foods.
- For the client with hypophosphatemia, discuss the importance of avoiding phosphorus-binding antacids. Provide a list of foods high in phosphorus.

HOME CARE CONSIDERATIONS

- A referral to a dietitian may be appropriate.

For more information, see the following pages in Medical-Surgical Nursing *by LeMone and Burke:*
Hyperphosphatemia, p. 144
Hypophosphatemia, p. 143

Pleural Effusion

OVERVIEW

- Pleural effusion occurs when there is an accumulation of excess fluid in the pleural space, which lies between the visceral and parietal pleural membranes.
- The effusion may be transudative or exudative fluid, pus, blood, or chyle and indicates that a fluid's formation is greater than its removal.
- A *transudate* is the accumulation of a fluid low in protein; usually it results from conditions that increase filtration from pulmonary vessels, or that block lymphatics, which drain pleural fluid.
- An *exudate* is the accumulation of a fluid rich in protein (LDH); it is associated with inflammatory or malignant conditions.
- *Pus* (empyema) accompanies bacterial infection.
- Blood results from trauma.
- Chyle comes from an obstructed thoracic duct.
- There are more than one million cases of pleural effusion each year in the United States.
- The prognosis is poor if signs and symptoms are present; permanent damage is extensive. The disease is progressive.
- Complications include respiratory failure.

P

CAUSES

Transudative

- Congestive heart failure (left-sided) is most common cause
- Pericardial disease
- Cirrhosis with ascites
- Nephrotic syndrome
- Pulmonary embolus

Exudative

- Neoplasms: mesothelioma, metastasis
- Infections: bacterial (empyema), tubercular, viral, fungal, parasitic
- Pulmonary embolus

- Gastrointestinal disorders: esophageal rupture, hiatal hernia, intra-abdominal surgery/abscess
- Collagen vascular disease: systemic lupus erythematosus, drug-induced lupus, rheumatoid pleuritis, Sjögren's syndrome
- Other: sarcoidosis, uremia, radiation, electrical burns, chylothorax

Signs & Symptoms

- Progressive dyspnea
- Cough
- Chest pain, pleuritic
- Decreased breath sounds, decreased tactile fremitus, dullness with percussion
- S/S of heart failure if due to heart failure
- Fever if infectious or malignant cause
- Diaphoresis
- Weight loss if due to tuberculosis or malignancy

Diagnostics

- Chest x-ray can show effusions of >300 mL, or mediastinal shift.
- Thoracentesis to obtain aspirated fluid; analysis will determine type of effusion.
- Biopsy assists in determining cause.

MEDICAL INTERVENTIONS

- Thoracentesis to remove the fluid is the treatment of choice for significant pleural effusion.
- Recurrent pleural effusions, often due to cancer, may be prevented by instilling an irritant such as tetracycline into the pleural space to cause adhesion of the parietal and visceral pleura.

SELECTED NURSING DIAGNOSES

- Risk for Injury
- Impaired Gas Exchange
- Activity Intolerance

SELECTED NURSING INTERVENTIONS

- Prepare for the thoracentesis procedure by assuring that the client has signed an informed consent form, providing client teaching, obtaining a thoracentesis tray and supplies, and placing the client in an upright position, leaning forward, with the arms and head supported on an anchored over-bed table.

- Following a thoracentesis:
  1. Monitor the client's pulse, color, vital signs, and respiratory status frequently.
  2. Assess the puncture site for bleeding or presence of crepitus.
  3. Apply a dressing over the puncture site and position the client on the unaffected side for 1 hour.
  4. Label the obtained specimen with the client's name, date, source, and diagnosis. Send the specimen to the laboratory for analysis.
  5. Obtain a chest x-ray.
  6. If chest tube is inserted, monitor client for signs and symptoms of respiratory distress. Encourage coughs and deep breathing. Document the color and amount of drainage.

CLIENT TEACHING

- Teach the client abdominal breathing technique and encourage its use.
- Teach the client about the disease process, its relationship to the client's underlying disorder, and treatments, including thoracentesis procedure and medication regimen.
- Instruct the client to report to the physician increasing dyspnea or shortness of breath, cough, hemoptysis, and pleuritic pain.

HOME CARE CONSIDERATIONS

- A referral to a smoking cessation program may be appropriate.
- The client may obtain information from the American Lung Association and the American Cancer Society.

For more information on Pleural Effusion, see Medical-Surgical Nursing *by LeMone and Burke,* p. 1470.

Pneumonia

Bacterial
Viral

OVERVIEW

- Pneumonia is an infection of the respiratory bronchioles and alveoli, called the *lung parenchyma.*
- Although almost any type of organism can cause pneumonia, it is most commonly caused by bacteria; the second most common cause is viruses.
- Bacterial pneumonia is generally more serious than viral pneumonia.
- Bacterial infection is characterized by intra-alveolar accumulation of polymorphonuclear leukocytes (PMNs), fibrin deposition, and edema, all contributing to a consolidation of the involved lung tissue.
- The consolidation pattern can be either lobar or bronchial.
- *Lobar* consolidation involves at least one entire lung lobe and is the more serious form.
- *Bronchopneumonia* shows a patchy pattern of consolidation; normal lung units are interspersed among consolidated areas.
- Viral pneumonia is characterized by a bilateral, panlobular pattern; interalveolar accumulation of lymphocytes; inflammation of alveolar septum; necrosis of type I pneumocytes; and hyperplasia of type II pneumocytes in areas of lung parenchyma.

CAUSES

Bacterial

- *Haemophilus influenzae*
- *Streptococcus pneumoniae*
- *Escherichia coli*

Viral

- Influenza virus
- Adenovirus
- Respiratory syncytial virus

- Cytomegalovirus
- Childhood disease viruses: measles, varicella
- Risk factors for pneumonia include:
  1. upper respiratory infection
  2. smoking/pollutants
  3. immunodepression
  4. debilitating disease
  5. prolonged immobility
  6. advanced age/newborns

Signs & Symptoms

- Fever is usually higher with bacterial pneumonia
- Dyspnea
- Cough and, with bacterial pneumonia, rust-colored or purulent sputum
- Chest pain
- Auscultation reveals rales, rhonchi

Diagnostics

- Chest x-ray will show type of infection and monitor progress.
- Sputum Gram stain and culture and sensitivity are used to detect the causative organism and direct therapy.
- A complete blood count (CBC) with white blood cell (WBC) differential is performed. In acute bacterial pneumonia, the WBC is generally elevated to 15,000 to 21,000/μL.
- Arterial blood gases (ABGs) may be ordered to determine blood oxygen and carbon dioxide levels.
- Blood culture is done to rule out sepsis.

MEDICAL INTERVENTIONS

- Medications include antibiotics to eradicate the causative organism and bronchodilators to reduce bronchospasm and facilitate ventilation. An agent to break up mucus or reduce its viscosity may be prescribed.
- Oxygen therapy may be prescribed if the client is tachypneic or if blood measurements reveal hypoxemia.

P

- Chest physiotherapy, postural drainage, and endotracheal suctioning may be prescribed.

SELECTED NURSING DIAGNOSES
WITH INTERVENTIONS

Ineffective Airway Clearance

- Assess the client's respiratory status, including vital signs, breath sounds, and skin color, at least every 4 hours.
- Assess cough and sputum.
- Monitor ABGs and pulse oximetry readings.
- Position the client in Fowler's position. Encourage frequent turning, sitting, and ambulation.
- Assist the client to cough, deep breathe, and use assistive devices. Provide endotracheal suctioning using aseptic technique as prescribed.
- Provide a fluid intake of at least 2500 to 3000 mL per day.
- Work with the physician and respiratory therapist to provide pulmonary hygiene measures.
- Administer prescribed medications and monitor for their effects.
- Administer oxygen therapy as prescribed.

Ineffective Breathing Pattern

- Assess the client's respiratory rate, depth, and lung sounds every 4 hours or more frequently.
- Place the client in an upright or semi-upright position.
- Provide for periods of rest.
- Assess and document pleuritic discomfort. Administer analgesics as prescribed.
- Provide reassurance when the client is experiencing respiratory distress.
- Administer oxygen as prescribed.
- Teach the client to use slow abdominal breathing.
- Teach the client relaxation techniques such as visualization and meditation.

Activity Intolerance

- Assess the client's level of activity tolerance, noting any increase in pulse, respirations, dyspnea, diaphoresis, or cyanosis.
- Assist the client with self-care activities such as bathing.

- Schedule activities, planning for rest periods.
- Provide assistive devices such as an overhead trapeze.
- Enlist the help of significant others to minimize the client's level of anxiety.
- Perform active or passive range-of-motion exercises.
- Provide emotional support and reassurance that the client's strength and activity level will return to normal.

CLIENT TEACHING

- Preventive teaching includes encouraging clients in high-risk groups to obtain immunizations against influenza and pneumococcal pneumonia.
- Stress the importance of following the prescribed medication regimen and completing the entire prescription.
- Instruct the client to limit activity and increase rest. Explain the importance of maintaining a high fluid intake.
- Tell the client to report to the physician any increase in or recurrence of shortness of breath, dyspnea, temperature, fatigue, headache, sleepiness, or confusion. Stress the importance of keeping all follow-up appointments.

HOME CARE CONSIDERATIONS

P

- A referral to a smoking cessation program may be appropriate.
- Provide information on obtaining influenza and pneumococcal pneumonia vaccinations.
- Home health care may be appropriate for elderly clients or those with additional chronic conditions.

For more information, see the following pages in Medical-Surgical Nursing *by LeMone and Burke:*
Bacterial Pneumonia, p. 1392
Viral Pneumonia, p. 1393

Pneumothorax

OVERVIEW

- Pneumothorax is an accumulation of air in the pleural space that results in compression and lung collapse.
- It can be caused by an opening of the parietal pleura (chest wall) or through the visceral pleura (lung rupture).
- A *spontaneous pneumothorax* happens unexpectedly due to rupture of an air-filled bleb, or blister, on the lung surface. Air accumulates in the pleural space until pressures are equalized or until collapse of the involved section causes the leak to seal.
- A *secondary pneumothorax* is characterized by overdistention and rupture of an alveolus. It occurs as a result of some pre-existing condition, usually chronic obstructive pulmonary disease (COPD).
- A *traumatic pneumothorax* occurs secondary to penetrating chest trauma.
- A *tension pneumothorax* results when air enters the chest with inspiration, but is unable to exit with expiration, and is trapped in the chest cavity. The lung on the affected side collapses, and pressure on the mediastinum causes thoracic organs to shift to the unaffected side, placing pressure on the opposite lung as well. Ventilation is severely compromised and venous return to the heart is impaired. Tension pneumothorax is a medical emergency.

CAUSES

- Trauma, chest aspiration, surgery
- Rupture of lung bleb/diaphragm
- Erosion by malignancy
- Positive pressure ventilation
- Air embolism due to decompression
- Bronchopleural fistula

Signs & Symptoms

- Visceral chest pain that is severe, sharp, and stabbing

- Severe dyspnea/shortness of breath
- Cyanosis
- Weakness
- Asymmetric chest contour
- S/S of shock: weak, rapid pulse; rapid, shallow breathing; pallor; anxiety
- Auscultation: diminished/absent breaths sounds
- Severe: tracheal deviation to unaffected side; distended neck veins; subcutaneous emphysema; hypotension

Diagnostics

- Chest x-ray shows air in the pleural space, its location and amount, and mediastinal shift, if present.
- Arterial blood gases show:
  1. pH <7.35
  2. Po_2 <80 mm Hg
  3. $Paco_2$ >45 mm Hg

MEDICAL INTERVENTIONS

- The treatment of choice is placement of a chest tube with water-seal drainage and suction to allow the lung to reexpand.
- A thoracotomy may be performed to excise blebs in clients with recurrence of spontaneous pneumothorax.

SELECTED NURSING DIAGNOSES WITH INTERVENTIONS

Impaired Gas Exchange
- Assess and document vital signs and respiratory status, including respiratory rate, depth, and lung sounds, at least every 4 hours.
- Evaluate chest wall movement, position of the trachea, and neck veins frequently.
- Place the client in Fowler's or high-Fowler's position.
- Administer oxygen as prescribed.
- Provide emotional support, particularly in early stages and during chest tube placement.
- Monitor drainage and function of chest tube.

- Help the client with position changes and ambulation as tolerated.
- Provide for rest periods.

Risk for Injury

- Assess chest tube and drainage system at least every 2 hours.
- When turning the client or providing care, ensure that tension is not placed on chest tubes.
- Secure a loop of drainage tubing to the sheet or client's gown.
- When turning the client to the affected side, be sure that neither the chest tube nor drainage tubing is kinked or occluded under the client.
- Teach the client how to ambulate with the drainage system, keeping the system lower than the chest. In most cases, suction can be discontinued during ambulation.
- Observe the insertion site for redness, swelling, pain, or drainage. Report any signs of infection, including fever, to the physician.
- Should a connection come loose, reconnect it as soon as possible.
- For clients who have an open pneumothorax or who have inadvertently removed a chest tube, seal the wound as soon as possible with a sterile occlusive dressing. Tape the dressing on three sides only.

CLIENT TEACHING

- Teach the client with spontaneous pneumothorax about their future risk, which is 50%. Stress the importance of avoiding smoking to reduce the risk. The client should also avoid exposure to high or low altitudes (e.g., mountain climbing, scuba diving). Also advise the client to avoid contact sports.
- Tell the client that exercise and activity can and should be increased gradually to previous levels.
- Tell the client to report to the physician any upper respiratory tract infection, fever, cough, or difficulty breathing; sudden, sharp chest pain; or redness, pain, swelling, tenderness, or drainage from the chest tube puncture wound.

HOME CARE CONSIDERATIONS

- Provide the client with a referral to a smoking cessation program as appropriate.
- A referral to the local chapter of the American Lung Association may be helpful for information and support.

For more information on Pneumothorax, see Medical-Surgical Nursing *by LeMone and Burke, p. 1472.*

Poliomyelitis

Acute Infection
Postpolio Syndrome

OVERVIEW

- Poliomyelitis is an infection of motor neurons with the poliovirus. It especially affects the anterior horn cells in the spinal cord.
- Infection is usually mild and self-limiting, producing a transitory meningitis with no sequelae. Less commonly, infection results in the complication of paralytic poliomyelitis.
- Poliovirus enters and replicates in the nasopharynx and gastrointestinal mucosa, often from drinking fecally contaminated water. A viremia spreads the organisms to the spinal cord.
- Acute infection is endemic in underdeveloped nations, but is close to eradication in developed countries. It occurs more commonly in warm months (summer, autumn).
- Postpolio syndrome is estimated to emerge in approximately half of clients who had the acute disease. Manifestations may emerge years after the initial infection. Most postpolio syndrome clients are between the ages of 45 and 65. The incidence is slightly higher in women.

- The mortality rate is 5% to 10% for clients with the paralytic form of disease, usually from respiratory arrest. Residual deficits parallel the extent of the original infection.

CAUSES

- Acute episode is caused by infection with poliovirus.
- Cause of postpolio syndrome is unknown.

Signs & Symptoms

Acute Infection

- Fever, malaise
- Nausea, vomiting
- Generalized muscle pain
- Spasms in unaffected muscle groups
- Decreased deep tendon reflexes
- Paralysis may follow above or may be first symptom: asymmetric; flaccid type; may affect muscles of respiration, cranial nerves, or somatic motor nerves
- Sensory changes: hypersensitivity to touch, paresthesias
- S/S of meningeal irritation: headache, stiff neck, Brudzinski's sign, Kernig's sign

Postpolio Syndrome

- Fatigue
- Muscle and joint weakness
- Loss of muscle mass
- Respiratory distress
- Pain
- Cold intolerance
- Dizziness
- Headache
- Urinary incontinence
- Sleep disorders

Diagnostics

- Viral cultures of the throat and stool will identify poliovirus.

- Cerebrospinal fluid (CSF) analysis will reveal excess leukocytes; pressure and protein may be slightly elevated.
- Other diagnostic studies include nerve conduction, muscle strength, and pulmonary function.

MEDICAL INTERVENTIONS

- Treatment is symptomatic.
- Analgesics may be prescribed to relieve pain.
- Respiratory status is carefully monitored and supported as indicated.
- Physical therapy also may be indicated.

SELECTED NURSING DIAGNOSES WITH INTERVENTIONS

Risk for Infection (Client Contacts)

- Collect fecal and nasopharyngeal specimens for laboratory analysis.
- Employ enteric precautions.
- Participate in follow-up of client contacts to ensure immunization.
- Make a report to the local health authority.

Ineffective Breathing Pattern

- Monitor client for dyspnea.
- Initiate ventilatory assistance if needed.
- Monitor for inability to swallow.
- Feed the client via a nasogastric tube if necessary.

Impaired Physical Mobility

- Position the client in a dorsal position with the extremities extended (maintain body alignment).
- Turn the client every 2 hours, or more often as needed.
- Perform range-of-motion (ROM) exercises every 8 hours.

Self-Care Deficit

- Feed the client, and increase diet from fluids to solids as tolerated.
- Assist with bowel and bladder elimination.
- Refer client to home health care prior to discharge.

P

CLIENT TEACHING

- Preventive teaching includes information about immunization with Sabin or Salk vaccines.
- Teach the client about the disease process, treatments, including activity restrictions, medication regimen, use of braces and other assistive devices, and prognosis.
- Teach the client how to prevent fatigue, promote optimal respiratory function, meet self-care needs, modify activities of daily living (ADLs), and maintain safety.
- Stress the importance of follow-up care with nurses, physicians, physical therapists, respiratory therapists, and psychologic counselors as indicated.

HOME CARE CONSIDERATIONS

- Emphasize the importance of lifelong follow-up with the physician. Long-term physcial therapy also may be necessary.
- Referral to a support group can make a positive difference in the client's ability to cope with the disorder. March of Dimes and Polio Network News provide information and support for clients and families.

For more information on Poliomyelitis, see Medical-Surgical Nursing *by LeMone and Burke, p. 1871.*

Polycystic Renal Disease

OVERVIEW

- Polycystic renal disease is a genetic disorder that changes renal parenchymal structures and eventually leads to renal failure.
- Cysts may be solitary or multiple.
- Adult and infantile types exist; the infantile type is extremely rare.

- Functional nephrons in the kidney are changed into fluid-filled cysts, which then impinge on remaining normal nephrons, altering their function.
- In the adult type, the process of cyst formation is bilateral and progressive; the infantile type is present at birth.
- It is associated with liver cysts, berry aneurysm formation, and/or floppy mitral valve; renal calculi and urinary tracy infection often develop.
- About 10% of all cases of chronic renal failure are due to polycystic renal disease.

CAUSES

- Genetic: adult type is autosomal dominant; infantile type is autosomal recessive
- Rarely may occur due to spontaneous mutation
- Faulty gene is located on the short arm of chromosome 16

Signs & Symptoms

- Flank pain
- Palpable kidneys
- Hematuria: gross or occult
- S/S of renal insufficiency: proteinuria, polyuria, nocturia, hypertension, azotemia
- S/S of renal failure: see Renal Failure, Chronic
- S/S of renal calculi: see Renal Calculi
- S/S of urinary tract infection: see Urinary Tract Infection

Diagnostics

- Serum may show elevations in creatinine, blood urea nitrogen (BUN), and uric acid.
- Urinalysis shows dilute urine and/or blood.
- Ultrasonography shows enlarged kidneys and cysts.
- Computed tomography (CT) scan shows cysts.
- Intravenous pyelography shows cysts as well as the extent of kidney involvement.

P

MEDICAL INTERVENTIONS

- Pharmacologic agents include analgesics for pain, antibiotics for infection, and antihypertensive agents and diuretics to control hypertension.
- When pain, infection, or bleeding cannot be controlled, clients with polycystic renal disease require hemodialysis or kidney transplantation.

SELECTED NURSING DIAGNOSES

- Risk for Fluid Volume Imbalance
- Risk for Constipation
- Anticipatory Grieving
- Anxiety
- Risk for Infection

SELECTED NURSING INTERVENTIONS

- Administer analgesics, antihypertensives, diuretics, or other medications as prescribed. Avoid aspirin products, which could cause bleeding.
- Monitor intake and output carefully. Record daily weight and abdominal girth. Notify the physician of any abnormalities.
- Increase intake of fluid and fiber to prevent constipation, unless contraindicated.
- Administer stool softeners or bulk-forming agents as prescribed.

CLIENT TEACHING

- Teach the client self-measurement of blood pressure, and advise the client to measure blood pressure daily.
- Tell the client to monitor temperature if fever is suspected.
- Teach salt and protein limitations as indicated for symptom management. Stress the importance of maintaining fluid intake of at least 2500 mL per day.
- Teach measures to prevent urinary tract infection.
- Explain to the client the need for lifelong follow-up care, and tell the client to notify the physician if the urine becomes foul-smelling or contains blood, if the client experiences pain or other symptoms of urinary tract infection, or if the client develops a persistent headache or visual disturbances.

- Explain the importance of checking with the physician before taking any new drug, including over-the-counter medications, as some may be toxic to the kidneys.

HOME CARE CONSIDERATIONS

- Discuss genetic counseling and screening of family members for evidence of the disease.
- Refer the client to the Polycystic Kidney Research Foundation, the National Kidney Foundation, and the American Association of Kidney Patients for further information and support.

For more information on Polycystic Renal Diseases, see Medical-Surgical Nursing *by LeMone and Burke, p. 950.*

Polycythemia

OVERVIEW

- Polycythemia is an increase in the red blood cell (RBC) count.
- Polycythemia can be relative (related to decreased plasma volume) or absolute (related to increased RBC mass).
- Polycythemia vera is a neoplastic stem-cell disorder characterized by the overproduction of RBCs and, to a lesser extent, certain white blood cell (WBC) elements. It is rare.
- Secondary polycythemia is excess erythropoiesis that arises as a response to either an abnormal increase in the secretion of erythropoietin or prolonged hypoxemia. It is relatively common.
- Polycythemia vera is an idiopathic myeloproliferative disease.
- The prognosis depends on causative factors.
- Complications include thrombus formation and thromboembolism.

P

CAUSES

- Relative polycythemia may be caused by hemo-concentration due to low fluid intake, marked plasma extravasation, profuse vomiting, diarrhea, or sweating.
- Absolute polycythemia may be caused by increased RBC mass due to primary or secondary etiology.
- Secondary polycythemia may be caused by increased erythropoietin secretion due to neoplasms, renal lesions, or familial erythrocytosis. It also may be caused by hypoxia from lung disease, cardiac disease, high altitude, smoking, or abnormal hemoglobin. It is also seen with Cushing's syndrome.

Signs & Symptoms

- Initially may be symptomless, and clients may be diagnosed during routine blood tests
- Skin color: plethoric, ruddy, or cyanotic
- Dizziness
- Headache or "full feeling" in head
- Epistaxis
- Splenomegaly
- Signs and symptoms of embolism

Diagnostics

- RBC count is elevated.
- WBC count is elevated in polycythemia vera.
- Hemoglobin and hematocrit may be elevated.
- Arterial blood gases will show decreased PaO_2 if polycythemia is due to hypoxia.
- Erythropoietin levels will be increased in the secondary forms.
- Bone biopsy will determine if symptoms are due to polycythemia vera.

MEDICAL INTERVENTIONS

- Phlebotomy may be performed repeatedly to keep blood volume and viscosity within normal levels.
- In polycythemia vera, radioactive phosphorus or chemotherapy can be used to suppress marrow function. However, these increase the chance for developing leukemia.

SELECTED NURSING DIAGNOSES

Altered Tissue Perfusion

- Report early signs of bleeding to the physician.
- Explain all necessary procedures; avoid invasive procedures when possible.
- Prepare the client for phlebotomy or apheresis therapy as indicated.

Pain

- Assess the client's level of pain on a scale of 0 to 10, including location, duration, and severity.
- Monitor effectiveness of prescribed analgesics.
- Place the client in a position of comfort.
- Assist the client when changing position.
- Use a bed cradle.
- Teach the client nonpharmacologic measures for pain relief, such as meditation, imagery, and progressive relaxation.
- Maintain a quiet environment.

Risk for Impaired Skin Integrity

- Monitor the client's skin and mucous membranes for cuts, scratches, and mouth sores.
- Instruct clients to avoid restrictive clothing.
- Keep the client's nails short and manicured to prevent scratches.

Knowledge Deficit

- Provide the client with information about his or her condition and progress.
- Discuss symptoms of recurrence and complications to report to the physician.
- Teach the client how to assess skin and peripheral pulses.
- Discuss trauma prevention.
- Explain the importance of regular follow-up care.

CLIENT TEACHING

- Teach the client about the disease process, treatment, and prognosis.
- Encourage the client to drink at least 3000 mL of fluids each day.
- Tell the client to avoid tight or constrictive clothing, especially garters or girdles.

- Tell the client to keep the feet elevated when sitting, to wear support hose while awake and ambulating, and to exercise according to physician's instructions.
- Suggest the client use an electric razor rather than razor blades to shave; a soft-bristled toothbrush; no floss; and to report signs of bleeding to the physician.
- Caution the client to avoid aspirin and aspirin-containing products.
- Emphasize the importance of smoking cessation to clients who smoke.

HOME CARE CONSIDERATIONS

- A referral for a smoking cessation program may be appropriate.
- Tell the client to contact the physician at the first signs of infection or bleeding.

For information on Polycythemia, see Medical-Surgical Nursing *by LeMone and Burke, p. 1286.*

Polyneuropathy

OVERVIEW

- Polyneuropathy is a widespread disorder of all peripheral nerves that results in motor, sensory, or autonomic malfunction.
- Peripheral impairment may result from damage to motor neurons, axons, or the myelin sheath. It is usually secondary to another condition.
- It may be due to genetic, nutritional, metabolic, toxic, ischemic, neoplastic, infectious, or immune processes.
- It may be acute (over days), subacute (over months), or chronic (over years).
- The prognosis depends on control of the underlying process; it is usually good with treatment.

- Complications include disability, respiratory paralysis, pneumonia, and possibly respiratory failure.

CAUSES

- Genetic: amyloidosis (genetic type), Fabry's disease, amyotrophic lateral sclerosis
- Nutritional: alcoholism; vitamin B_1, B_6, or B_{12} deficiency; malabsorption syndromes
- Metabolic: most frequent cause is complication of diabetes mellitus, uremia, porphyria, hypothyroidism
- Toxic: acrylamide, arsenic, lead, organic phosphates, thallium
- Drugs: hydralazine, isoniazid, metronidazole, nitrofurantoin, nucleosides, phenytoin, platinum, megadoses of pyridoxine (B_6), vincristine
- Ischemic: small vessel disease
- Neoplastic: carcinomas, lymphomas, multiple myeloma
- Infectious: Lyme disease, diphtheria, poliomyelitis, HIV
- Immune: Guillain-Barré syndrome (demyelination), Sjögren's syndrome
- Other: trauma, radiation, posthypothermia, frostbite

Signs & Symptoms

P

Motor

- Weakness, distal
- Muscle atrophy
- Decreased deep tendon reflexes

Sensory

- Paresthesias
- Numbness/hypesthesia: stocking-glove pattern
- Pain: peripheral; along nerve route

Autonomic

- Constipation
- Incontinence
- Postural hypotension
- Impotence

Diagnostics

- Electromyography detects whether polyneuropathy is due to axonal degeneration or demyelination.
- Cerebrospinal fluid analysis may indicate an infectious process.

MEDICAL INTERVENTIONS

- Treatment consists of identifying and treating the underlying cause and providing supportive care.

SELECTED NURSING DIAGNOSES

Risk for Injury

- Teach clients with decreased sensation in their legs and feet proper foot care, including daily washing, moisturizing with lanolin lotion, wearing clean cotton socks, and inspecting feet and legs. The client also should wear well-fitting shoes and avoid going barefoot.
- Teach the client to avoid extremes of temperature, hot baths or dishwater, heating pads and electric blankets, and sitting too close to radiators. The client should exercise caution when cooking to avoid burns.

Risk for Ineffective Breathing Pattern

- Encourage the client to cough and perform deep-breathing exercises every 2 hours.
- Position the client to optimize respiratory excursion.

Altered Nutrition: Less than Body Requirements

- Assess the client's food preferences, including likes and dislikes.
- Encourage the involvement of significant others in meals.
- Offer high-protein, high-kilocalorie drinks such as Ensure.

Constipation

- Determine the client's normal elimination patterns and maintain them as much as possible.

- Provide natural bowel stimulants (e.g., coffee, prune juice).
- Encourage the intake of high-fiber foods.

Sexual Dysfunction

- Encourage the client to talk about feelings and concerns related to changes in sexuality.
- Provide supportive counseling services to client, when receptive.

Noncompliance

- Explore the client's willingness to participate in self-help and support groups.
- Avoid a punitive attitude.

CLIENT TEACHING

- Encourage clients who smoke to quit.
- Teach clients with postural hypotension to rise slowly from a sitting or lying position to a standing position and to wear support or antiembolism stockings to minimize pooling of blood in the legs.

HOME CARE CONSIDERATIONS

- A referral to a dietitian may be appropriate to assist the client in maintaining adequate nutrition.
- Referral to a smoking cessation program may be appropriate.
- Refer the client to social services, clergy, physical therapist, occupational therapist, or home health care for support, assistance, and care.

P

For more information on Polyneuropathy, see Medical-Surgical Nursing *by LeMone and Burke, p. 729.*

Potassium Imbalance

Hyperkalemia
Hypokalemia

OVERVIEW

- Potassium, the primary intercellular cation, plays a vital role in cell metabolism and helps determine the membrane potential of nerve and muscle cells.
- The ratio of intracellular potassium to extracellular potassium helps determine the resting membrane potential of nerve and muscle cells; either a deficit or an excess of potassium can adversely affect neuromuscular and cardiac function.
- The largest reservoir of body potassium is within the intracellular space (approximately 3500 mEq, or 90%). The intracellular fluid (ICF) potassium concentration is 140 to 150 mEq/L; the plasma concentration of the extracellular fluid (ECF) fluctuates from 3.5 to 5 mEq/L.
- The ECF potassium depends on such variables as pH, body fluid content, the concentration of certain hormones (aldosterone, glucocorticosteroids, insulin), or any condition that causes potassium to be liberated or shifted from the ICF space.
- Regulation of potassium is achieved primarily by the kidneys. Even when potassium intake is stopped, the kidneys continue to excrete it. Although dietary intake and renal output affect serum potassium levels, movement of potassium into and out of the cells is potentially a greater source of serum potassium changes. Aldosterone assists the kidneys in controlling the level of potassium concentration in the body through a feedback mechanism.
- The normal serum potassium level is 3.5 to 5.0 mEq/L.

CAUSES

Hyperkalemia (Serum [Potassium] >5.0 mEq/L)

- Potassium retention
  1. renal failure

2. Addison's disease
- Potassium shifting (ICF to ECF)
    1. acidosis
    2. insulin deficiency
    3. massive tissue damage (hemolysis, crush injury)
    4. catabolic states
    5. hyperuricemia
- Increased intake of foods containing potassium, including salt substitutes
- Potassium-sparing diuretics
- Factitious: old blood sample

Hypokalemia (Serum [Potassium] <3.5 mEq/L)
- Potassium shifting (ECF to ICF)
    1. alkalosis
    2. high insulin levels
    3. massive tissue repair periods (post trauma, burns)
- Potassium loss
    1. drug therapy: potassium-wasting diuretics, gentamicin, amphotericin B
    2. endocrine disorders: hyperaldosteronism, Cushing's syndrome
    3. GI losses: diarrhea, laxative abuse, vomiting, GI suction, ostomies
    4. diaphoresis
    5. renal tubular dysfunction (potassium wasting)
- Reduced intake of foods containing potassium (as in starvation, crash diets, etc.)
- Water intoxication (dilutional)

Signs & Symptoms

Hyperkalemia
- Overall, increased excitability of nerve and muscles (all types)
- Cardiac S/S: slow, weak pulse; EKG changes (prolonged P-R, wide QRS, ST depression, tall T waves); hypotension; cardiac arrest
- Abdominal muscle cramps
- Diarrhea

- Skeletal muscle spasms
- Weakness
- Irritability/anxiety

Hypokalemia

- Overall, reduced excitability of nerve and muscles (all types)
- Paralytic ileus: reduced bowel sounds, abdominal distension, anorexia
- Skeletal muscle S/S: weakness, paralysis, poor tone
- Cardiac S/S: fast, then slow pulse; dysrhythmias; EKG changes (ST depression, flat T wave, U wave); cardiac arrest
- Respiratory S/S: shallow respirations, shortness of breath
- Paresthesias

Diagnostics

- Serum potassium level is outside normal range.
- Arterial blood gases reveal acidosis, pH <7.35; or alkalosis, pH >7.45.
- EKG will show specific patterns.

MEDICAL INTERVENTIONS

Hyperkalemia

- Measures that favor the intracellular shift of potassium include IV administration of hypertonic dextrose, administration of regular insulin, and IV administration of sodium bicarbonate. Slow IV administration of calcium gluconate is used to suppress temporarily the toxic effects of potassium on the heart.
- To remove potassium from the body, drugs such as sodium polystyrene sulfonate may be administered orally or rectally. In the client with renal failure, hemodialysis and peritoneal dialysis are used to manage hyperkalemia.

Hypokalemia

- Administration of parenteral and/or oral potassium may be prescribed.

SELECTED NURSING DIAGNOSES WITH INTERVENTIONS

Hyperkalemia

Decreased Cardiac Output

- Monitor the EKG rate and rhythm for indications of hyperkalemia, such as development of peaked, narrow T waves, prolongation of the P-R interval, depression of the ST segment, widened QRS interval, and loss of the P wave. Notify the physician of changes.
- Monitor clients receiving sodium bicarbonate closely for fluid volume excess.
- Monitor the administration of calcium gluconate closely, particularly in patients who may be receiving digitalis.

Hypokalemia

Decreased Cardiac Output

- Monitor vital signs at regular intervals, including peripheral pulses.
- Monitor clients taking digitalis for digitalis toxicity. Monitor clients taking antidysrhythmics for resistance to the effects of these drugs.
- In clients on EKG rate and rhythm monitors, observe for the characteristic pattern indicating hypokalemia.
- Monitor the rate of IV potassium administration closely. IV potassium should be diluted and administered via an electronic infusion device. Do not administer undiluted potassium directly into the vein. The usual concentration is 20 to 40 mEq/L. The rate of infusion should not exceed 20 to 40 mEq per hour. Evaluate the client's serum potassium level and clinical symptoms frequently during replacement therapy. In clients receiving rapid potassium replacement, monitor the EKG for evidence of deadly cardiac effects.
- IV potassium administration is painful. Control discomfort over the infusion site. Discomfort may be controlled by applying an ice pack.

CLIENT TEACHING

- Teach the client about the disease process, treatment, and strategies for preventing recurrence.
- Provide the client with a list of potassium-rich foods, salt substitutes, and medications that contain potassium, with individualized instructions.
- Teach the client to measure potassium levels at regular intervals, and to monitor the rate, rhythm, and quality of peripheral pulses daily.

HOME CARE CONSIDERATIONS

- Provide a referral to a dietitian if appropriate.

For more information, see the following pages in Medical-Surgical Nursing *by LeMone and Burke:*
Hyperkalemia, p. 133
Hypokalemia, p. 127

Prostate Cancer

OVERVIEW

- Prostate cancer is a primary malignant neoplasm of the prostate gland.
- Although there are several types of prostate cancer, 95% are adenocarcinomas that arise in the acini, usually at the periphery of the gland.
- Without treatment the tumor invades local tissues, including the seminal vesicles.
- Spread of the neoplasm can occur by direct extension or via the lymph or blood.
- Prostate cancer is the most common malignancy in males, with about 184,500 new cases and 39,200 deaths per year.
- The disease rarely strikes men younger than 50 years of age; incidence rises with age.

CAUSES

- Unknown
- Risk factors:
    1. advanced age; rare in young men
    2. race: African Americans, followed by European Americans, followed by Asian Americans
    3. possibly heredity and diet

Signs & Symptoms

- Asymptomatic in early stages
- First S/S are usually related to urinary obstruction:
    1. dysuria
    2. retention
    3. recurrent urinary tract infection (UTI)
    4. hematuria; painless gross or occult
- Bone pain is a late symptom

Diagnostics

- Digital rectal examination reveals an enlarged, hard, irregularly shaped gland.
- Prostatic specific antigen (PSA) is a sensitive test for detection of early prostate cancer.
- Transrectal sonography will show densities in the peripheral portion of the gland.
- Magnetic resonance imaging (MRI) can localize the tumor for biopsy and show spread.
- Computed tomography (CT) scan can localize the tumor for biopsy and show spread.
- Biopsy is diagnostic for the specific type of cancer.

MEDICAL INTERVENTIONS

- Hormone and chemotherapy therapy is used to treat metastatic prostate cancer.
- Surgery for clients with prostate cancer includes several types of prostatectomies and transurethral resection of the prostate.
- Radiation therapy is used in treatment of prostate cancer and also for palliative care.

P

SELECTED NURSING DIAGNOSES WITH INTERVENTIONS

Altered Urinary Elimination

- Assess the client for the degree of incontinence and its impact on lifestyle.
- Teach the client exercises designed to help restore continence.
- Teach the client methods to control dampness and odor from stress incontinence.
- Teach the client to control occasional episodes of incontinence with absorbent pads worn inside the underwear and changed as needed. Most pads are made with a polymer gel that controls odor.
- Explore options with the client who has total incontinence.
- Help the client to verbalize his feelings about the impact of incontinence on his quality of life.

Sexual Dysfunction

- Assess the client's pretreatment sexual function.
- Teach the client about the impact of therapy on sexual function.
- Assist the client in choosing therapeutic options for erectile dysfunction.

Pain

- Assess the intensity, location, and quality of the client's pain.
- Teach the client and family methods of pain control.
- Instruct the client and significant others about the use of analgesic drugs to control pain.
- Monitor the client's pain status.

CLIENT TEACHING

- Provide information about the disease process, the types of treatment, their side effects, and the prognosis, and listen to the client's concerns.
- Because of the high incidence of prostate cancer metastasis to the spinal cord, clients need to be taught early warning symptoms of spinal cord compression, such as back pain and lower extremity weakness.

- Following surgery, tell clients to avoid strenuous activity, including sexual intercourse, for 6 to 8 weeks. Encourage long walks, and tell the client to continue dorsiflexion exercises done in the hospital to prevent blood clots in the legs. The client may drive after 2 weeks. Tub baths should be avoided while the catheter is in place.
- Tell the client about possible complications to watch for, including excessive bleeding, chills, fever, abdominal pain, swollen or tender scrotum, pain in one calf, chest pain, or difficulty breathing. These should be reported to the physician promptly.

HOME CARE CONSIDERATIONS

- Provide the names and addresses of local cancer support groups. Special prostate cancer support groups may be available in the client's area.
- Emphasize the critical nature of keeping all regularly scheduled follow-up appointments to detect metastasis or local recurrence.

For more information on Prostate Cancer, see Medical-Surgical Nursing *by LeMone and Burke, p. 1977.*

P

Psoriasis

OVERVIEW

- Psoriasis is a chronic inflammatory skin condition characterized by red, scaling plaques.
- Plaques form mostly over the dorsal surfaces and joints.
- Psoriasis represents an abnormally increased rate of epidermal proliferation with polymorphonuclear (PMN) leukocyte infiltration.
- It often occurs in a paroxysmal pattern; exacerbations may be precipitated by skin trauma, infection, or stress.

- Psoriasis is very common, affecting 1% to 2% of the population; it can occur at any age, but usually begins in young adults.

CAUSES

- The cause is unknown; however, some evidence suggests it may be an autoimmune disorder.
- Exacerbating factors include:
  1. sunlight
  2. seasonal changes
  3. hormone fluctuations
  4. steroid withdrawal
  5. certain drugs
- Trauma to the skin from surgery, sunburn, or excoriation are common precipitating factors.

Signs & Symptoms

- Skin lesions: well demarcated, reddish plaques covered by silvery scales
- Lesion locations: over extensor skin surfaces of elbows, knees; on scalp or trunk
- Bleeding: punctate, if scales scraped off
- Nails: pitted, discolored, thickened
- Joint pain, if arthritis is a feature

Diagnostics

- Skin biopsy will distinguish between clinically similar disorders.
- Ultrasonography may be performed to measure skin thickness.

MEDICAL INTERVENTIONS

- Topical corticosteroids, tar preparations, anthralin, and retinoids are typically used to decrease inflammation, prolong the maturity time of keratinocytes, and increase remission time.
- Photochemotherapy is the preferred treatment for severe psoriasis.
- Ultraviolet light therapy may also be used to treat psoriasis.

SELECTED NURSING DIAGNOSES WITH INTERVENTIONS

Impaired Skin Integrity

- Demonstrate methods to reduce injury to the skin when taking therapeutic baths or treatments:
  1. Use warm, not hot, water.
  2. Gently rub lesions with a soft washcloth, using a circular motion.
  3. Blot the skin dry with a soft towel.
  4. Keep the skin lubricated at all times.
- Demonstrate application of topical medications:
  1. Apply the medication in a thin layer.
  2. Avoid getting medication in the eyes, on mucous membranes, or in skinfolds.
  3. Apply a covering over the medicated areas as prescribed. Usually, the covering is applied for only 12 hours, often during the evening and night. Choose some type of plastic wrap that covers the area well.
- Teach the client and significant others the manifestations of infection and to contact the physician if these occur.
- Teach the client and significant others to assess for the complications of treatment: excoriation, increased erythema, increased peeling, blister formation.

Body Image Disturbance

- Establish a trusting relationship by expressing acceptance of the client, both verbally and nonverbally.
- Encourage the client to verbalize feelings about self-perception in view of the chronic nature of psoriasis, and to ask questions about the disease and its treatment.
- Promote social interaction through family involvement in care, referral to support groups, and referral to the National Psoriasis Foundation.

P

CLIENT TEACHING

- Teach the client to eat a healthy, well-balanced diet, to use relaxation techniques to reduce stress, to get adequate rest and exercise, and to avoid exposure to contagious illnesses.
- Tell the client to avoid extremely cold or hot temperatures.
- Encourage the client to expose the skin to sunlight, but to avoid sunburn.
- Stress the importance of avoiding trauma to the skin. Tell the client to use only an electric shaver.

HOME CARE CONSIDERATIONS

- Tell the client to discuss all medications, including nonprescription drugs, with the physician. Some medications may precipitate exacerbations of psoriasis.
- Provide the client with simply written instructions on self-care.
- Refer the client to the National Psoriasis Foundation and local support groups for people with chronic skin conditions.

For more information on Psoriasis, see Medical-Surgical Nursing *by LeMone and Burke, p. 571.*

Pulmonary Edema

OVERVIEW

- Pulmonary edema is the accumulation of excessive fluid within the lungs.
- Fluid first collects in the interstitial spaces, then spills into the alveoli.
- It has multiple causes, and is often classified as cardiac or noncardiac.
- Excess fluid may be secondary to elevations in pulmonary capillary pressure, decreased plasma oncotic pressure, more negative intra-pleural pres-

sure, lymphatic insufficiency, or increased capillary permeability.
- As fluid accumulates, the lungs become increasingly stiffer and more difficult to inflate, producing a restrictive lung disorder, with its characteristic rapid and shallow breathing pattern.

CAUSES

Cardiac

- Left ventricular heart failure (most common cause)
- Valve disease: usually mitral stenosis

Noncardiac

- Adult respiratory distress syndrome (ARDS) due to:
  1. pneumonia
  2. inhaled toxins
  3. aspiration/near drowning
  4. immune reactions
  5. disseminated intravascular coagulopathy (DIC)
- Pulmonary embolism
- Lymphatic metastasis
- Silicosis
- High altitude
- Narcotic overdose
- Toxemia of pregnancy
- Excess IV fluids
- Nephrotic syndrome
- Central nervous system disorders
- Following:
  1. anesthesia
  2. cardiopulmonary bypass
  3. cardioversion
  4. lung transplant
  5. radiation

Signs & Symptoms

- Dyspnea on exertion, orthopnea, paroxysmal nocturnal dyspnea
- Cough: early, nonproductive; advanced, frothy and/or bloody expectorations

P

- Rapid and shallow breathing pattern
- Auscultation: dependent rales, rhonchi
- Diastolic (S_3) gallop
- Neck vein distention
- S/S of shock: rapid, thready pulse; hypotension; cold, clammy, pale skin

Diagnostics

- Arterial blood gases show:
  1. hypoxemia (PaO_2 <80 mm Hg)
  2. early, respiratory alkalosis (pH >7.45, $PaCO_2$ <35 mm Hg)
  3. with respiratory failure, respiratory acidosis (pH <7.35, $PaCO_2$ >45 mm Hg)
- Chest x-ray shows diffuse haziness.

MEDICAL INTERVENTIONS

- Oxygen therapy is instituted for the client in acute pulmonary edema.
- Morphine sulfate is the drug of choice for treating acute pulmonary edema. Potent loop diuretics are administered intravenously to promote rapid diuresis.

SELECTED NURSING DIAGNOSES WITH INTERVENTIONS

Ineffective Airway Clearance

- Ensure airway patency; assess the effectiveness of respiratory efforts and airway clearance.
- Auscultate the client's lungs anteriorly and posteriorly to evaluate airway clearance.
- Encourage the client to cough up secretions; provide nasotracheal suctioning if needed. Assess the color, consistency, and amount of sputum. Teach the client coughing and deep-breathing techniques to facilitate removal of secretions.
- Have emergency equipment readily available in case of respiratory arrest.
- Be prepared to assist with intubation and initiation of mechanical ventilation.

Impaired Gas Exchange

- If the client's blood pressure is adequate, place the client in high-Fowler's position with the legs dangling.
- Provide oxygen and administer IV diuretics and other medications as prescribed.
- Carefully monitor intake and output, catheterizing if necessary for accurate measurement. Expect increased output 5 to 15 minutes after administration of IV diuretic. Restrict fluids as prescribed.
- Continuously monitor the client's blood pressure, pulse, respiratory rate, and cardiac rhythm, as well as the client's subjective feelings about being able to breathe. Monitor trends in the client's arterial blood gases and report any abnormalities to the physician.

Anxiety

- Acute pulmonary edema is a frightening experience. Explain all procedures and the reasons for them to the client and significant others.
- Maintain close contact with the client and significant others, providing reassurance that recovery is often as dramatic as onset.
- Answer questions and provide accurate information in a caring manner.

CLIENT TEACHING

P

- During the acute period, teaching focuses on care measures being performed and their purpose. Keep information brief and to the point. Use short sentences and a reassuring tone to decrease anxiety.
- After resolution of the acute episode, teach the client about the disease process, medications, dosage, effects, and side effects.
- Discuss the need for lifestyle alterations, such as changes in diet and physical activity, to decrease demand on heart and lungs.

HOME CARE CONSIDERATIONS

- A home care referral for assistance with activities of daily living and prescribed medical regimen may be appropriate.

- Referral to a dietitian for consultation regarding a low-sodium diet also may be appropriate.
- Provide the client with the address and phone number of the American Heart Association for educational materials and support groups in the community.

For more information on Pulmonary Edema, see Medical-Surgical Nursing *by LeMone and Burke,* *p. 1137.*

Pulmonary Embolism

OVERVIEW

- Pulmonary embolism (PE) is an obstruction of a pulmonary artery resulting in disruption of blood supply to the lung parenchyma.
- Obstruction can be due to a blood clot, air, or any particulate matter that gains access to the peripheral venous circulation.
- Affected lung portions form areas that are ventilated but not perfused (dead space units).
- Reduced blood flow causes surfactant production by type II pneumocytes to cease; atelectasis follows.
- Pulmonary vascular resistance and pressure increases and may lead to cor pulmonale.
- PE is the most common pulmonary complication, and cause of sudden death, in the hospitalized patient.

CAUSES

- Deep vein thrombosis (DVT) due to:
  1. leg trauma
  2. surgery
  3. prolonged bed rest
  4. clotting disorders
  5. pregnancy
  6. oral contraceptives, especially in smokers

- Fat embolism due to fracture of large bones
- Amniotic fluid embolism
- Air embolism (scuba diving accidents)
- Foreign matter: contaminated IV solutions; injection drug abuse

Signs & Symptoms

- Dyspnea: sudden onset; usually earliest symptom
- Breathlessness
- Tachypnea
- Tachycardia
- Fever: low grade
- S/S of shock: rapid, thready pulse; hypotension; cold, clammy, pale, skin
- If infarction: pleuritic, anginal pain; hemoptysis

Diagnostics

- Ventilation/perfusion lung scan may identify perfusion defect without ventilation defect.
- Arterial blood gases show hypoxemia and respiratory alkalosis (pH >7.45, Po_2 <80 mm Hg, $Paco_2$ <35 mm Hg).
- Fibrin split products may be elevated.
- Chest x-ray may show pleural effusion, areas of atelectasis, or infarction.
- EKG shows tall, spiked P wave; right-shifted QRS, and ST or T-wave abnormalities.
- Computed tomography (CT) scan with contrast media may show central emboli.
- Pulmonary angiography detects emboli as small as 3 mm in diameter.

MEDICAL INTERVENTIONS

- Anticoagulant therapy is used in low doses to prevent pulmonary emboli in clients at risk. Higher doses are used in the client with pulmonary embolism. Thrombolytic therapy may be instituted for clients with a massive pulmonary embolus and hypertension.
- When anticoagulant therapy fails to prevent recurrent emboli or is contraindicated, surgical placement of a filter in the inferior vena cava may be performed.

P

SELECTED NURSING DIAGNOSES WITH INTERVENTIONS

Impaired Gas Exchange

- Conduct and record respiratory assessment frequently, including depth, rate, effort, and lung sounds.
- Monitor and record the client's level of consciousness, mental status, and skin color.
- Place the client in Fowler's or high-Fowler's position, with the lower extremities dependent.
- Start oxygen per nasal cannula or mask as prescribed.
- Monitor arterial blood gas results, and report abnormal findings as indicated. Maintain pulse oximetry and arterial line, if in place.
- Administer vasopressors and other medications as prescribed.
- Maintain bed rest.

Decreased Cardiac Output

- Assess and record vital signs frequently as indicated.
- Auscultate heart sounds every 2 to 4 hours, and report any abnormalities.
- Monitor and record intake and output hourly.
- Assess skin color and temperature.
- Place the client on a cardiac monitor.
- Carefully monitor the response to prescribed vasopressors.
- Monitor pulmonary artery and wedge pressures, neck vein distention, and peripheral edema. Report findings as indicated.
- Maintain intravenous and arterial access sites as well as central lines.
- Provide frequent skin care.
- Instruct the client to report any chest pain or other symptoms.

Fear

- Assess the client's level of anxiety.
- Provide reassurance and emotional support, listening to the client's fears. Do not negate the client's fear of dying, but reassure the client that treatment is generally effective to restore respiratory function.
- Remain with the client as much as possible.

- Explain procedures and treatments, using short, simple sentences.
- Reduce environmental stimuli, and use a calm, reassuring manner.
- Allow calm, supportive family members to remain with the client as much as possible.
- Administer morphine sulfate as ordered to reduce pain and anxiety.

CLIENT TEACHING

- Teach the client about the disease process, prevention measures, and treatment, including the importance of early ambulation and regular exercise such as walking. Teach the client about the prescribed medication regimen.
- For clients on anticoagulants, discuss measures to prevent bleeding, such as using a soft toothbrush, and the need to monitor stool, urine, and sputum for blood. Explain the need to avoid taking aspirin without checking with the physician. Advise the client to wear a MedicAlert bracelet or necklace, and provide information on obtaining one.
- Discuss symptoms that could indicate a recurrence, such as chest pain, shortness of breath, and possibly bloody sputum.
- Stress the need to avoid smoking.

P

HOME CARE CONSIDERATIONS

- Provide a referral to a smoking cessation program as appropriate.
- The client may be in need of a referral for psychologic counseling to help cope with a near-death experience.

For more information on Pulmonary Embolism, see Medical-Surgical Nursing *by LeMone and Burke, p. 1451.*

Pyelonephritis

Acute
Chronic

OVERVIEW

- Pyelonephritis is an inflammation of the renal tubules and interstitial tissues; it may be acute or chronic.
- *Acute* pyelonephritis is a sudden infection of the renal tubules and interstitium by bacteria; usually ascending gram-negative species.
- *Chronic* pyelonephritis is a long-standing tubulointerstitial inflammatory process that results in permanent renal scarring, fibrosis, and eventually renal failure.

CAUSES

Acute

- Bacterial infection: usually ascending from lower urinary tract infection (UTI); possibly traumatic, hematologic, or lymphatic route
- Bacterial species: *Escherichia coli* (80%), *Proteus, Pseudomonas, Staphylococcus saprophyticus* or *aureus, Streptococcus faecalis*
- Risk factors:
  1. catheters
  2. urinary tract surgery, instrumentation, or trauma
  3. stasis
  4. neurogenic bladder
  5. sexual activity (women)
  6. pregnancy

Chronic

- Recurrent or untreated bouts of acute pyelonephritis
- Tubulointerstitial kidney disease: hereditary (polycystic kidney, Alport's syndrome); toxic (extrinsic, metabolic); immune (hypersensitivity, amyloidosis, transplant rejection); vascular (sickle cell

nephropathy, nephrosclerosis); neoplastic (lymphoma, leukemia, multiple myeloma)
- Vesicoureteral reflux
- Urinary obstruction

Signs & Symptoms

Acute

- S/S of UTI: dysuria; frequency; urgency; nocturia; hematuria (occult); cloudy, foul-smelling urine
- Fever: 102 F (38.9C) or greater
- Shaking chills
- Pain: flank; costovertebral angle tenderness
- Anorexia
- Malaise

Chronic

- S/S of UTI: dysuria; frequency; urgency; nocturia; hematuria (occult); cloudy, foul-smelling urine
- S/S of renal insufficiency: proteinuria, polyuria, nocturia, hypertension, azotemia
- S/S of chronic renal failure: see Renal Failure, Chronic

Diagnostics

- Urinalysis in acute condition will show greater than 100,000 bacteria per mL urine; it will be cloudy, with red blood cells (RBCs), white blood cells (WBCs), and pyuria.
- The serum WBC count will be elevated.
- Culture and sensitivity will identify specific organism and treatment.
- X-ray of the kidneys, ureters, and bladder may show or rule out calculi, tumors, and cysts.
- Intravenous pyelogram may show a swollen (acute) or shrunken (chronic) kidney.

MEDICAL INTERVENTIONS

- Pharmacologic agents include antibiotics, analgesics, and urinary antiseptics.
- Surgery is indicated if there are structural defects in the kidney that may cause obstruction, or if the infection becomes intractable, at which time a nephrectomy may be performed.

P

SELECTED NURSING DIAGNOSES WITH INTERVENTIONS

Pain

- Assess pain parameters: timing, quality, intensity, location, duration, and aggravating and alleviating factors.
- Provide comfort measures. Nonpharmacologic relief measures include warm sitz baths, warm packs or heating pads, balanced rest and activity. Systemic analgesics, urinary analgesics, or antispasmodics may be administered as prescribed.
- Increase fluid intake unless contraindicated by therapeutic regimen.

Altered Urinary Elimination

- Monitor urinary output and color, clarity, and character of urine, including odor.
- Provide for easy access to a bedpan, urinal, commode, or bathroom.
- Teach the client to avoid caffeinated drinks and alcohol.

Knowledge Deficit

- Collaborate with the client to develop a plan for taking medications, such as taking them with meals (unless contraindicated) or setting out all doses for the day in the morning.
- Instruct the client to complete the full course of antibiotic therapy even if symptoms resolve rapidly.
- Instruct the client to keep appointments for follow-up and urine culture.

CLIENT TEACHING

- Teach the client about the disease process, causes, treatments, and prevention strategies. Review the medication regimen and stress the importance of completing all prescribed antibiotics.
- If surgery was performed, provide postoperative teaching, including the importance of avoiding heavy lifting and manual labor for the prescribed time.
- Teach the signs and symptoms of recurrence and stress the importance of reporting these immediately to the health care provider.

HOME CARE CONSIDERATIONS

- Schedule a follow-up appointment with the physician as prescribed, and stress the importance of follow-up care for any signs of recurrence.
- Information is available from the National Kidney Foundation and the American Urological Association.

For more information on Pyelonephritis, see Medical-Surgical Nursing *by LeMone and Burke, p. 956.*

P

Raynaud's Phenomenon

OVERVIEW

- Raynaud's phenomenon is an arterial vasospastic condition of the distal extremities that is usually initiated by exposure to cold.
- Attacks are paroxysmal, initiated by exposure to cold or stress, and have two phases with three color changes; there is usually bilateral distribution.
- In the early, *ischemic,* stage, small arterial vessels in the fingers and toes spasm, blanching the digits and making them cold to the touch; venous dilation accompanies, and as oxygen is extracted from venous blood, cyanosis develops.
- The *hyperemic* phase follows, as the previously contracted arterioles fully dilate (reactive hyperemia), increasing perfusion to such an extent that the digits turn bright red (rubor) and feel warm.
- Raynaud's phenomenon may be secondary to a number of conditions or follow several traumatic injuries; the primary form is idiopathic and referred to as Raynaud's disease.

CAUSES

Primary

- Idiopathic: possibly due to intrinsic imbalance in sympathetic control

Secondary

Associated with:

- Occlusive arterial disorders: acute arterial occlusion, atherosclerosis, Buerger's disease (thromboangiitis obliterans), thoracic outlet syndrome
- Collagen vascular disorders: rheumatoid arthritis, systemic lupus erythematosus, progressive systemic sclerosis/scleroderma, dermatomyositis, polymyositis
- Pulmonary hypertension
- Trauma: frostbite, vibration damage, electric shock, occupational (typing, hammering, jackhammering, playing music)

- Neurologic conditions: carpal tunnel syndrome, herniated nucleus pulposus, spinal cord tumors, stroke, polio, syringomyelia
- Blood dyscrasias: cold antibody disease; myelo-proliferative disorders
- Drugs: beta-adrenergic blockers, bleomycin, cis-platin, ergot compounds, methylsergide, vin-blastin

Signs & Symptoms

Ischemic Phase
- Blanching: of fingers, possibly toes
- Cyanosis: follows blanching
- Coldness of digits accompanies blanching and cyanosis
- Paresthesias may accompany blanching and cyanosis

Hyperemic Phase
- Rubor
- Rewarming of digits

Long-Term Changes
- Trophic changes in skin, nails, connective tissue, muscle
- Gangrene (possible)

Diagnostics

- An arteriogram may identify plaques.

R

MEDICAL INTERVENTIONS
- Conservative treatment measures include wearing gloves when outside in cold weather, stress reduction, exercise, smoking cessation, and maintaining a healthy body weight.
- Vasodilators are sometimes prescribed for symptom relief, and analgesics may be prescribed for pain.

SELECTED NURSING DIAGNOSES
- Altered Tissue Perfusion: Peripheral
- Risk for Impaired Skin Integrity

- Chronic Pain
- Self-Esteem Disturbance

SELECTED NURSING INTERVENTIONS

- Assess and record objective signs of an episode, including signs of color changes and swelling, and record subjective reports of numbness, coldness, tingling, and pain.
- Assist client to identify precipitating events, and to develop strategies for preventing or minimizing future occurrences.

CLIENT TEACHING

- Review the disease process, treatment, including medications, and strategies for preventing further attacks.
- Teach the client that the primary prevention strategy is to protect the extremities from exposure to temperature extremes (including cold water) and from trauma.
- Encourage lifestyle habits that contribute to vascular health, including limiting dietary fat, increasing activity level, maintaining healthy body weight, stopping smoking, and managing stress effectively.

HOME CARE CONSIDERATIONS

- Referrals to smoking cessation, weight reduction, and stress management programs may be appropriate.

For more information on Raynaud's Phenomenon, see Medical-Surgical Nursing *by LeMone and Burke, p. 1228.*

Renal Calculi (Nephrolithiasis, Kidney Stones)

OVERVIEW

- Renal calculi are masses of crystals, composed of materials normally excreted in the urine, that form within the renal calyces or pelvis.
- They cause hematuria, obstruct urine flow, and can lead to hydronephrosis.
- Stones can be composed of calcium salts, or uric acid; cystine or struvite ($MgNH_4PO_4$).
- Men most frequently form calcium-salt stones; women more commonly form struvite stones secondary to urinary tract infection (UTI) with bacteria of the *Proteus* species.
- When stones enter a ureter, they cause obstruction, bleeding, and severe pain.

CAUSES

- Hypercalciuria: idiopathic; prolonged bed rest; hyperparathyroidism
- Hyperuricemia: gout; renal disease, dehydration, malignancy, high protein diet
- Infection: *Proteus,* urease-producing
- Hereditary cystinuria

Signs & Symptoms

- Hematuria: gross or occult; usually precedes all other symptoms
- Renal colic is the pain due to stone entrapment in the ureter
  1. flank area, radiates to groin/scrotum
  2. severe and sharp or dull and aching
  3. intermittent or constant
  4. visceral type
- S/S of shock: rapid, thready pulse; hypotension; cold, clammy, pale, skin; nausea

R

- S/S of UTI: dysuria, frequency, urgency, nocturia, hematuria (occult)
- S/S of renal insufficiency: proteinuria, polyuria, nocturia, hypertension, azotemia

Diagnostics

- Urinalysis may be positive for blood; possibly positive for white blood cells (WBCs) and pyuria.
- Urine studies may detect elevated calcium or uric acid levels or abnormal metabolites.
- Chemical analysis of stones may determine the type or whether they are due to metabolic disease.
- X-rays of the kidneys, ureters, and bladder will show most types of stones.
- Ultrasonography can detect obstructive changes such as hydroureter and hydronephrosis.
- Intravenous pyelogram may determine the size and exact location of stones.

MEDICAL INTERVENTIONS

- Narcotic analgesics are used to provide analgesia and moderate the ureteral spasms. Drugs with anticholinergic activity may be used adjunctively to help relieve ureteral spasm. A thiazide diuretic, frequently prescribed for calcium calculi, acts to reduce urinary calcium excretion and is very effective in preventing further stones.
- Dietary changes include increased fluid intake regardless of stone composition. For calcium stones, the recommended diet restricts foods rich in calcium and is high in acid-ash foods. A diet low in purines is recommended for clients with uric acid stones. Organ meats, sardines, and other high-purine foods are eliminated from the diet. Clients with uric acid and cystine stones require increased amounts of alkaline-ash foods.
- Stones that are too large to be passed spontaneously may require surgical intervention. The newest procedure for destruction and removal of renal calculi is extracorporeal shock-wave lithotripsy (ESWL).

SELECTED NURSING DIAGNOSES
WITH INTERVENTIONS

Pain

- For all complaints of pain, assess the intensity, quality, location, timing, aggravating and relieving factors, and associated symptoms.
- Administer pain-relief measures as prescribed.
- Unless contraindicated, increase fluid intake and encourage ambulation in the client with ureteral colic.
- Use nonpharmacologic measures such as positioning, moist heat, relaxation techniques, guided imagery, and diversion as adjunctive therapy for pain relief.
- For the client who has had surgery, monitor urinary output, catheters, incision, and wound drainage.

Altered Patterns of Urinary Elimination

- Monitor urinary output for quantity, pattern, and presence of stones. Measure all urine. If the client is catheterized, measure hourly. Document the presence of hematuria, dysuria, frequency, urgency, and pyuria. Strain all urine for stones, saving any recovered stones for laboratory analysis.
- Maintain patency and integrity of all catheter systems in place. Secure catheters well, label as indicated, and use sterile technique for all prescribed irrigations or other procedures.

R

CLIENT TEACHING

- Teach the client about all diagnostic and therapeutic procedures. If the client is to be discharged prior to stone passage, teach the client to collect and strain all urine, saving any stones; to report stone passage to the physician and bring the stone in for analysis; and to observe the amount and character of urine, reporting any changes.
- Instruct the client in measures to prevent further renal calculi: increase fluid intake to 2500 to 3500 mL per day; follow recommended dietary guidelines; maintain an activity level that will prevent urinary stasis and bone resorption; and take medications as prescribed.

- When the client is discharged with dressings, a nephrostomy tube, or a catheter, both the client and significant others need to know how to change dressings and manage the drainage systems. Teach sterile technique for dressing changes, and teach wound care.
- Tell the client to report recurrent stone symptoms to the physician immediately, and to return to the physician periodically for continued monitoring.

For more information on Renal Calculi (Nephrolithiasis, Kidney Stones), see Medical-Surgical Nursing *by LeMone and Burke, p. 908.*

Renal Failure

Acute
Chronic

OVERVIEW

- Renal failure is the cessation of normal renal function; it may be acute or chronic.
- *Acute renal failure (ARF)* is classified according to cause as prerenal, intrarenal, or postrenal; the onset is rapid and potentially reversible.
- *Chronic renal failure (CRF)* is progressive and usually takes years to reach the end stage.
- The stages of acute versus chronic renal failure are different.

Acute Renal Failure

- Stage I—onset: precipitating event until oliguria; development of azotemia (decreased blood urea nitrogen [BUN], creatine); lasts hours to days
- Stage II—oliguric: urine output >400 mL/24 hours; continued azotemia; edema develops; lasts one to several weeks

- Stage III—diuretic: urine output above normal, to 10 L/day; asotemia resolving
- Stage IV—recovery: slow return to normal renal function; not always a feature; may convert to CRF

Chronic Renal Failure

- Stage I—decreased renal reserve: begins when 50% of nephron units are destroyed (glomerular filtration rate [GFR] is 50%); normal units compensate; asymptomatic
- Stage II—renal insufficiency: GFR is 20% to 35% of normal; anemia, azotemia, hypertension, and polyuria develop
- Stage III—renal failure: GFR is 5% to 20% of normal; anemia, azotemia, hypertension, and polyuria worsen; edema develops; acid-base and electrolyte disturbances begin; activities of daily living (ADLs) are reduced; systemic S/S begin
- Stage IV—end-stage renal disease (ESRD) (uremia): GFR is less than 5% of normal; all S/S listed above worsen; all body systems become involved; oliguria leading to anuria; without dialysis or transportation, death ensues

CAUSES

Acute Renal Failure

Prerenal: Mechanism is decreased renal perfusion

- Shock:
    1. Cardiogenic
    2. Hypovolemic:
        a. hemorrhage
        b. dehydration
        c. third spacing: the movement of a significant amount of fluid from the blood into a third space (i.e., space not usually containing this much fluid)
- Renal artery obstruction:
    1. Spasm
    2. Strictures
    3. Thrombus
    4. Embolus
    5. Neoplasm

R

Intrarenal: Mechanism is intrinsic nephron disease

- Acute tubular necrosis:
    1. Acute pyelonephritis
    2. Prerenal ischemia >30 minutes
    3. Nephrotoxins
    4. Acute transplant rejection
- Acute glomerulonephritis
- Intratubular obstruction

    1. Hemolysis (hemoglobin)
    2. Rhabdomyolysis (myoglobin)
    3. Multiple myeloma (immunoglobulin)
    4. Uric acid crystals

Postrenal: Mechanism is postrenal obstruction

- Uretral obstruction:
    1. Calculi
    2. Strictures
    3. Neoplasms
- Bladder obstruction

    1. Benign prostate hypertrophy (BPH)
    2. Prostate cancer
    3. Pelvic neoplasms
    4. Bladder caluli
    5. Neurogenic bladder
- Urethral obstruction

    1. Strictures
    2. Neoplasms
    3. Foreign bodies
    4. Swelling

Chronic Renal Failure

- Can develop from any of the above, if left untreated or controlled
- Additional cases include:
    1. Immune-mediated glomerulonephropathies (glomerulonephritis)—the most common cause
    2. Hereditary renal diseases
    3. Diabetes mellitus, complications of
    4. Hypertension, complications of

Signs & Symptoms

Acute Renal Failure

- Azotemia: a recent rise in nitrogenous wastes
- Oliguria, leading to anuria (rare), leading to polyuria, leading to a return to normal output
- Edema: generalized, pitting
- Hypertension
- Gastrointestinal S/S:
  1. Nausea, vomiting, anorexia
  2. Hematemesis
  3. Constipation
  4. Stomatitis
  5. Uremic fetor (breath)
- Central nervous system S/S:
  1. Headache
  2. Drowsiness
  3. Irritability
  4. Confusion
  5. Seizures
  6. Coma
- S/S of metabolic acidosis: Kussmaul's respirations (hyperventiltion)

Chronic Renal Failure

- Renal/urologic S/S
  1. Stages II/III: polyuria (nocturia), leading to salt wasting, leading to hypokalemia/hyponatremia, leading to volume contraction, leading to hypotension
  2. Stage IV: oliguria, leading to salt retention, leading to hyperkalemia/hypernatremia, leading to volume expansion, leading to hypertension; hypocalcemia; hyperphosphatemia; azotemia; continuous rise in creatine, BUN, uric acid, metabolic acidosis
- Cardiovascular S/S
  1. Hypertension
  2. Left ventricular hypertrophy
  3. Myopathy
  4. Uremic pericarditis/friction rub/effusion

R

5. S/S of left ventricular congestive heart failure (CHF)

    a. pulmonary edema
    b. dyspnea
    c. dyspnea on exertion
    d. orthopnea
    e. paroxysmal nocturnal dyspnea
    f. frothy expectoration
    g. wet rales
    h. cyanosis

6. S/S of right ventricular CHF:

    a. peripheral edema, ascites
    b. jugular vein distention
    c. hepatomegaly
    d. weight gain
    e. abdominal distress
    f. increased central venous pressure
    g. cyanosis

- Hematologic S/S

    1. Anemia: normocytic, normochromic; hemolysis
    2. Leukopenia: increased susceptibility to infection
    3. Thrombocytopenia/decreased clotting factors: abnormal bleeding

- Respiratory S/S

    1. Uremic lung: pneumonitis, pleura pain/friction rub, increased susceptibility to pulmonary infection
    2. S/S of compensatory response to metabolic acidosis:

        a. Kussmaul's respirations (hyperventilation)
        b. deep sighing/yawning

    3. S/S of pulmonary edema:

        a. dyspnea
        b. dyspnea on exertion
        c. orthopnea
        d. paroxysmal nocturnal dyspnea
        e. frothy expectoration
        f. wet rales

- Gastrointestinal S/S

    1. Nausea, vomiting, anorexia
    2. Hematemesis

        3. Constipation/diarrhea
        4. Uremic gastritis
        5. Stomatitis
        6. Uremic fetor (breath)
        7. Metallic taste
- Neurologic S/S

        1. Headache
        2. Drowsiness
        3. Irritability
        4. Inability to concentrate
        5. Confusion
        6. Seizures
        7. Coma
        8. Peripheral neuropathy
        9. Paresthesias
        10. Muscle twitching, tremors
        11. Slurred speech
- Musculoskeletal S/S

        1. Muscle: weakness, twitching, spasms
        2. Bone: osteodystrophy, pain, pathologic fracture
- Endocrinologic S/S

        1. Hyperparathyroidism
        2. Hyperaldosteronism
        3. Hypogonadism (see below)
        4. Carbohydrate intolerance
- Dermaologic S/S

        1. Pallor; yellow-gray skin tint
        2. Ecchymosis/purpura
        3. Dry skin
        4. Severe pruritis (due to uric acid crystals)
        5. Uremic frost (due to uric acid crystal precipitates; rare today with dialysis)
        6. Skin breakdown (soft tissue calcification)
- Reproductive S/S

        1. Females: amenorrhea, reduced libido, infertility
        2. Males: reduced libido, impotence, infertility

Diagnostics

- Serum creatinine shows azotemia (elevations in creatinine, BUN, uric acid); elevated potassium; low hemoglobin.

- Urinalysis may show casts, cellular debris; altered specific gravity; proteinuria; hematuria.
- Arterial blood gases show respiratory acidosis (pH <7.35, $Paco_2$ >45 mm Hg).
- Ultrasonography can show renal and renal pelvic anatomy; masses/obstruction; hydronephrosis.
- Renal scan can estimate renal perfusion.
- X-rays of the kidneys, ureters, and bladder can show size, shape, or some types of obstruction.
- Intravenous pyelogram can show size, shape, and perfusion pattern of kidneys.
- Renal biopsy will delineate underlying pathologic process.

MEDICAL INTERVENTIONS

Acute Renal Failure

- Dopamine is useful to increase renal blood flow. A loop or osmotic diuretic may be administered along with fluid resuscitation. All drugs that are nephrotoxic or that may interfere with renal perfusion are discontinued. Histamine H_2-receptor antagonists may be administered to prevent gastrointestinal hemorrhage. A potassium-binding exchange resin may be administered to treat hyperkalemia, and aluminum hydroxide, an antacid, may be used to treat hyperphosphatemia.
- Once any impairment of renal perfusion is corrected and vascular volume is restored, fluid intake is generally restricted during the oliguric phase.
- The client in ARF needs an adequate intake of nutrients and calories to prevent catabolism: proteins are limited to minimize azotemia, and carbohydrates are increased.
- The client in ARF who cannot be managed conservatively may require dialysis.

Chronic Renal Failure

- Diuretics may be prescribed to reduce the volume of extracellular fluid. Antihypertensive agents are often employed to maintain the blood pressure within normal levels and slow the progress of renal failure. Other pharmacologic agents may be used to manage the electrolyte imbalances and acidosis accompanying CRF. Folic acid and iron supplements are useful to combat the anemia associated with CRF.

- Water and sodium intake is regulated to maintain the extracellular fluid volume at normal levels. Potassium intake is carefully regulated to avoid serum levels that put the client at risk for lethal cardiac rhythm disruptions. Regulation of protein intake is indicated for the client in CRF.
- When conservative management is no longer effective, dialysis or renal transplantation are considered.

SELECTED NURSING DIAGNOSES WITH INTERVENTIONS

Acute Renal Failure

Fluid Volume Imbalance

- Assess and document intake and output hourly.
- Weigh the client at the same time each day or more frequently as indicated. Use the same scale and have the client wear the same clothes or drapes.
- Monitor and record vital signs at least every 4 hours.
- Frequently assess breath sounds for the presence of rales and heart sounds for the presence of an S_3 or S_4 gallop. Assess the degree of peripheral edema and distention of neck veins.
- If not contraindicated by other factors, place the client in semi-Fowler's position.
- Monitor serum electrolytes; report abnormal results and signs and symptoms of electrolyte imbalance.
- Restrict fluids as prescribed. Provide frequent mouth care and encourage the use of hard candies to decrease the thirst response.
- Administer medications with meals.
- Turn the client frequently and provide good skin care.
- Administer diuretics as prescribed and monitor the client's response.

Altered Nutrition: Less than Body Requirements

- Monitor and document food intake, including both the amount and type of food consumed.

R

- Weigh the client at the same time daily, documenting weight accurately.
- Arrange for consultation with a dietitian to plan a diet that meets the therapeutic requirements and takes the client's food preferences into account.
- Engage the client in planning daily menus.
- Allow the client's family to prepare meals within the dietary restrictions and encourage family members to eat with the client.
- Provide frequent, small meals or between-meal snacks.
- Administer antiemetic agents as prescribed and provide mouth care prior to meals.
- Administer and monitor parenteral nutrition as prescribed for the client who is unable to eat or tolerate enteral nutrition.

Chronic Renal Failure

Altered Tissue Perfusion

- Regularly monitor intake and output; vital signs, including orthostatic blood pressures, and weight.
- Restrict fluids as prescribed, usually to 500 mL per day plus an amount equivalent to the previous 24-hour urinary output unless the client is undergoing dialysis.
- Monitor respiratory status, including lung sounds, at least every 8 hours.
- Monitor laboratory results for BUN, serum creatinine, pH, electrolytes, and CBC.
- Assess the client for evidence of electrolyte imbalances, including cardiac dysrhythmias and other EKG changes, muscle tremors and possible tetany, and Kussmaul's respirations.
- Administer aluminum hydroxide gel, calcium carbonate, sodium bicarbonate, and sodium polystyrene sulfonate as prescribed.
- Monitor the client carefully for desired and adverse effects of all medications administered.
- Monitor blood pressure carefully and administer antihypertensive medications as prescribed.
- Time activities and procedures to allow for periods of rest.

Risk for Infection

- Use standard precautions and good hand-washing techniques at all times.
- Use strict aseptic technique when handling ports, catheters, and incisions.
- Monitor the client's temperature and vital signs at least every 4 hours.
- Monitor the client's WBC count and differential.
- Culture urine, peritoneal dialysis fluid, and other drainage as indicated.
- Provide good oral hygiene at least every 4 hours.
- Provide good respiratory hygiene including position changes, coughing, and deep breathing.
- Restrict visits from obviously ill visitors. Educate the client and significant others about the risk for infection and measures to reduce the spread of infection.

CLIENT TEACHING

- Teach the client about the nature of the disease, diagnostic tests and therapeutic procedures, and treatment options, including dietary and fluid restrictions. Instruct the client about the signs and symptoms of complications. Teach the client how to monitor weight, blood pressure, and pulse.
- Instruct the client to avoid nephrotoxic drugs.
- The client on hemodialysis needs to know how to assess and protect the fistula or shunt, and, if dialysis is to be done at home, how to perform the procedure and care for the catheter. If possible, a significant other should also be instructed fully in the hemodialysis procedure.
- When a renal transplantation has been done, provide teaching about medications, adverse effects and their management, infection prevention, and the signs and symptoms of organ rejection.

HOME CARE CONSIDERATIONS

- The client with ARF or CRF may need a referral for home care.
- Local chapters of the National Kidney Foundation and the American Association of Kidney Patients

R

on Hemodialysis and Transplantation may be able to provide information and support for clients.

For more information, see the following pages in Medical-Surgical Nursing *by LeMone and Burke:*
Acute Renal Failure, p. 979
Chronic Renal Failure, p. 990

Respiratory Failure

OVERVIEW

- Respiratory failure is a state characterized by:
  1. inadequate oxygenation of the blood (hypoxemia);
  2. inadequate carbon dioxide removal (hypercapnia/hypercarbia); and
  3. respiratory acidosis.
- There are three patterns by which respiratory failure can develop:
  1. *hypoxemic failure,* or inadequate oxygen reaching the blood (Pao_2 <50 mm Hg);
  2. *hypercapnic failure,* or hypoventilation, $Paco_2$ >50 mm Hg); or
  3. *hypoxemic-hypercapnic failure,* ($Paco_2$ <50 mm Hg and $Paco_2$ >50 mm Hg).

CAUSES

Hypoxic (Oxygenation) Failure

- Reduced fraction of inspired o_2
- Pneumonia
- Pneumothorax
- Pulmonary embolism
- Pulmonary edema, acute
- Pulmonary hypertension
- Ventilation/perfusion mismatching leading to right-to-left shunt
- Adult respiratory distress syndrome (ARDS)
- Abnormal hemoglobin

Hypercapnic (Ventilation) Failure

- Hypoventilation:
  1. respiratory muscle fatigue/paralysis
  2. mechanical deformation of chest wall
  3. central respiratory center depression
  4. severe pain

Hypoxic-Hypercapnic (Combination) Failure

- Obstructive disorders:
  1. asthma
  2. chronic obstructive pulmonary disease (COPD)
- Left ventricular congestive heart failure

Signs & Symptoms

- S/S of pulmonary edema: dyspnea, dyspnea on exertion, orthopnea, paroxysmal nocturnal dyspnea, frothy expectoration, wet rales
- Ventilation pattern changes: rapid, shallow; slow, shallow
- S/S of hypoxia: headache; anxiety/agitation, confusion, coma, cor pulmonale
- S/S of hypercapnia: shock, respiratory acidosis
- S/S of shock: rapid, thready pulse; hypotension; cold, clammy, pale skin

Diagnostics

- Arterial blood gases (ABGs) show respiratory acidosis: pH <7.35, Po_2 <80 mm Hg, $Paco_2$ >45 mm Hg.
- Chest x-ray may show the cause of failure as pneumonia, pulmonary edema, chest-wall deformity, pneumothorax, or ARDS.

MEDICAL INTERVENTIONS

- Pharmacologic management consists primarily of bronchodilators to reverse airway spasm and constriction, and antibiotics to treat infection.
- Oxygen therapy is vital to reverse hypoxemia.
- Clients who do not readily respond to supplemental oxygen therapy, who have an upper airway obstruction, or who need positive-pressure mechanical ventilation require intubation with an endotracheal

R

tube. Mechanical ventilation is indicated for acute respiratory failure.

SELECTED NURSING DIAGNOSES WITH INTERVENTIONS

Ineffective Breathing Pattern

- Assess and document the client's respiratory rate and other vital signs every 15 to 30 minutes.
- Assess the client for other signs of respiratory distress, including nasal flaring, use of accessory muscles, intercostal retractions, cyanosis, increasing restlessness, anxiety, or a decreased level of consciousness.
- Monitor ABG results and pulse oximetry readings for evidence of improving or worsening respiratory status. Report changes promptly.
- Administer oxygen as prescribed, monitoring the client's response. Observe closely for signs of respiratory depression, especially in clients with COPD.
- Place the client in Fowler's position.
- Minimize activities and energy expenditures by assisting the client with care, spacing procedures and activities, and allowing uninterrupted rest periods.
- Avoid sedatives and respiratory depressant drugs.
- Prepare for endotracheal intubation and mechanical ventilation.
- Explain the procedure and its purpose to the client, providing reassurance that this is a temporary measure to reduce the work of breathing and allow the client to rest. Tell the client that talking is not possible while the endotracheal tube is in place, and establish a means of communication.

Ineffective Airway Clearance

- Assess the client's respiratory status frequently, including rate, ventilator settings, chest movement, and lung sounds.
- Assess coordination of respiratory efforts with ventilator. Be sure to count the client's respiratory rate, not that of the ventilator.
- Monitor and assess oxygen saturation and ABGs.
- Suction the client as needed to maintain a patent airway.
- Obtain a specimen for culture if the sputum appears purulent or develops an odor.

- Perform percussion, vibration, and postural drainage as indicated.
- Use minimal occluding volume technique, minimal leak technique, or measured pressures of 20 to 25 mm Hg in the cuff of the endotracheal tube.
- Firmly secure the endotracheal tube. Provide adequate slack to prevent tension when turning or positioning.
- Assess the client's fluid balance, and maintain adequate hydration.
- Change the client's position frequently, using semi-Fowler's and Fowler's positions if tolerated.

Risk for Injury

- Assess the client frequently.
- Do not bypass or turn off any ventilator alarms.
- Turn and reposition the client frequently.
- Keep skin and linens clean, dry, and wrinkle-free. Moisturize and massage pressure points frequently.
- Perform passive range-of-motion (ROM) exercises every 4 to 8 hours.
- Keep side rails up and use soft restraints as needed.
- Administer histamine H_2 blockers and antacids as prescribed.

CLIENT TEACHING

- Teach the client about the disease process. Provide explanations for all procedures, monitors, tubes, machines, and alarms.
- Teach the client alternative communication strategies. Explain to significant others that the client, although not able to speak, is able to hear and understand. Emphasize the importance of talking to the client, not above or about the client. Explain that mechanical ventilation is a temporary measure.
- Teach the client measures to prevent future respiratory failure. Teach effective coughing, and pulmonary hygiene measures such as percussion, vibration, and postural drainage.
- Clients with end-stage COPD and recurrent respiratory failure may choose terminal weaning rather than face a future of further disability. Discuss the terminal weaning process with the client and significant others, and explain that support services,

R

such as clergy, psychotherapists, and so on, are available to the client and loved ones.

HOME CARE CONSIDERATIONS

- Referral to a smoking cessation program may be appropriate.
- Encourage the client to obtain influenza and pneumococcal vaccinations.
- The client may require a referral to a long-term-care facility, or a home health nurse.

For more information on Respiratory Failure, see Medical-Surgical Nursing *by LeMone and Burke,* p. 1484.

Rheumatoid Arthritis

OVERVIEW

- Rheumatoid arthritis (RA) is a chronic, progressive, systemic inflammatory disease.
- RA displays a wide variety of symptoms between clients, but almost always produces an inflammatory synovitis, usually in the small joints of the hands and feet.
- The immunologic activity of RA includes infiltration and proliferation of T lymphocytes or T cells in the synovial membrane, initiating an immune response. Many of the inflammatory features of RA appear to result from the release of cytokines, which further stimulate macrophage activity. B cells are then stimulated to produce autoantibodies known as rheumatoid factors, which are the hallmark of the disease. The end stage of this immune process is the release of lysosomal enzymes that destroy joint tissue.
- Inflammation causes hyperemia and pannus formation, which erodes articular cartilage, followed by scarring, fibrosis, and bony ankylosis of the affected joint.

- RA can affect people at any age but is most frequently diagnosed between 35 and 50 years of age.
- RA affects about 1% of the population, with a female-to-male ratio of 3 to 1.
- The course is highly variable, but most clients experience progression at a moderate rate.

CAUSES

- Unknown, but probably autoimmune
- Genetic factors associated with certain HLA types
- Possible environmental triggers: Mycoplasma, Epstein-Barr virus, cytomegalovirus, parvovirus, rubella virus, "superantigens"

Signs & Symptoms

Early

- Fever, malaise
- Anorexia, weakness
- Joint swelling and pain: usually distal joint of hands and feet, but varies; symmetric pattern; worse in morning
- Decreased range-of-motion (ROM)
- May be accompanied by lymphadenopathy or splenomegaly
- Possible systemic manifestations: rheumatoid nodules, skeletal muscle atrophy, rheumatoid vasculitis (can lead to mono/polyneuritis), pleural fibrosis, constrictive pericarditis, scleritis, osteoporosis, Felty's syndrome (splenomegaly, neutropenia, anemia, thrombocytopenia)

Late

- Knobby joint deformity
- Ulnar drift of fingers
- Contractures

Diagnostics

- Rheumatoid factor is positive in 70% to 80% of cases.
- Erythrocyte sedimentation rate typically is elevated.
- Complete blood count (CBC) often shows anemia.
- X-ray of affected joints as the disease progresses

R

may show osteoporosis around the joint, joint space narrowing, and erosions.

MEDICAL INTERVENTIONS

- Aspirin, other nonsteriodal anti-inflamatory drugs (NSAIDs), and analgesics are used to reduce the inflammatory process and manage signs and symptoms. If necessary, low-dose corticosteroids are added to the regimen.
- Disease-modifying drugs including gold salts, anti-malarial agents, sufasalazine, and D-penicillamine, can decrease disease activity.
- For clients with severe RA, immunosuppressive or cytotoxic drugs may be employed.
- Surgeries such as synovectomy, arthrodesis, or arthroplasty may be performed for severe cases.

SELECTED NURSING DIAGNOSES WITH INTERVENTIONS

Pain

- Assess the level of pain and duration of morning stiffness.
- Encourage the client to relate pain to activity level and adjust activities accordingly. Teach the importance of joint and whole-body rest.
- Teach the use of heat and cold applications to provide pain relief.
- Teach about the use of prescribed anti-inflammatory medications and the relationship of pain and inflammation.
- Encourage the client to use other nonpharmacologic pain-relief measures such as visualization, distraction, and meditation.

Fatigue

- Encourage the client to balance rest and activity.
- Stress the importance of planned rest periods during the day.
- Help the client prioritize activities, performing the most important ones early in the day.
- Encourage the client to engage in regular physical activity in addition to prescribed ROM exercises.
- Refer the client to counseling or support groups.

Altered Role Performance

- Discuss the effects of the disease on the client's career and other life roles. Encourage the client to identify changes brought on by the disease.
- Encourage the client and family to discuss their feelings about role changes and grieve lost roles or abilities.
- Listen actively to concerns expressed; acknowledge the validity of concerns about the disease, prescribed treatment, and prognosis.
- Help the client and family identify strengths they can use to cope with role changes.
- Encourage the client to make decisions and assume personal responsibility for disease management.
- Encourage the client to maintain life roles as far as the disease allows.

CLIENT TEACHING

In addition to the above:

- Teach the client about the disease process, including systemic effects such as stiffness, fatigue, anorexia, and weight loss.
- Emphasize the importance of taking medications as prescribed, and not on an as-needed basis. Encourage the client to take aspirin or other NSAIDs with food or milk to mimimize gastric distress and to report GI symptoms or black stools to the physician promptly.
- Discuss the use of asssistive devices and where to obtain them.
- Stress the importance of keeping all follow-up appointments with the physician.

HOME CARE CONSIDERATIONS

- Refer the client to a dietitian, physical therapist, or occupational therapist as necessary.
- The client may require a referral to social services or a home health nurse.

For more information on Rheumatiod Arthritis, see Medical-Surgical Nursing *by LeMone and Burke, p. 1639.*

Scoliosis

OVERVIEW

- Scoliosis is a lateral deviation of the thoracic, lumbar, or thoracolumbar spine; it may curve left or right.
- As scoliosis emerges, the muscles and ligaments shorten on the concave side of the curvature. Over time, progressive deformities of the vertebral column and ribs develop, causing one-sided compression of the vertebral bodies.
- Twisting of the spine axis can also occur and may result in a compromised rib cage.
- Scoliosis is associated with lordosis (swayback) and kyphosis (humpback).

CAUSES

- Hereditary: possibly autosomal dominant or polygenic; later in life
- Congenital vertebral deformity: present at birth
- Secondary: asymmetric paralysis, cerebral palsy, or muscle disease
- Functional: poor posture; inequality in limb lengths

Signs & Symptoms

- Visible curvature of spine
- Unequal hip, shoulder, elbow heights
- Asymmetric back muscles
- Backache, fatigue
- Possible dyspnea if chest volume is decreased

Diagnostics

- Upright anterior-posterior and lateral x-rays of the spine will show deformity. The degree of curvature is measured by determining the amount of lateral deviation to the left or right.

MEDICAL INTERVENTIONS

- Conservative treatment for adults with scoliosis may include weight reduction, active and passive exercises, and the use of braces for support.

- Surgery for severe scoliosis involves attaching metal reinforcing rods to the vertebrae.

SELECTED NURSING DIAGNOSES WITH INTERVENTIONS

Risk for Injury

- Assess the environment for safety hazards.
- Teach the client ways to reduce irritation of skin surfaces beneath the brace.
- Teach the client to loosen the brace during meals and for the first 30 minutes after each meal.
- Instruct the client in the importance of maintaining body alignment.
- Turn the client by using the log-rolling technique.
- Use a fracture bedpan when the client needs to urinate or defecate.
- Teach the client how to apply the brace and explain ambulatory restrictions.
- Instruct the client who has been on extended bed rest to change slowly from a reclining position to sitting position.
- Instruct the client to sit on the edge of the bed for a few minutes prior to ambulating.

Risk for Peripheral Neurovascular Dysfunction

- Following spinal surgery, assess the movement and sensation of lower extremities every 2 hours for the first 8 hours, then every shift and as needed.

CLIENT TEACHING

In addition to the above:

- Teach the client about the disease process, contributing factors, treatment, and prognosis.
- Following spinal surgery, teach the client activity restrictions as prescribed.

HOME CARE CONSIDERATIONS

- Following surgery, the client may require social services or a home health nurse.

For more information on Scoliosis, see Medical-Surgical Nursing by LeMone and Burke, p. 1557.

Shock

Cardiogenic
Postcardiac
Hypovolemic
Distributive

OVERVIEW

- Shock, no matter what the initiating event, represents a series of hemodynamic changes that ultimately reduce systemic perfusion below the level required for basic function of organ systems.
- There are four major categories of initiating events associated with the development of shock: cardiogenic, postcardiac, hypovolemic, and distributive.
- *Cardiogenic shock* occurs when intrinsic cardiac disease reduces the pumping force generated by the myocardium.
- *Postcardiac* shock occurs when the heart is forced to work against such afterloads that flow in downstream vascular segments is inadequate.
- *Hypovolemic shock* results from inadequate intravascular volume (loss greater than 10%–15%), when pressure within the vessels is inadequate to drive flow.
- *Distributive shock* occurs in response to any condition that causes a generalized vasodilation and/or increased permeability of blood vessels; it is most often due to the release of mediators.

CAUSES

Cardiogenic

- Myocardial infarction (MI)
- Cardiac dysrhythmia/arrest
- Cardiomyopathy
- Electrolyte imbalance: potassium; calcium; magnesium
- Cardiac valve disease
- Ventricular aneurysm

Postcardiac

- Pericarditis
- Cardiac tamponade
- Pulmonary embolism
- Pulmonary hypertension
- Coarctation of the aorta

Hypovolemic

- Hemorrhage
- Dehydration
- Third spacing

Distributive

- Sepsis: endotoxin
- Anaphylaxis: histamine, leukotrienes, kinins, prostaglandins
- Neurogenic: central vasomotor center malfunction

Signs & Symptoms

All Types

- Hypotension: mean arterial pressure less than 60 mm Hg (nonhypertensive adult)
- Tachycardia, with weak, thready pulse
- Cool, clammy, mottled skin
- Oliguria
- Clouded sensorium

Cardiogenic

- Dysrhythmias
- Elevated filling pressures
- Gallop rhythm

Postcardiac

- Murmurs
- S/S of pericardial effusion: pulsus paradoxus; muffled heart sounds

Hypovolemic

- Accompanying/previous vomiting, diarrhea, diaphoresis
- Poor skin turgor

S

Distributive

- Septic: will have accompanying fever, chills, malaise; bleeding disorders (petechiae)
- Anaphylactic: may have accompanying bronchoconstriction with wheezing and dyspnea

Diagnostics

All Types

- Arterial blood gases early on will reveal respiratory alkalosis; later, they will show metabolic acidosis.
- Pulmonary wedge pressure via Swan-Ganz catheter will be reduced.

Septic

- Blood cultures are done to rule out or identify bacteria in blood.
- White blood cell (WBC) count may be elevated early but reduced if overwhelming infection is present.
- Coagulation studies may show abnormal bleeding times.

Hypovolemic

- Serum electrolytes, blood urea nitrogen (BUN), hemoglobin and hematocrit are all elevated.
- Urine is concentrated and shows increased specific gravity.

MEDICAL INTERVENTIONS

- Emergency care of the client in shock focuses on maintaining a level of tissue perfusion adequate to sustain life. Administration of IV fluids and blood is the most effective treatment for a client in hypovolemic shock. In addition, establishing and maintaining a patent airway and ensuring adequate oxygenation are critical interventions.
- Military antishock trousers are a device used to treat hypovolemic shock resulting from trauma and hemorrhage. The device facilitates an increase in arterial pressure.
- Vasoactive and inotropic drugs may also be used to treat shock. Other pharmacologic agents may be

used specific to the type of shock; for example, antibiotics may be given to suppress organisms responsible for septic shock.

SELECTED NURSING DIAGNOSES WITH INTERVENTIONS

Decreased Cardiac Output

- Assess and monitor cardiovascular function, including blood pressure, heart rate and rhythm, capillary refill time, peripheral pulses, and hemodynamic monitoring of pulmonary artery pressures and central venous pressures.
- Measure and record intake and output hourly.
- Monitor bowel sounds, abdominal distention, and abdominal pain.
- Monitor for sudden, sharp chest pain, dyspnea, cyanosis, anxiety, and restlessness.
- Maintain the client on bed rest, and provide to the extent possible a calm, quiet environment.
- Position the client in a supine position with the legs elevated to about 20°, trunk flat, and head and shoulders elevated higher than the chest.

Altered Tissue Perfusion

- Monitor skin color, temperature, turgor, and moisture.
- Monitor cardiopulmonary function by assessing blood pressure, rate and depth of respirations, lung sounds, capillary refill, peripheral pulses, jugular vein distention, and central venous pressure measurements.
- Monitor body temperature.
- Monitor urinary output per Foley catheter hourly, using a urimeter.
- Assess mental status and level of consciousness.

CLIENT TEACHING

- Provide information about the current setting to both the client and significant others.
- Provide significant others with information about resources that are available such as pastoral services, social services, temporary housing, meals, and so on.

497

- Provide anticipatory guidance to prepare for recovery or death and to support realistic hope.

HOME CARE CONSIDERATIONS

- Depending on the cause of the episode, the client may require referrals for home health care, social services, financial assistance, rehabilitation services, a long-term-care facility, or psychologic counseling.

For more information, see the following pages in Medical-Surgical Nursing *by LeMone and Burke:*
Cardiogenic shock, p. 170
Hypovolemic shock, p. 169

Sickle Cell Anemia

OVERVIEW

- Sickle cell anemia is a genetically determined abnormality in the structure of hemoglobin.
- The inheritance pattern is classic Mendelian.
- Heterozygotes have *sickle cell trait* while homozygotes have two abnormal S genes, and have *sickle cell disease.*
- The HbS crystallizes under conditions of deoxygenation, thus deforming the entire red blood cell (RBC) into an elongated, crescent shape.
- Such cells become trapped in capillaries, producing ischemia and/or necrosis of tissues; hemolysis of trapped RBCs results in anemia.
- Individuals with sickle cell trait experience few clinical problems and have a normal life expectancy; RBCs sickle only under conditions of extremely low Pao_2.
- Those with sickle cell disease experience recurrent episodes of *sickle cell crisis,* require multiple hospitalizations and transfusions, and have significantly higher mortality rates than normal persons. The mutation arose in Africans and imparted protection against malaria to heterozygotes.

- About 10% of African Americans carry the sickle cell trait; 0.15% have the disease.

CAUSES

- Point mutation in hemoglobin gene produces abnormal hemoglobin S.
- Trait is passed genetically to offspring.

Signs & Symptoms

- S/S of anemia: pallor, fatigue, shortness of breath, tachycardia
- Chronic tissue/organ damage in heart, lung, kidney, spleen, liver, gall bladder, skin, eye, nerve
- Sickle cell crisis may be precipitated by viral or bacterial infection, changes in environmental temperatures, or any condition producing decreased Pao_2, such as asthma
- Pain is ischemic and may be located anywhere, but most often is in the abdomen, chest, joints, or back
- Jaundice

Diagnostics

- Complete blood count (CBC) shows decreased hemoglobin, hematocrit, and RBC count.
- Peripheral blood smear will show characteristic RBC sickle morphology.
- Sickle cell prep will be positive with either the trait or the disease (no distinction).
- Hemoglobin electrophoresis will provide a definitive diagnosis.

S

MEDICAL INTERVENTIONS

- Folic acid is administered to meet the increased demands of the bone marrow.
- Hydration therapy is administered to clients in sickle cell crisis to improve blood flow, reduce pain, and prevent renal damage. Analgesics are given for pain.
- Blood transfusions may be necessary in severe cases and for pregnant women.
- Genetic counseling is important for clients and significant others at risk for sickle cell anemia.

SELECTED NURSING DIAGNOSES WITH INTERVENTIONS

Pain

- Ask the client to rate the pain on a scale of 0 to 10. Also assess the client's nonverbal cues indicating pain.
- Administer analgesics as prescribed, and assess the client's response.
- Teach the client alternative, nonpharmacologic measures to reduce pain, such as meditation, guided imagery, and distraction.

Altered Tissue Perfusion

- Administer oxygen as prescribed for the client in sickle cell crisis.
- Ensure adequate hydration by offering noncaffeinated beverages and administering normal saline IV, as prescribed.
- Encourage the client to wear loose, nonconstrictive clothing.
- Tell the client to avoid flexion of the knees and hips to promote venous return.
- Maintain a room temperature of at least 72F.
- Avoid taking blood pressure with an external cuff. Avoid use of tourniquets for extended periods of time.
- Perform neurovascular checks of extremities every hour, including pulse oximetry of fingers and toes.

CLIENT TEACHING

- Teach the client the disease process, the genetic component, treatment options, and how to avoid conditions that lead to crisis.
- Discuss manifestations that signal the need for prompt medical treatment.

HOME CARE CONSIDERATIONS

- Discuss the hereditary nature of the disease, and refer the client for prenatal testing and genetic counseling as appropriate.
- Stress the need for lifelong medical supervision of the disease and its manifestations.

- A referral to a support group or other information resource may be helpful in increasing the client's coping skills.

For more information on Sickle Cell Anemia, see Medical-Surgical Nursing *by LeMone and Burke, p. 1272.*

Skin Cancer, Nonmelanoma

OVERVIEW

- Nonmelanoma skin cancer may be classified as either basal cell carcinoma or squamous cell carcinoma.
- These are the most frequently occurring cancers in the United States, with about one million new cases diagnosed each year; basal cell carcinoma accounts for about 75%, and squamous cell for 25%.
- *Basal cell carcinoma (BCC)* arises from epidermal basal cells and is locally invasive but usually does not metastasize.
- *Squamous cell carcinoma (SCC)* arises from keratinizing epidermal cells; it invades the dermis, can grow rapidly, and can metastasize via local lymphatics.

CAUSES

Basal Cell Carcinoma

- Unknown
- Risk factors include age, fair complexion, sun (UV) exposure, immunosuppression, xeroderma pigmentosa (defective DNA repair)

Squamous Cell Carcinoma

- Unknown
- Risk factors include age; sun (UV) exposure; xeroderma pigmentosa (defective DNA repair); or history of ionizing radiation exposure, burns (scars), industrial carcinogen exposure, arsenic exposure, or draining lesions (fistulas, osteomyelitis)

S

Signs & Symptoms

Basal Cell Carcinoma—Skin Lesion

- Early: dome-shaped papule or nodule; pearly white, pink with telangiectasis on surface or plaques (may be pigmented)
- Late: painless, central ulceration with raised, rolled borders (rodent ulcer)
- Typically located on sun-exposed areas of face, chest, arms

Squamous Cell Carcinoma—Skin Lesion

- In situ: keratotic, scaly, red plaques
- Invasive: red, raised, ulcerative nodules with central necrosis and edematous border
- Typically located on sun-exposed areas of face, scalp, ears, lips, hands; burn scar areas; draining lesion areas

Diagnostics

- Skin biopsy establishes the diagnosis of either type of cancer.

MEDICAL INTERVENTIONS

- Nonmelanoma skin cancers may be removed through surgical excision or through Mohs micrographic surgery.
- Cryosurgery is a noninvasive technique that may be used to freeze and destroy the tumor tissue.
- Radiation usually is used only for lesions that are inoperable because of their location or size.

SELECTED NURSING DIAGNOSES

- Impaired Skin Integrity
- Risk for Infection
- Anxiety
- Risk for Body Image Disturbance

SELECTED NURSING INTERVENTIONS

- Monitor the client for manifestations of infection: fever, tachycardia, malaise, and incisional erythema, swelling, pain, or drainage that increases or becomes purulent.

- Keep the incision line clean and dry by changing dressings as necessary.
- Follow principles of medical and surgical asepsis when caring for the client's incision. Teach the client and significant others the importance of careful hand washing. Maintain universal precautions if drainage is present.
- Encourage and maintain adequate kilocalorie and protein intake in the diet.
- Provide accurate information about the illness, treatment, and expected length of recovery.
- Encourage discussion of expected physical changes and ways to minimize disfigurement through cosmetics and clothing.
- Provide strategies for participating in the recovery process and minimizing the risk of future recurrences.

CLIENT TEACHING

- Teach the client primary prevention behaviors recommended by the American Cancer Society and the Skin Cancer Foundation:
  1. Minimize exposure to the sun between the hours of 10 AM and 3 PM
  2. Cover up with a wide-brimmed hat, sunglasses, long-sleeved shirt, and long pants when in the sun.
  3. Use a waterproof sunscreen with an SPF of 15 or more.
  4. Avoid tanning booths.
- Teach the client how to conduct a monthly skin self-examination.

HOME CARE CONSIDERATIONS

- Provide the client with a brochure describing types of skin cancers and prevention behaviors, and showing photographs of lesions.
- Refer the client to the American Cancer Society for further information.

For more information on Skin Cancer, Nonmelanoma, see Medical-Surgical Nursing *by LeMone and Burke, p. 604.*

Sodium Imbalance

Hypernatremia
Hyponatremia

OVERVIEW

- Sodium (Na^+) is the major extracellular fluid (ECF) cation.
- The sodium in the ECF is critical for maintaining normal:
  1. ECF osmolality (ECF osmolality can be estimated by doubling the serum sodium value);
  2. ECF volume;
  3. function of excitable tissue throughout the body (nerve and all types of muscle); and
  4. acid-base balance (substitutes for hydrogen at the renal tubule)
- Regulation of sodium is achieved by input mechanisms such as salt hunger or thirst as well as output mechanisms involving the kidneys via the hormones aldosterone, antidiuretic hormone (ADH), and atrial natriuretic hormone.
- ADH is secreted by the hypothalamus in response to high serum osmolality and acts to restore normal osmolality by causing thirst, thus increasing input, and by reabsorbing water at renal collecting duct, reducing output. Both mechanisms lower sodium and osmolality.
- Aldosterone is secreted by cells in the adrenal cortex in response to reduced sodium, high potassium, or increased levels of angiotensin. Aldosterone reduces sodium excretion in the distal renal tubule, reducing sodium output, thus helping to maintain ECF volume.
- Atrial natriuretic hormone (ANH) is secreted by atrial myocytes in response to hypervolemia. ANH acts to reduce total body sodium content and circulating volume by increasing the glomerular filtration rate and producing natriuresis and diuresis.

CAUSES

Hypernatremia (Serum Sodium >147 mEq/L)

Water deficit (dehydration)

- Diaphoresis: fever, heat stroke
- Vomiting
- GI tube suction
- Diarrhea
- Diuretic therapy
- Water deprivation: strandings, coma
- Diabetes insipidus
- Diabetes mellitus

Sodium excess

- Excess hypertonic IVs
- Cushing's syndrome
- Conn's disease
- Excess ingestion: table salt; salt water ingestion/near drowning; sodium bicarbonate ingestion or IV treatment; Kayexolate treatment

Hyponatremia (Serum Sodium <137 mEq/L)

Hypovolemic

- History of GI losses: vomiting, diarrhea, suctioning; draining fistulas
- History of renal losses: diuretics; tubular polyuria; Addison's disease
- History of third spacing: burns; wound drainage

Normovolemic or hypervolemic

- Syndrome of inappropriate ADH secretion (SIADH)
- Excess ingestion of water: water intoxication, primary psychogenic polydipsia
- Excess hypotonic IV therapy
- Tap water enemas
- Edema due to: congestive heart failure, renal failure, cirrhosis with ascites

Signs & Symptoms

Hypernatremia

- Thirst: intense
- Central nervous system S/S: fatigue, restlessness, agitation, coma

S

- Increased deep tendon reflexes
- Increased muscle tone/spasms
- S/S of dehydration (water loss): fever; flushed, dry skin; poor skin turgor; rough, dry tongue; soft eyeballs; postural hypotension; oliguria
- S/S of pulmonary edema (sodium gain): dyspnea, dyspnea on exertion; orthopnea; paroxysmal nocturnal dyspnea; frothy expectoration; wet rales

Hyponatremia

Hypovolemic

- Postural hypotension
- CNS S/S: irritability, anxiety, personality changes, tremors, seizures, coma
- S/S of shock: rapid, thready pulse; hypotension; cold, clammy, pale skin
- Oliguria

Hypervolemic

- Headache
- Hypertension
- CNS S/S: fatigue, weakness; confusion, depression

Diagnostics

- Serum sodium will show increased or decreased levels.
- Serum osmolality will show elevation or reduction.
- Urine sodium will show increased or decreased levels.
- Urine specific gravity will show elevation or reduction.

MEDICAL INTERVENTIONS

- Treatment for hypernatremia aims to reduce serum sodium by restoring fluid balance using IV infusions of dextrose in water. Occasionally, diuretics are used in combination with water replacement.
- Hyponatremia is treated by fluid volume replacement with sodium-containing fluids. Loop diuretics also may be used.

SELECTED NURSING DIAGNOSES WITH INTERVENTIONS

Hypernatremia

Risk for Injury

- Monitor and maintain oral and IV fluid replacement to within the prescribed limits. Monitor serum sodium levels and osmolality; report rapid declines in serum sodium and osmolality.
- Monitor neurologic function, assessing for altered mental status, lethargy, headache, nausea, vomiting, elevated blood pressure, and decreased pulse rate.
- Institute safety precautions as necessary: keep the bed in its lowest position, side rails up and padded, and airway at the bedside.
- Keep clocks, calendars, and familiar objects at the bedside. Provide orientation, and tell the client and significant others that disorientation is usually temporary.

Hyponatremia

Risk for Fluid Volume Imbalance

- Monitor for signs of circulatory overload.
- For clients requiring fluid restriction, explain why fluid intake must be limited, how much fluid is allowed over 24 hours, and how to measure fluid volumes.
- Monitor intake and output, weigh daily, and calculate 24-hour fluid balance.

Risk for Sensory/Perceptual Alterations

S

- Assess the client for neurologic changes such as lethargy, altered level of consciousness, confusion, and convulsions. Monitor behavior, mental status, and orientation.
- Assess neuromuscular status for changes in muscle strength, tone, and deep tendon reflexes.
- Maintain a quiet environment, and institute safety precautions for clients at high risk for injury from seizure.

CLIENT TEACHING

- Discuss the need for dietary restrictions or increases of sodium and how to incorporate them.
- Teach the client about the disease process, manifestations of hyper- and hyponatremia, and strategies for prevention of recurrences.
- Teach the client prone to hyponatremia the importance of drinking liquids containing sodium and other electrolytes at frequent intervals when perspiring heavily or when experiencing diarrhea.
- Stress the importance of having regular laboratory tests to monitor electrolytes, especially if the client is taking a potent diuretic or is on a low-sodium diet.

HOME CARE CONSIDERATIONS

- A referral to a dietitian may be appropriate.

For more information, see the following pages in Medical-Surgical Nursing *by LeMone and Burke:*
Hypernatremia, p. 124
Hyponatremia, p. 121

Syndrome of Inappropriate Antidiuretic Hormone Secretion (SIADH)

OVERVIEW

- Syndrome of inappropriate ADH secretion (SIADH) is a condition in which secretion of ADH (vasopressin) is in excess even though the plasma osmolality is low.
- Since ADH increases water reabsorption, the syndrome produces water retention, extracellular fluid (ECF) volume expansion, and hyponatremia (dilutional).
- Excess ADH may be secreted secondary to a direct affect of disease, drugs, or trauma on the neurohypophysis or to secretion from an ectopic focus.

CAUSES

Excess release from neurohypophysis:

- Head injury: skull fracture, subdural hematoma, subarachnoid hemorrhage
- Cerebrovascular accident
- Acute encephalitis
- Meningitis: bacterial, tuberculous
- Cerebral atrophy
- Systemic lupus erythematosus
- Guillain-Barré syndrome

Ectopic release:

- Malignancies:
    1. small (oat) cell carcinoma of the lung
    2. carcinoma of the pancreas
    3. carcinoma of the duodenum
    4. thymoma
    5. lymphomas: lymphosarcoma, Hodgkin's lymphoma, reticulum cell sarcoma
- Drugs:
    1. carbamazepine
    2. chlorpropamide
    3. general anesthetics
    4. narcotics
    5. oxytocin
    6. tricyclic antidepressants
    7. chemotherapeutics: cyclophosphamide, vincristine, vinblastine
- Hypothyroidism
- Mechanical respiration

S

Signs & Symptoms

- Anorexia, nausea, vomiting
- Increased body weight
- Tachycardia
- Hypothermia
- S/S of cerebral edema: headache, irritability, anxiety, hostility, personality changes, confusion, tremors, seizures, coma
- Decreased deep tendon reflexes

Diagnostics

- Serum sodium will be less than 135 mEq/L and falling.
- Serum osmolality will be greater than 300 mOsm/L.
- Plasma or urine arginine vasopressin levels will be elevated.

MEDICAL INTERVENTIONS

- Medical care is aimed at treating the underlying causes, treating the hyponatremia with IV hypertonic saline, and restricting oral fluid intake to less than 800 mL per day.
- Diuretics may be prescribed if the client has symptoms of congestive heart failure from fluid overload.

SELECTED NURSING DIAGNOSES

- Fluid Volume Excess
- Risk for Injury
- Nausea

SELECTED NURSING INTERVENTIONS

- Restrict fluid intake as instructed, typically to less than 800 mL per day. Provide ice chips (if allowed, as part of the fluid allowance), hard candy, and/or lemon-glycerin swabs to relieve mouth dryness. Provide frequent mouth care.
- Carefully monitor intake and output. Notify the physician of any abnormalities.
- Weigh the client daily at the same time of day and in the same clothes. Notify the physician of any weight gain.
- Administer diuretics and other medications as prescribed.
- Monitor the client's neurological status, including level of consciousness, motor and sensory functions, and so on. Institute seizure precautions, providing interventions for client safety (such as padding bed rails, keeping bed in low position, etc.). In the event of a seizure, provide interventions to maintain a patent airway.

CLIENT TEACHING

- Teach the client and significant others about the disease process, treatment, medication regimen, and prognosis.
- Teach the client and significant others how to recognize signs of recurrence and how to cope with seizure activity. Stress the importance of maintaining a safe home environment.

HOME CARE CONSIDERATIONS

- Tell the client and significant others to maintain prescribed fluid restrictions, and explain the rationale to increase compliance.
- Emphasize the importance of weighing the client daily at the same time of day and in the same clothing, and of reporting any weight gain to the physician.
- Tell the client to avoid nonsteroidal anti-inflammatory drugs and aspirin, which may contribute to hyponatremia.

For more information on Syndrome of Inappropraite ADH (SIADH), see Medical-Surgical Nursing *by LeMone and Burke, p. 714.*

Syphilis

S

OVERVIEW

- Syphilis is a sexually transmitted disease (STD) caused by the spirochete *Treponema pallidum,* which begins locally and causes a systemic infection.
- The incubation period averages about 3 weeks.
- Untreated syphilis passes through three stages:
  1. *Primary* lesion (chancre) occurs on genitalia.
  2. *Secondary* lesions form on skin and mucous membranes.

3. *Tertiary* lesions form in the central nervous system; granulomatous lesions (gummas) form in blood vessels (especially the thoracic aorta), visceral organs, and skin.

- If not treated, syphilis can lead to blindness, paralysis, mental illness, cardiovascular damage, and death.
- Congenital syphilis is passed transplacentally to the embryo or fetus.
- Syphilis is most often seen in teens or young adults.

CAUSES

- Sexually or congenitally transmitted spirochete, *T. pallidum*

Signs & Symptoms

- *Primary syphilis* is the earliest stage and its presence is announced by the formation of a chancre, a painless, raised, indurated papule with an ulcerated center located on external genitalia or within the rectum or on the cervix; spontaneously resolves; latency period follows
- *Secondary syphilis* is heralded by the appearance of:
  1. generalized skin rash: non-itchy; symmetric; macular/papular, possibly pustular; on face, scalp, trunk, palms, soles
  2. condyloma lata: broad, moist, white/gray lesions, surrounded by redness; found on mucous membranes or wet skin areas
  3. alopecia: scalp, eyebrows, beard
  4. lymphadenopathy
  5. other: headache, fever, malaise; sore throat, weight loss
- A period of latency also follows secondary syphilis
- *Tertiary syphilis* can present in numerous ways:
  1. neurosyphilis: paresis, ataxia, meningeal syphilis, cranial neuropathies, incontinence, impotence, optic atrophy with blindness
  2. cardiovascular syphilis: aortic vasculitis with medial necrosis; aneurysm formation, aortic regurgitation

3. gumma formation: multiple, diffuse or solitary inflammatory, granulomatous lesions of skin, skeletal system; mucosa of respiratory, gastrointestinal tracts or any visceral organ; locally destructive

- *Congenital syphilis* may result in fetal demise, stillbirth, prematurity, condyloma lata, runny nose (loaded with spirochetes), bullae, abnormal bone formation, hepatomegaly, splenomegaly, lymphadenopathy, anemia, petechiae

Diagnostics

- Venereal disease research laboratory (VDRL) serology test will be positive (false positives are possible).
- Rapid plasma reagin (RPR) serology test will be positive.
- Fluorescent treponemal antibody-absorbed serum (FTA-ABS) test will be positive.

MEDICAL INTERVENTIONS

- The treatment of choice for syphilis is benzathine penicillin G, given intramuscularly. It is very effective in the early stages, less so in later stages.
- Tetracycline or doxycycline is used in penicillin-sensitive clients.

SELECTED NURSING DIAGNOSES WITH INTERVENTIONS

Risk for Injury

- Teach the importance of taking any prescribed oral medication.
- Encourage the client to refer any partner(s) for evaluation and any necessary treatment.
- Teach the client to abstain from sexual contact until client and partner(s) are cured and to use condoms to prevent future infections.
- Emphasize the importance of returning for follow-up testing at 3- and 6-month intervals for early syphilis, and 6- and 12-month intervals for late latent syphilis.
- Provide information about the signs and symptoms of reinfection.

S

Anxiety

- Emphasize that syphilis can be effectively treated, thus preventing the serious complications of late-stage disease.
- Teach the pregnant client that taking medications as directed and returning each month for follow-up testing will help ensure the well-being of her baby.

Self-Esteem Disturbance

- Create an environment where the client feels respected and safe to discuss questions and concerns about the disease and its effect on the client's life.
- Provide privacy and confidentiality.
- Let the client know that the nurse and other health care providers care about him or her and the successful outcome of the disease.

CLIENT TEACHING

- Emphasize that syphilis is a chronic disease and can be spread to others even when no symptoms are present.
- Clients need to understand the importance of:
  1. taking any and all prescribed medication;
  2. referring sexual partners for evaluation and treatment;
  3. abstaining from all sexual contact for a minimum of 1 month after treatment;
  4. using a condom to avoid transmitting or contracting infections in the future;
  5. returning for follow-up testing at 3- and 6-month intervals for early syphilis, and 6- and 12-month intervals for late latent syphilis.

HOME CARE CONSIDERATIONS

- Provide a referral to social services, a psychologic counselor, or a couples counselor as appropriate.

For more information on Syphilis, see Medical-Surgical Nursing *by LeMone and Burke, p. 2077.*

Systemic Lupus Erythematosus (SLE)

OVERVIEW

- Systemic lupus erythematosus (SLE) is a chronic inflammatory connective-tissue disease of autoimmune origin.
- The pathophysiology of SLE involves the production of a large variety of autoantibodies against normal body components such as nucleic acids, erythrocytes, coagulation proteins, lymphocytes, and platelets.
- Inflammation with SLE damages joints, blood cells/vessels, neurons, serosal surfaces, and organs such as the heart, lung, kidneys, intestines, eyes, and skin.
- The disease is often difficult to diagnose as manifestations vary considerably in different clients. In some clients, only one or two systems are affected, while in others, many systems are affected.
- The course is highly variable, with severity ranging from mild to intermittent to rapidly fulminating; most clients experience multiple exacerbations and remissions, spread over years.

CAUSES

- Autoimmune (Type II & III mechanisms)
- Believed to be caused by multi-gene genetic predisposition coupled with environmental factors.
- Risk factors:
  1. female gender; 90% of cases are women, usually those in the reproductive years
  2. race: African American greater than Latino, and Asian American greater than European American
  3. family history; higher concordance rates in identical versus fraternal twins; 10% increase in frequency in relatives
  4. SLE is also seen with greater frequency in individuals with certain HLA tissue types

S

Signs & Symptoms

- General: fever, malaise, fatigue, anorexia, weight loss
- Dermatologic: "butterfly" rash, a fixed, red, macular or papular rash over malar surface is classic; may be generalized, or may also occur in areas of sun exposure (photosensitive), usually seen during an exacerbation; alopecia accompanies
- Musculoskeletal: arthralgia, symmetric joint swelling, synovitis, avascular bone necrosis (due to glucocorticoid therapy), myalgia
- Hematologic: S/S of anemia such as pallor, fatigue, shortness of breath, tachycardia, S/S of thrombocytopenia such as abnormal bleeding, ecchymosis, petechiae
- Neurologic: headache, changes in cognition and/or mood, personality changes, cranial neuropathy, retinal vasculitis, blindness, ataxia, seizures, cerebrovascular accident
- Endocrinologic: syndrome of inappropriate ADH secretion
- Vascular: vasculitis, thrombosis
- Cardiac: pericarditis with effusion or tamponade, dysrythmias; myocardial infarction, sudden cardiac arrest, heart failure
- Pulmonary: pneumonitis; pleuritis, with effusion; pulmonary hypertension; adult respiratory distress syndrome
- Renal: glomerulonephritis, with S/S of renal insufficiency/failure such as proteinuria, polyuria, nocturia, hypertension, azotemia, oliguria
- Gastrointestinal: nausea, vomiting, diarrhea, cramping, obstruction, perforation

Diagnostics

- Virtually all clients with SLE have positive antinuclear antibody tests.
- Complete blood count (CBC) may show anemia, and white blood cell (WBC) count may show leukopenia and lymphopenia.
- Erythrocyte sedimentation rate typically is elevated.
- Serum complement levels are usually decreased.

- Urinalysis shows mild proteinuria, hematuria, and blood cell casts during exacerbations of the disease.

MEDICAL INTERVENTIONS

- Aspirin and other NSAIDs can manage mild arthralgia, fatigue, fever, and arthritis. Skin and arthritis manifestations may be treated with antimalarial drugs. Severe SLE requires corticosteroid therapy. Immunosuppressive agents also may be employed.
- Clients with SLE who progress to end-stage renal disease are treated with dialysis and kidney transplantation.

SELECTED NURSING DIAGNOSES WITH INTERVENTIONS

Impaired Skin Integrity

- Assess the client's knowledge of the disease and its possible effects on the skin.
- Discuss the relationship between sun exposure and disease activity, both dermatologic and systemic. Help the client identify strategies to limit sun exposure.
- Keep the skin clean and dry. Apply therapeutic creams or ointments to lesions as prescribed.

Altered Protection

- Wash hands on entering the client's room and before providing client care.
- Use strict aseptic technique in caring for IV lines and indwelling catheters or performing any wound care.
- Assess the client frequently for signs and symptoms of infection. Monitor temperature and vital signs every 4 hours. Assess for signs of cellulitis, including tenderness, redness, swelling, and warmth. Report signs of infection to physician promptly.
- Monitor laboratory values, including CBC and tests of organ function, and report changes to physician.
- Initiate reverse or protective isolation procedures as indicated by the client's immune status.
- Instruct visitors to avoid contact with the client when they are ill.

S

- Help ensure an adequate nutrient intake, offering supplementary feedings as indicated or maintaining parenteral nutrition if necessary.
- Teach the client the importance of good hand washing after using the bathroom and before eating.
- Provide good mouth care.
- Monitor for potential adverse effects of medications.

CLIENT TEACHING

- Teach the client about the disease and its potential effects. Promote an optimistic outlook, stressing that the majority of clients do not require long-term corticosteroid therapy and that the disease may improve over time.
- Discuss the importance of skin care, including avoidance of harsh chemicals and of sun exposure.
- Stress the importance of avoiding exposure to infection, and getting adequate rest and nutrition.
- Emphasize the importance of following the prescribed treatment plan, including medication regimen and follow-up appointments. Tell the client to report the following symptoms to the physician: fever, chills, rash, increased fatigue and malaise, arthralgias, arthritis, urinary manifestations, chest pain, cough, or neurologic symptoms.

HOME CARE CONSIDERATIONS

- Encourage the client to wear a MedicAlert bracelet or necklace and provide information on how to obtain one.
- Discuss family planning with the client and spouse as appropriate. The use of oral contraceptives may be contraindicated. The pregnant client requires close monitoring for acute episodes.
- A referral to national and community agencies for support and education is important.

For more information on Systemic Lupus Erythematosus, see Medical-Surgical Nursing *by LeMone and Burke, p. 1654.*

Testicular Cancer

OVERVIEW

- Testicular cancer is a primary malignant neoplasm of the testis, usually of sperm cell precursors (e.g., germ cells).
- Local spread to the epididymis or spermatic cord is inhibited by the outer covering of the testicles, the tunica albuginea. Therefore, spread by lymphatic and vascular channels to other organs often causes distant disease before large masses develop in the scrotum.
- Bilateral presentation of testicular cancer is unusual.
- Testicular cancer is the most common cancer in men between the ages of 20 and 35; the cure rate is nearly 100% for men with early-stage disease.

CAUSES

- Unknown
- Risk factors:
  1. 48 times higher in clients with a history of cryptorchidism
  2. age: late teens to thirties
  3. race: European Americans greater than African Americans or Asian Americans

Signs & Symptoms

- Palpable mass in testis
- Swollen testis
- Pain and/or pulling sensation, may be sporadic

Diagnostics

- Biopsy will identify and classify malignancy.
- Serum studies will show elevated levels of tumor markers. Serum human chorionic gonadotropin (HCG) may be elevated.

MEDICAL INTERVENTIONS

- The client with advanced disease may receive platinum-based combination chemotherapy.

- Radical orchiectomy is the definitive treatment used in all forms and stages of testicular cancer.
- Radiation therapy also may be indicated.

SELECTED NURSING DIAGNOSES WITH INTERVENTIONS

Altered Tissue Perfusion

- Provide routine pre- and postoperative care. Provide both verbal and written instructions for pain control, wound care, signs of complications, and so on, since most orchiectomy clients are discharged within 24 hours of the procedure.
- Prepare the client for an extensive surgical procedure when retroperitoneal lymph node dissection is to be performed.
- Assess frequently for complications of surgery, including vital signs, wound care, and so on.
- Administer pain medications as prescribed. Ice bags and scrotal support may also reduce pain.

Altered Sexuality Patterns

- Assess the client's prediagnosis sexual functioning.
- Clarify possible effects of treatment on sexual functioning.
- Discuss the possibility of preserving sperm in a sperm bank. If the client has chemotherapy and retroperitoneal surgery, the chance of preserving reproductive function is remote.
- Help the client to cope with his feelings about altered sexual function. Use active listening skills, and recommend male support groups and couple's counseling.

CLIENT TEACHING

- Teach the client about the disease process, treatment options, and prognosis.
- Teach the client methods to control pain. In addition to analgesics, ice bags may be applied to the scrotum. A scrotal support provides relief, especially when the client ambulates.
- Teach the client the signs of complications. If the incision gapes open, or if there is bleeding beyond slight oozing after 24 hours, the client should call

the physician. Scrotal edema, which may be caused by bleeding from the stump of the spermatic cord, also requires prompt intervention.

- Reinforce the client's knowledge concerning the effects of surgery on sexuality. If the treatment involves only a radical orchiectomy, there should be no lasting effects on the client's sexual or reproductive function. If the client has had chemotherapy and retroperitoneal surgery, the chance of preserving reproductive function is remote. Include the client's sexual partner as appropriate in discussions of sexual and reproductive function.
- Teach the client with a high risk for recurrence the importance of surveillance with periodic physical examinations, chest x-rays, tumor marker tests, and CT scans. Stress the importance of monthly testicular self-examination on remaining testis.

HOME CARE CONSIDERATIONS

- Provide the names and addresses of local cancer support groups. Refer the client to the American Cancer Society for information and support services.
- A referral for psychologic or sexual therapy may be important.

For more information on Testicular Cancer, see Medical-Surgical Nursing *by LeMone and Burke,* *p. 1987.*

Tetanus

OVERVIEW

- Tetanus (commonly called "lockjaw") is an acute condition characterized by severe, uncontrolled skeletal muscle spasms caused by a toxin secreted from the anaerobic bacteria, *Clostridium tetani*, which lives in soil. Spores enter the body through open wounds contaminated with dirt or feces.

- The toxin, called tetanospasmin, ascends nerves leading to the spinal cord and blocks neurons that inhibit muscle contraction; spasms result.
- Tetanus is rare in developed countries owing to regular vaccination programs; however, it is seen in adults whose immunity has been lost.

CAUSES

- Infection with the anaerobic bacteria *Clostridium tetani.*
- Infectious agent usually gains access to the body via a deep puncture wound or laceration and grows best in body regions with low Po_2 (for example, the foot).

Signs & Symptoms

- Initially, stiffness and pain occur in the jaw or trunk
- Backward, arching spasms of head, back, extremities
- Mask-like grin
- Symptoms progress to generalized spasms of most body muscles: respiratory spasms are the most dangerous

Diagnostics

- There are no definitive laboratory or diagnostic tests for tetanus. The diagnosis is based on the clinical manifestations and history.

MEDICAL INTERVENTIONS

- Tetanus is completely preventable by active immunization.
- Pharmacologic agents for clients with tetanus include antibiotics to destroy the organism and chlorpromazine or diazepam to control muscle spasms and seizures. Anticoagulants also may be used.

SELECTED NURSING DIAGNOSES

- Risk for Injury
- Ineffective Breathing Pattern

- Impaired Gas Exchange
- Altered Nutrition: Less than Body Requirements

SELECTED NURSING INTERVENTIONS

- Place the client in a quiet, darkened room to decrease stimuli that cause muscle spasms and seizures.
- Provide only necessary physical care, and do so during periods of maximal sedation to decrease tactile stimulation that causes muscle spasms.
- Maintain oxygenation through mechanical ventilator and frequent suctioning of secretions.
- Maintain intravenous access for the administration of fluids and medications.
- Administer prescribed antibiotics, anticonvulsants, and sedatives.
- Provide adequate nutrition through prescribed nutritional support.
- Monitor respiratory and cardiovascular status and provide immediate interventions for respiratory or cardiovascular failure.
- Monitor fluid and electrolyte status. Ensure adequate fluid intake to maintain hydration and urinary output.
- Monitor urinary output, which should be maintained at 1.5 to 2 L per day.
- Monitor for the hazards of immobility, including constipation, pneumonia, deep vein thrombosis, and pressure ulcers.

CLIENT TEACHING

- Teach clients about the disease process, treatments, including medication regimen, and prognosis.
- Prevention teaching focuses on promoting immunizations for children and educating adults about the need for booster doses. It is also important to teach the proper care of wounds. Tell clients that all wounds, no matter how small, should be thoroughly washed with soap and water, all foreign material carefully flushed out or removed with tweezers or other devices, and protected from dirt while healing. Medical care should be sought promptly for large or contaminated wounds.

T

- Teach the client with tetanus and significant others about safety measures, seizure precautions, and symptoms that require further medical attention.

HOME CARE CONSIDERATIONS

- Teach clients how to take the prescribed antibiotic (e.g., either with food or on an empty stomach; the dosage and timing; and potential side effects).
- Instruct the client and significant others to monitor the wound site for S/S of infection.
- Review seizure precautions with the client and significant others prior to discharge.

For more information on Tetanus, see Medical-Surgical Nursing *by LeMone and Burke, p. 1869.*

Thromboangiitis Obliterans (Buerger's Disease)

OVERVIEW

- Buerger's disease is an inflammatory, occlusive vascular disorder that involves small- and medium-sized arteries and veins.
- Thrombi formation follows inflammation, occluding blood flow.
- The disease usually affects the distal upper and lower extremities, but may involve cerebral, visceral, and coronary vessels.
- Ulceration and eventually gangrene may result.

CAUSES

- Genetic/familial: highest incidence in Asians and Jewish males
- Smoking: associated with heavy smoking

Signs & Symptoms

- Intermittent claudication, especially of calves and feet, aggravated by exercise, relieved by rest

- Color changes: elevation of extremities or exposure to cold temperatures causes cyanosis followed by rubor (redness) upon lowering extremity or warming (reactive hyperemia)
- Sensory changes: elevation or exposure to cold causes coldness and numbness followed by excessive warmth upon lowering (reactive hyperemia), and tingling
- Weak peripheral pulses
- Muscle atrophy
- Ulceration/gangrene

Diagnostics

- Doppler ultrasonography may show diminished peripheral perfusion.
- Plethysmography may show diminished peripheral perfusion.
- Arteriography locates lesions and rules out atherosclerosis.

MEDICAL INTERVENTIONS

- Complete smoking cessation is the most important therapy in the conservative management of Buerger's disease.
- Buerger-Allen exercises involving raising and lowering the extremities may significantly improve peripheral-vascular circulation. The exercises are repeated three to four times daily.
- Pharmacologic intervention in Buerger's disease is limited. Calcium channel–blocking agents provide some relief.
- A sympathectomy or arterial bypass graft may be indicated. Amputation is necessary if irreversible damage to the arterial bed has occurred and irreparable gangrene is present.

SELECTED NURSING DIAGNOSES WITH INTERVENTIONS

Altered Tissue Perfusion: Peripheral

- Assess peripheral pulses, capillary refill, and temperature and color of digits and extremities every shift and more often if changes occur.

- Teach client and significant others the importance of smoking cessation.
- Promote activities that improve arterial circulation.

Pain

- Assess the client's pain every shift and as needed.
- Place affected extremities in dependent position, and change position every 2 hours or more often if needed.
- Help the client make lifestyle choices that reduce pain.
- Provide time for the client to discuss issues related to pain.

Impaired Physical Mobility

- Explain the physiologic basis for rest.
- Provide diversional activities to combat boredom from prolonged rest.
- Encourage the client to follow the collaborative plan of care.
- Encourage the client to turn every 2 hours and to perform progressive range-of-motion (ROM) exercises at least every shift.

Risk for Injury

- Inspect extremities every shift and more often if changes in color, sensitivity, or skin continuity are apparent.
- Teach the client the importance of meticulous foot care.

CLIENT TEACHING

- Teach the client that avoiding smoking is absolutely imperative. Alcohol also should be avoided.
- Instruct the client to exercise caution with applications of heat (e.g., electric blankets) and to avoid prolonged exposure to cold.
- Stress the importance of carrying out daily foot care, seeking health care follow-up, and reducing stress.

HOME CARE CONSIDERATIONS

- Smoking cessation must be continued throughout the client's life.

- Discuss with the client the importance of long-term medical follow-up care.

For more information on Thromboangiitis Obliterans, see Medical-Surgical Nursing *by LeMone and Burke, p. 1223.*

Thrombocytopenia

OVERVIEW

- Thrombocytopenia is a less than normal platelet count; the normal count is 150,000 to 400,000/μL.
- When platelets fall to about 10,000/μL, abnormal, spontaneous bleeding occurs.
- Idiopathic thrombocytopenic purpura (ITP) is an acute or chronic condition in which platelet destruction is accelerated. It is believed that the body's immune system destroys the platelets.
- Secondary thrombocytopenia is a condition in which there is a defect in platelet production.

CAUSES

- Disseminated intravascular coagulopathy
- Leukemia/metastatic cancer
- Aplastic anemia
- Cancer chemotherapy
- AIDS
- Overwhelming infection
- Splenomegaly
- Transfusions
- Drugs: meprobamate, methyldopa, quinidine, thiazide diuretics
- ITP: autoimmune

Signs & Symptoms

- Petechiae and/or purpura on skin and mucous membranes
- Ecchymosis with little trauma
- Prolonged bleeding following minimal injury

T

- Bleeding gums
- Epistaxis
- Melena
- Hematuria
- Menorrhagia

Diagnostics

- Platelet count will be <150,000/μL.
- Bone marrow biopsy is definitive.
- Platelet autoantibodies will be positive with ITP.

MEDICAL INTERVENTIONS

- Corticosteroids are administered to suppress the immune response and decrease the number of antibodies targeted for the platelets. They also reduce bleeding time.
- Platelet transfusion may be necessary.
- A splenectomy may be necessary if the client does not recover following more conservative treatment. The spleen is the site of platelet destruction and antibody production.

SELECTED NURSING DIAGNOSES

- Risk for Injury: Bleeding
- Fatigue
- Anxiety
- Risk for Infection

SELECTED NURSING INTERVENTIONS

- Assess all body systems for manifestations of bleeding every shift.
- Monitor vital signs as well as platelet counts every 4 hours.
- Avoid the following invasive procedures, if possible:
  1. use of rectal suppositories or taking of rectal temperature
  2. use of vaginal douches, suppositories, or tampons
  3. urinary catheterizations
  4. parenteral injections
- Diagnostic procedures such as biopsy or lumbar puncture should not be done if the platelet count is less than 50,000.

- Apply pressure to puncture sites for 3 to 5 minutes; apply pressure to arterial blood gas sites for 15 to 20 minutes.
- Use soft toothbrushes or sponges for oral hygiene.
- Administer corticosteroids and other medications as prescribed.
- Administer platelet transfusions for acute, life-threatening bleeding, as prescribed.

CLIENT TEACHING

- Teach the client about the disease process, manifestations, treatments, and self-care. Tell the client to taper off medications at the direction of the physician, and caution the client against stopping medications abruptly.
- Teach the client to avoid the following:
  1. picking crusts from the nose.
  2. blowing the nose forcefully.
  3. straining to have a bowel movement.
  4. forceful coughing or sneezing.

HOME CARE CONSIDERATIONS

- Stress the importance of avoiding people with bacterial and viral infections.
- Emphasize the need for long-term follow-up care with the hematologist for continued management.

For more information on Thrombocytopenia, see Medical-Surgical Nursing *by LeMone and Burke,*
p. 1291.

T

Thrombophlebitis

OVERVIEW

- Thrombophlebitis is an acute inflammation with thrombus formation of deep veins (called DVT, or deep vein thrombophlebitis) or superficial veins (called SVT, or superficial vein thrombophlebitis), usually in the lower extremities.

- Inflammation of the vein (phlebitis) usually precedes thrombus formation; spontaneous thrombus formation is called phlebothrombosis. It is rare.
- SVT usually affects small veins and resolves spontaneously.
- DVT can affect small veins but usually affects large veins such as the femoral, iliac, and vena cava.
- DVT is much more likely than SVT to progress in size and/or result in pulmonary embolus.

CAUSES

Deep Vein Thrombophlebitis

- Reduced tissue perfusion: bed rest, cardiac disease, cerebrovascular accident
- Hyperreactive clotting factors: perinatal period, oral contraceptive use, disseminated intravascular coagulopathy, sepsis
- Endothelial cell damage: infection, trauma, fracture, surgery
- Neoplasms
- Idiopathic

Superficial Vein Thrombophlebitis

- Infection
- Inflammation: IV therapy, IV drug abuse
- Trauma

Signs & Symptoms

Deep Vein Thrombophlebitis

- Severe pain at site of DVT
- Positive Homan's sign
- Swelling of affected limb
- Cyanosis of affected limb may or may not be present
- Fever/chills
- Malaise

Superficial Vein Thrombophlebitis

All S/S along the course of the affected vein:

- Pain
- Redness
- Heat
- Swelling

Diagnostics

- Doppler ultrasound shows reduced perfusion patterns.
- Ascending phlebography shows reduced filling and/or alternate flow patterns.
- Plethysmography shows reduced flow distal to the DVT.

MEDICAL INTERVENTIONS

- Pharmacologic agents most commonly prescribed for clients with thrombophlebitis include anti-inflammatory agents, anticoagulants, thrombolytics, and antibiotics.
- For clients with SVT, the application of warm, moist compresses and the use of anti-inflammatory drugs are usually sufficient.
- For clients with DVT, anticoagulation therapy is initiated, and clients are placed on strict bed rest until symptoms resolve. Thrombolytics may be used simultaneously.
- Surgery may be indicated to remove the thrombus or to control the potential spread of thrombi throughout the system.

SELECTED NURSING DIAGNOSES WITH INTERVENTIONS

Pain

- Assess the client's level of pain regularly on a scale of 0 to 10.
- Measure the diameter of the calf and thigh of the affected extremity on admission and daily thereafter. Report increases promptly.
- Apply warm, moist heat to the affected extremity at least four times daily, using warm, moist compresses or an aqua-K pad.
- Maintain bed rest and teach the client the rationale for it.

Altered Tissue Perfusion: Peripheral

- Assess peripheral pulses, skin integrity, capillary refill times, and color of the extremities at least once each shift. Report changes promptly.

T

- If extremity is swollen, measure and document circumference.
- Elevate extremities at all times, keeping knees slightly flexed and legs above the level of the heart.
- Maintain use of prescribed antiembolic stockings, removing them for short periods (30–60 minutes) during daily hygiene.
- Administer and monitor the effectiveness of analgesics, anticoagulants, thrombolytics, and antibiotics.
- Encourage position changes every 2 hours while the client is awake.

Impaired Physical Mobility

- Encourage active or passive range-of-motion (ROM) exercises at least once each shift.
- Encourage the client to turn, cough, and breathe deeply at least four times during each shift while awake.
- Encourage the client to increase intake of fluids and dietary fiber.
- Provide progressive ambulation within prescribed guidelines.

CLIENT TEACHING

- Teach prescribed collaborative therapy and prevention of complications and future thrombotic episodes. Thoroughly explain the disease process, and treatment, including medications and activity restrictions, and the importance of follow-up visits.
- Teach the client to avoid sitting for long periods in any one position, to avoid crossing the legs or ankles when sitting, and to follow prescribed exercise plan.
- Clients requiring surgery should be informed before surgery of the nature and extent of the surgery, the risks involved, the prognosis for improvement, and their role in the recovery process.

HOME CARE CONSIDERATIONS

- Tell the client to report any signs of bleeding, especially in the urine or stools. Clients should also report unusual bruising, altered level of consciousness, and joint pain.

- Tell the client to check with the physician before using any over-the-counter medications, especially those containing aspirin.
- Suggest the client obtain and wear a MedicAlert bracelet or necklace at all times.
- A referral to a smoking cessation or weight reduction program may be helpful.

For more information on Thrombophlebitis, see Medical-Surgical Nursing *by LeMone and Burke, p. 1240.*

Tonsillitis

OVERVIEW

- Tonsillitis is an inflammation of the tonsils and nasopharynx that is usually caused by infection. Usually it is acute.
- Acute tonsillitis lasts about 1 week and is most often caused by bacteria of the *Streptococcus* genus or by viruses.
- It is frequently encountered in children, especially between the ages of 5 and 10.

CAUSES

- *Streptococcus*, especially beta-hemolytic
- Bacteria: other strains
- Viruses

Signs & Symptoms

- Sore throat: mild to severe; pain may be referred to ear area
- Dysphagia, increased swallowing
- Lymphadenopathy: cervical and submandibular nodes
- Fever, chills
- Anorexia, malaise
- Headache

T

Diagnostics

- Culture and sensitivity of the throat will grow offending bacteria.
- White blood cell (WBC) count is elevated.

MEDICAL INTERVENTIONS

- Antipyretics and mild analgesics are used to provide symptomatic relief.
- Antibiotics are administered for at least 7 to 10 days.
- A peritonsillar abscess may be drained by needle aspiration or by incision and drainage.
- Surgical removal of the tonsils may be performed if the client fails to respond to more conservative therapies.

SELECTED NURSING DIAGNOSES

- Hyperthermia
- Pain
- Risk for Fluid Volume Imbalance
- Ineffective Airway Clearance

SELECTED NURSING INTERVENTIONS

- Administer antipyretics, analgesics, and/or antibiotics as prescribed.
- Encourage the client who is having difficulty swallowing to follow a liquid or soft diet, increase fluid intake, and use saline gargles, moist inhalations, and an ice collar to reduce pain.
- Following a tonsillectomy, ensure a patent airway by positioning the client with the head toward the side for drainage of secretions from the mouth and pharynx.
- Apply an ice collar to reduce swelling and pain.
- Monitor the client for hemorrhage.

CLIENT TEACHING

- Teach the client about the disease process, treatment, and medication regimen. Stress the importance of completing the full course of antibiotics.
- Teach pain-reducton strategies such as applying an ice collar, gargling with warm saline every 1 to 2

hours, and drinking ice-cold fluids. Anesthetic lozenges may also reduce pain.

HOME CARE CONSIDERATIONS

- Instruct the client or significant others to monitor temperature in the morning and evening and to report an elevation to the physician.

For more information on Tonsillitis, see Medical-Surgical Nursing *by LeMone and Burke, p. 1352.*

Trigeminal Neuralgia

OVERVIEW

- Trigeminal neuralgia (also called tic douloureux) is an idiopathic mononeuropathy of one or more of the three branches of the trigeminal nerve. It causes severe facial pain.
- Trigeminal neuralgia occurs in attacks of excruciating pain usually following the maxillary and mandibular branches of the nerve; sometimes the ophthalmic branch is affected.
- Attacks are generally of short duration (a few seconds to a few minutes) but are extremely intense, producing a facial tic.
- Attacks occur sporadically, and may be initiated when "trigger zones" on the face, such as lips, cheeks, chin, or tongue, are stimulated, as by washing the face or brushing the teeth.

CAUSES

- Local disease, infection, or trauma involving the jaw, teeth, sinuses
- Demyelination of trigeminal nerve root
- Lesions near nerve root: aneurysms, redundant vessels, neurofibromas, meningiomas
- Arteriosclerotic changes of an artery close to the nerve

Signs & Symptoms

- Excruciating pain along the route of the nerve; usually fleeting; appears in paroxysmal attacks; triggered by facial stimulation
- Sensory loss may also be present if due to local lesions

Diagnostics

- X-rays of sinuses, teeth, and face to rule out primary disease.
- Computed tomography (CT) to rule out primary disease.

MEDICAL INTERVENTIONS

- Anticonvulsants are used to control the pain. These include the tricyclic carbamazepine (Tegretol) and phenytoin (Dilantin). Baclofen, a skeletal muscle relaxant, also may be used.
- Surgery may be performed when pharmacologic therapy is ineffective. Percutaneous rhizotomy destroys part of the trigeminal nerve. A total severing of the sensory root of the trigeminal nerve through a retrogasserian rhizotomy is done less often now than in the past.

SELECTED NURSING DIAGNOSES WITH INTERVENTIONS

Pain

- Identify factors that trigger an attack and discuss with the client strategies to avoid precipitating factors.
- Determine the client's usual response to pain.
- Assess factors that affect the client's ability to tolerate the pain, including knowledge of the cause of the pain, knowledge of pain management options, cultural factors, and client support system.
- Monitor the effects of the medication prescribed for the neuralgia.

Risk for Altered Nutrition: Less than Body Requirements

- Monitor dietary intake and weight loss at each visit, and ask the client to keep a record of weekly weight measurements.

- Discuss with the client the effect of temperature and consistency of foods.
- Suggest that the client chew on the unaffected side of the mouth.
- If the client is unable to tolerate oral food, tube feedings may be necessary.

CLIENT TEACHING

- Teach the client about the disease process, medications, and methods of reducing the incidence of attacks.
- Clients treated with surgery are at risk for injury as a result of deficits in the corneal reflex. Teach proper eye care:
  1. Do not rub eyes. Use artificial tears if the eyes are dry or irritated.
  2. Wear an eyepatch at night, and sunglasses or goggles when outside or working in areas where dust or other eye irritants may be present.
  3. Remember to blink frequently.
  4. Check the eyes for redness or swelling each day.
  5. Schedule regular eye examinations.
- Clients treated with surgery are at risk for injury as a result of loss of sensation in the involved side of the face. Teach face and mouth care:
  1. Chew on unaffected side of mouth.
  2. Avoid eating hot foods or drinking hot liquids.
  3. After each meal brush the teeth and inspect the mouth for food that may collect between the gums and cheek.
  4. Have regular dental examinations.
  5. Use an electric razor to shave.
  6. Protect the face from cold and wind.

T

HOME CARE CONSIDERATIONS

- Following surgery, referral to a physical therapist may be appropriate.

For more information on Trigeminal Neuralgia, see Medical-Surgical Nursing *by LeMone and Burke, p. 1864.*

Tuberculosis

OVERVIEW

- Tuberculosis (TB) is a chronic, infectious disease caused by *Mycobacterium tuberculosis*.
- *M. tuberculosis* is an aerobic, acid-fast bacillus that characteristically forms granulomas and cavities.
- TB is spread via respiratory droplets, grows within alveoli, and spreads via the bloodstream or lymphatics.
- Primary infection is in the lungs; large areas of caseous necrosis and cavitation are the most common lesions formed. In TB pneumonia, consolidation is lobar.
- Primary progressive TB or reactivation TB can be disseminated to any organ.
- Types of extrapulmonary tuberculosis include:
  1. Miliary TB results when the primary TB lesion erodes into a blood vessel and the bacilli spread via the bloodstream throughout the body.
  2. Genitourinary TB results when the organism spreads to the kidneys via the blood from the primary lesion in the lungs.
  3. Tuberculous meningitis results when TB spreads to the subarachnoid space.
  4. Skeletal TB typically occurs when the primary disease is contracted during childhood. Organisms spread via the blood to vertebrae, the ends of long bones, and joints.
- The rate of infection in the United States is presently about 12 per 10,000, but the incidence is rising, especially in high-risk groups such as those with AIDS. Rates are much higher in less developed countries.
- Previous primary infection is detectable via purified protein derivative (PPD).
- Strains of TB resistant to available antimicrobials are increasing.

CAUSES

- Infection with *M. tuberculosis*

Signs & Symptoms

Primary Infection
- Usually subclinical; subsides spontaneously

Primary Progressive TB or Reactivation TB
- Weight loss, anorexia
- Fatigue
- Low-grade afternoon fever, night sweats
- Cough that is dry initially and later becomes productive of purulent and/or blood-tinged sputum
- Fever, night sweats

Diagnostics

- Tuberculin testing is used to screen for TB infection. The amount of induration surrounding the injection site is used to determine infection.
- Sputum for acid-fast bacillus will be positive.
- Culture and sensitivity for *M. tuberculosis*.
- PPD will be positive.
- X-ray of chest will show cavitary lesions in lung.

MEDICAL INTERVENTIONS

- Chemotherapeutic medications are used both to prevent and treat TB.
- Surgical resection of infected lung tissue is rarely employed today. It may be used for clients with localized disease or cavitation when the infecting bacilli are resistant to several drugs.

SELECTED NURSING DIAGNOSES WITH INTERVENTIONS

Risk for Infection

The spread of TB is a risk in any facility housing many people. It is especially high in residential care facilities for the elderly and for persons with AIDS, in homeless shelters, and in drug treatment centers.

- Place the client in a private room with air flow control that prevents air within the room from circulating into the hallway or other rooms. A negative flow room and multiple fresh-air exchanges dilute the concentration of droplet nuclei within the room.

T

- Use universal precautions and TB isolation techniques as recommended by the CDC.
- Use personal protective devices to reduce the risk of transmission during client care. OSHA requires use of a HEPA-filtered respirator.
- Inform the client about the reasons for and importance of carrying out respiratory isolation procedures during hospitalization. For clients treated as outpatients, provide instruction about avoiding crowds and close physical contact, and maintaining ventilation in living facilities, particularly during the first 3 weeks of treatment.
- Place a mask on the client when transporting to other parts of the facility.
- Inform all personnel having contact with the client of the diagnosis.
- Assist visitors to mask prior to entering the client's room.

Ineffective Management of Therapeutic Regimen: Individual

- Assess the client's self-care abilities and support systems.
- Assess the client's level of knowledge and understanding of the disease, its complications, its treatment, and risks to others. Provide additional teaching and reinforcement as indicated.
- Work with the client to identify barriers or obstacles to managing the prescribed treatment.
- Assist the client to develop a plan for managing the prescribed regimen.
- Provide verbal and written instructions that are at the client's level of knowledge, literacy, and understanding.

CLIENT TEACHING

- Teach the client about the disease process, treatment, respiratory isolation and its purpose, and the medication regimen.
- Emphasize the importance of maintaining good general health by eating a well-balanced diet, balancing exercise with rest, and avoiding crowds and people with respiratory infections.
- Stress the importance of avoiding alcohol and other substances that damage the liver while taking chemotherapeutic drugs.

- Encourage fluid intake of 2.5 to 3 quarts of fluid per day.
- Teach the client measures to limit the transmission of TB:
  1. Always cough and expectorate into tissues.
  2. Dispose of tissues personally in a closed bag.
  3. If the client is unable to control respiratory secretions, as when sneezing, he or she should wear a mask.
- Teach the client how to collect sputum specimens.
- Teach the client the importance of complying with prescribed treatment for the entire course of the regimen.
- Tell the client to report to the physician chest pain, hemoptysis, or dyspnea; anorexia, nausea, or vomiting; yellow tint to skin or sclera; sudden weight gain, swollen feet, ankles, legs, or hands; hearing loss, tinnitus, or vertigo; and change in vision or difficulty discriminating colors.

HOME CARE CONSIDERATIONS

- Make referrals as appropriate to smoking cessation programs, alcohol and drug treatment groups or facilities, and hospice or residential care facilities.
- Provide active intervention for homeless people, including shelter placement or other housing, and ongoing follow-up by easily accessed health care providers.
- Refer clients who are unlikely to comply with the treatment regimen to the public health department for management and follow-up.

T

For more information on Tuberculosis, see Medical-Surgical Nursing *by LeMone and Burke, p. 1409.*

Ulcerative Colitis

OVERVIEW

- Ulcerative colitis is a chronic, inflammatory bowel disease (IBD) that usually affects the large bowel. It shares many characteristics with Crohn's disease.
- It usually begins in the distal rectum and ascends; the worst cases reach the ileocecal valve.
- The clinical course is variable; characterized by remissions and exacerbations.
- Pathologic features of ulcerative colitis include congestion, edema, and hemorrhagic inflammation that is confluent over the entire mucosal surface of the colon. Abscesses form in the crypts, ulcers may spread into deeper layers, and eventually the bowel mucosa becomes atrophic and rigid.
- Occurs at a rate of 4 to 12 per 100,000; there is an increased incidence in European Americans, especially in Jews; there is an increased incidence in those with relatives with the same diagnosis.

CAUSES

- Unknown
- There may be an autoimmune component; heredity, infection, dietary factors, smoking, and other environmental factors also may play a role in the disease; psychologic factors may affect the severity of the illness

Signs & Symptoms

Minimal Disease

- Diarrhea: several semiformed stools per day without gross blood
- Constipation if limited to lower rectum
- Abdominal pain: mild, crampy

Severe Disease

- Diarrhea: frequent liquid stools containing blood and pus
- Abdominal pain: severe
- Fever

- Dehydration
- Postural hypotension/tachycardia
- Weight loss

Extracolonic Manifestations
- Arthritis
- Uveitis
- Skin changes
- Liver disease

Diagnostics

- Stool culture to rule out infection or parasites.
- A decrease in the serum albumin level indicates serious protein loss via bowel.
- Serum alkaline phosphatase elevation indicates liver involvement.
- White blood cell (WBC) count is elevated, with a left shift.
- Erythrocyte sedimentation rate elevated.
- Sigmoidoscopy, colonoscopy, or rectal biopsy may be performed.

MEDICAL INTERVENTIONS

- Locally acting and systemic anti-inflammatory drugs are the primary medications used to manage ulcerative colitis. Antidiarrheal agents may be given to slow GI motility and reduce diarrhea.
- Dietary management may restrict milk products, caffeine, and raw fruits and vegetables. Bulk-forming agents may be prescribed.
- Surgical removal of the colon effects a cure for the client with ulcerative colitis and is recommended when the disease resists more conservative treatment.

U

SELECTED NURSING DIAGNOSES WITH INTERVENTIONS

Diarrhea
- Monitor the appearance and frequency of bowel movements using a stool chart.
- Monitor for the presence of blood in stools by testing for occult blood as well as observing for bright red bleeding.

- Assess and document the color, amount, and frequency of diarrhea and, if present, emesis. Maintain accurate fluid intake and output records.
- Assess and document vital signs every 4 hours.
- Record the client's weight daily.
- Assess the client for other indications of fluid deficit: warm, dry skin; poor skin turgor; dry, shiny mucous membranes; weakness, lethargy; complaints of thirst.
- Administer anti-inflammatory and antidiarrheal medications as prescribed.
- Maintain fluid intake by mouth or by parenteral means as indicated.
- Provide good skin care.
- Assess the perianal area for irritation or denuded skin from the diarrhea. Provide measures to protect the perianal area. Use gentle cleansing agents and a zinc oxide-based cream.

Body Image Disturbance

- Accept the client's feelings and perception of self.
- Encourage the client to discuss physical changes and their consequences that have affected his or her self-concept.
- Encourage discussion about concerns regarding the effect of the disease or treatment on close personal relationships.
- Encourage the client to make choices and decisions regarding care.
- Discuss possible effects of treatment options openly and honestly.
- Involve the client in care, providing teaching and instruction as needed.
- Provide care in an accepting, nonjudgmental manner.
- Arrange for interaction with other clients or groups of persons with ulcerative colitis or ostomies.
- Teach coping strategies (odor control, dietary modifications, and so on), and support the client's use of them.

CLIENT TEACHING

- Teach the client about the disease process, treatment, symptom management, exacerbating factors, and need for lifelong medical follow-up.

- Provide information about prescribed medications, including drug names, desired effects, schedules for tapering the doses if ordered, and possible side effects.
- Provide written and verbal information about the prescribed diet and emphasize the need to maintain a fluid intake of at least 2 to 3 quarts per day, and more when the weather is hot, during exercise or strenuous work, or if feverish.
- Provide information about the surgery performed, if appropriate, and follow-up care, including wound care and ostomy care.
- Discuss activity restriction for the postoperative period.

HOME CARE CONSIDERATIONS

- If surgery is performed, a referral to an enterostomal therapy nurse is appropriate. Provide the client with information on where to obtain ostomy supplies.
- Discuss the increased risk for colorectal cancer and stress the need for lifelong follow-up care with the surgeon and gastroenterologist.
- Refer the client to the local chapters of the Foundation for Colitis and Ileitis and the United Ostomy Association for visitor services, support groups, and education.

For more information on Ulcerative Colitis, see Medical-Surgical Nursing *by LeMone and Burke, p. 819.*

U

Urinary Tract Infection (UTI)

OVERVIEW

- Urinary tract infection is a term applied to an infectious process anywhere in the urinary tract: kidney, ureter, bladder, urethra.

- The most common site of infection is the bladder mucosa, producing *cystitis*.
- Infection can develop in the urethra and ascend into the bladder, or be deposited in the bladder directly by way of trauma, surgery, catheters, or other foreign bodies.
- *Pyelonephritis*, an upper urinary tract infection of the kidneys, can also develop via sepsis.
- Cystitis can occur at any age, and is much more common in women than men because of the shorter length of the female urethra.

CAUSES

- Bacterial infection: the most common organisms seen in UTI are gram-negative bacteria, including *Escherichia coli; Proteus* species; *Klebsiella; Pseudomonas; Serratia*
- Risk factors include: female gender; sexually active; pregnancy; uncircumcised males; urinary obstruction; instrumentation; incomplete bladder emptying (neural or muscular); diabetes mellitus; immunodepression; poor hygiene

Signs & Symptoms

- Cystitis is often asymptomatic
- Pyelonephritis usually displays obvious, and more serious, S/S

General S/S
- Fever, chills
- Malaise, anorexia
- Nausea, vomiting

S/S of Cystitis
- Dysuria, urgency
- Frequency, nocturia
- Hematuria (occult)

S/S of Pyelonephritis
- All of the above, with high fever and shaking chills; hematuria may be gross
- Tachycardia
- Flank pain/costovertebral angle tenderness

Diagnostics

- Urine microscopy can reveal heavy bacterial loads; presence of white blood cells (WBCs); pyuria; casts.
- Culture and sensitivity will establish exact causative organism and identify effective antibiotic for treatment.
- WBC count may be elevated.

MEDICAL INTERVENTIONS

- Traditional treatment of UTI involves administration of oral antimicrobial therapy for 7 to 10 days. Single-dose antibiotic therapy or a short, 3-day course is often prescribed for infections of the lower urinary tract.
- Surgery may be indicated for the client with recurrent UTI if diagnostic testing indicates the presence of calculi, structural anomalies, or strictures that contribute to the risk of infection.

SELECTED NURSING DIAGNOSES WITH INTERVENTIONS

Pain

- Assess pain parameters: timing, quality, intensity, location, duration, and aggravating and alleviating factors.
- Provide comfort measures. Nonpharmacologic relief measures include warm sitz baths, warm packs or heating pads, balanced rest and activity. Systemic analgesics, urinary analgesics, or antispasmodic medication may be administered as prescribed.
- Increase fluid intake unless contraindicated by therapeutic regimen.

Altered Urinary Elimination

- Monitor urinary output and color, clarity, and character of urine, including odor.
- Provide for easy access to a bedpan, urinal, commode, or bathroom. Make sure that lighting is adequate and that pathways are free of obstacles.
- Teach the client to avoid caffeinated drinks, including coffee, tea, and cola, and alcoholic beverages.

U

Knowledge Deficit

- Assess the client's level of knowledge about the disease process, risk factors, and preventive measures.
- Teach the client to follow the treatment regimen prescribed by the primary care provider.
- Teach measures to prevent future UTI:
  1. Empty the bladder at least every 2 to 4 hours while awake. Avoid voluntary urinary retention.
  2. Maintain intake of 2 to 2.5 quarts, or eight to ten glasses, of fluid per day.
  3. For women: cleanse perineal area front to back after voiding and defecating; void before and after sexual intercourse; avoid bubble baths, feminine hygiene sprays, and douches; wear cotton (not nylon) undergarments.
- Teach the client how to obtain a midstream clean-catch urine specimen.
- Unless contraindicated, teach the client measures to maintain acidic urine; for example, drink two glasses of cranberry juice per day; take ascorbic acid (vitamin C); avoid excess intake of milk and milk products, other fruit juices, and sodium bicarbonate (baking soda).

CLIENT TEACHING

- Teach the client about the disease process, causes, treatment, and prevention strategies listed above. Clients should be able to identify the early manifestations of UTI and state the importance of seeking medical intervention promptly.
- Make the client aware of the role of stressors in the development of infection to determine whether lifestyle changes may reduce the risk for future UTI.
- Stress the importance of completing all of the prescribed antibiotic regimen.

HOME CARE CONSIDERATIONS

- Advise the client to refrain from sexual intercourse until infection and inflammation have cleared.
- Tell the client to schedule a follow-up appointment with the physician, usually 10 to 14 days after initial treatment, and to seek medical care for any signs of recurrence.

- Information is available from the National Kidney Foundation, the Cystitis Foundation, and the American Urological Association.

For more information on Urinary Tract Infection (UTI), see Medical-Surgical Nursing *by LeMone and Burke, p. 895.*

Uterine Myoma (Fibroids, Leiomyomas)

OVERVIEW

- Uterine myomas are benign tumors of the uterine smooth muscle (myometrium).
- Uterine myomas are the most common of all female genital tract neoplasms.
- They are usually multiple and can vary in size from tiny to very large.
- Most form in the body of the uterus, but any location is possible.
- Location often determines the type and severity of symptoms.
- The incidence of myoma is about 20% of all women, with the rate in African American women three times higher than in European American women.
- Myomas are estrogen-dependent tumors that increase in size during pregnancy and regress following menopause.

U

CAUSES

- Unknown

Signs & Symptoms

- Hypermenorrhea
- Dysmenorrhea
- Pelvic pain
- Uterine enlargement on examination

- S/S of urinary bladder compression: frequency, urgency, nocturia
- S/S of bowel compression: constipation, obstruction
- S/S of anemia: pallor, fatigue, shortness of breath, tachycardia

Diagnostics

- Complete blood count (CBC) may show decreased hemoglobin, hematocrit.

MEDICAL INTERVENTIONS

- Surgical treatment for clients who have symptoms or are past childbearing age includes myomectomy, in which only the fibroids are removed, and hysterectomy or panhysterectomy.

SELECTED NURSING DIAGNOSES

- Pain
- Stress Incontinence
- Constipation
- Fatigue
- Fear
- Anxiety
- Anticipatory Grieving

SELECTED NURSING INTERVENTIONS

- Provide information about pharmacologic and nonpharmacologic methods of pain control, including nonnarcotic analgesics, use of a heating pad, acupuncture, meditation, or other stress-reduction techniques.
- Suggest use of perineal pads to absorb urine leakage, and reduction of caffeine intake to decrease urinary urgency and frequency.
- Recommend increased intake of fresh fruits and vegetables and other high-fiber foods.
- Encourage iron-rich foods in the diet, such as lean meats; dark, leafy green vegetables; eggs; whole grain and enriched breads and cereals; dried fruits; legumes; shellfish; and molasses.

- Suggest extra periods of rest and relaxation to relieve the fatigue, particularly when symptoms are most acute.
- Encourage the woman to express her feelings and fears.
- Explore previously used coping mechanisms and reinforce those appropriate to the situation.
- Emphasize that fibroids are benign and that there may be alternatives to hysterectomy.
- Provide information about surgical intervention, if necessary, including potential outcomes and self-care measures.
- Explore with the woman what her uterus means to her, and what childbearing means to her self-concept.

CLIENT TEACHING

- Teach the client about the disease process, treatment options, and prognosis.
- If surgery is deferred, explain the need for regular follow-up assessments to monitor tumor growth.
- If surgery is chosen, teaching emphasizes pain control techniques and appropriate preoperative and postoperative teaching.

HOME CARE CONSIDERATIONS

- Suggest a support group and/or a therapist if appropriate. This referral may include the client's partner as well.

For more information on Uterine Myoma (Fibroids, Leimyomas), see Medical-Surgical Nursing *by LeMone and Burke, p. 2025.*

U

Vaginitis

OVERVIEW

- Vaginitis is an inflammation of the vaginal mucosa, which can be due to several causes.
- In younger clients, inflammation usually results from an infectious agent, the three most common of which are bacterial vaginosis, candidiasis, and trichomonas.
- The low pH of vaginal secretions, normal vaginal flora, and estrogen provide protection against vaginal infections. Thus, alterations in these factors are conducive to the development of vaginal infection.
- In older women, atrophic vaginitis results from estrogen withdrawal at menopause.
- Less commonly, vaginitis may be due to parasites (pediculosis pubis) or to a hypersensitivity to feminine hygiene products.

CAUSES

- Bacteria: *Escherichia coli; Staphylococcus, Streptococcus*
- Protozoa: *Trichomonas vaginalis*
- Fungi: *Candida albicans*
- Parasites: *Pediculus pubis*
- Atrophic: lack of estrogen
- Hypersensitivity
- Risk factors include use of oral contraceptives or broad-spectrum antibiotics, obesity, diabetes, pregnancy, unprotected sexual intercourse, multiple sexual partners, and poor personal hygiene

Signs & Symptoms

- Burning
- Itching
- Edema
- Discharge

Diagnostics

- Vaginal smear with microscopy can identify trichomoniasis and candidiasis.

- Culture and sensitivity can identify specific bacterial species.

MEDICAL INTERVENTIONS

- Medical intervention is aimed at identifying the causative organism and prescribing a regimen of the appropriate antibiotic or antifungal agent

SELECTED NURSING DIAGNOSES WITH INTERVENTIONS

Pain

- Suggest the use of cool compresses and vinegar or povidone-iodine douches.
- Recommend sitz baths to alleviate discomfort and cleanse the perineal area.

Body Image Disturbance

- Discuss the client's sexual concerns openly and honestly.
- Assess for high-risk behaviors.
- Encourage the client to participate in self-care measures.

CLIENT TEACHING

- Explain to the client and her partner how the infection is transmitted. Many infections are transmitted most easily during certain times of the menstrual cycle; some can be transmitted by towels or other inanimate objects, or by certain types of sexual activity.
- Teach the client and her partner about the need for both of them to complete the full course of treatment. Incomplete treatment allows for recurrence of infection and reinfection of the partner.
- Educate the client and her partner about safe sex practices and improved genital hygiene techniques that can reduce the risk of recurrence. Unless contraindicated, encourage the client with repeated mild candidiasis infections to consume daily 8 ounces of yogurt containing live active cultures to help restore normal vaginal flora. Explain the negative effects of strong douches, feminine hygiene sprays, and perfumed powders in the genital area.

V

Tell the client to cleanse the perineum from front to back after urine and bowel elimination and to wear cotton underwear.

- Most postmenopausal women experience atrophic vaginitis due to thinning and drying of the vaginal mucosa that results from lack of estrogen. These clients should be taught about the use of topical estrogen creams to restore vaginal tissue, the use of water-soluble lubricants for sexual intercourse, and other methods of minimizing the undesirable effects of menopause.

HOME CARE CONSIDERATIONS

- Encourage follow-up visits if the client experiences any recurrence of symptoms. Also stress the importance of regular Pap smears.

For more information on Vaginitis, see Medical-Surgical Nursing *by LeMone and Burke, p. 2039.*

Valvular Heart Disease

Mitral Stenosis
Mitral Insufficiency (Regurgitation)
Mitral Valve Prolapse
Aortic Stenosis
Aortic Insufficiency (Regurgitation)

OVERVIEW

- All forms of valvular heart disease are characterized by alterations in the normal function of heart valves.
- Normal valves function to allow unrestricted blood flow in one direction, while preventing flow in the opposite, or retrograde, direction. The mitral (bicuspid) valve lies between the left atrium and ventricle and allows the free flow of blood *from* the left atrium *to* the left ventricle but prevents retrograde flow. The aortic valve lies between the left ventri-

cle and aorta and allows the free flow of blood *from* the left ventricle to the aorta but prevents retrograde flow.

- Two major types of valve defects are seen:
  1. A *stenotic* valve has a constricted opening and represents an area of high resistance to flow; forward direction of blood is impeded.
  2. An *insufficient (regurgitative)* valve is one that does not close completely and thus allows blood to flow backward.
- Both types result in an increase in cardiac workload for the overloaded chambers.
- Mitral valve prolapse is a minor valve defect that is neither stenotic nor insufficient; rather, it is a mitral valve with an increased compliance.
- Cardiac muscle can compensate for increased workloads, by dilation and hypertrophy, for a long time but serious defects eventually lead to heart decompensation and failure.
- Although there are four valves within the heart, valvular heart disease usually affects those valves on the left side of the heart, the mitral and aortic valves. Mitral valve lesions are most common; aortic, second; tricuspid, third; pulmonic lesions, rare.
- It is possible to have more than one valve affected (mixed lesion).

Mitral Stenosis

- Mitral stenosis prevents adequate flow from the left atrium to the left ventricle during atrial systole.
- The left atrium becomes overloaded, then dilates and hypertrophies to compensate.
- The left ventricle can be underloaded, resulting in reduced cardiac output.
- With left atrial decompensation, blood backs up into the pulmonary circulation causing pulmonary congestion and hypertension.
- If the left atrium fails, pulmonary edema results.
- The right ventricle may then fail.

Mitral Insufficiency (Regurgitation)

- Mitral insufficiency allows the free flow of blood from the left atrium to the left ventricle during

V

diastole, but then allows blood to flow in a retrograde fashion, from the left ventricle back to the left atrium during ventricular systole.
- The left atrium becomes overloaded, then dilates and hypertrophies to compensate.
- The left ventricle also becomes overloaded, then dilates and hypertrophies to compensate.
- With left atrial and/or ventricular decompensation, blood backs up into the pulmonary circulation, causing pulmonary congestion and hypertension.
- If the left atrium and/or ventricle fails, pulmonary edema results.
- The right ventricle may then fail.

Mitral Valve Prolapse
- The mitral valve closes at the onset of ventricular systole.
- Due to its increased compliance, the valve bulges backward into the left atrium, slightly increasing its volume.

Aortic Stenosis
- Aortic stenosis prevents adequate flow from the left ventricle to the aorta.
- The left ventricle becomes overloaded, then dilates and hypertrophies to compensate.
- The aorta can be underloaded, resulting in reduced cardiac output.
- With left ventricular decompensation, blood backs up into the pulmonary circulation, causing pulmonary congestion and hypertension.
- If the left atrium fails, pulmonary edema results.

Aortic Insufficiency (Regurgitation)
- Aortic insufficiency allows the free flow of blood from the left ventricle to the aorta during systole, but then allows blood to flow in a retrograde fashion, from the aorta back to the left ventricle during diastole.
- The left ventricle becomes overloaded, then dilates and hypertrophies to compensate.
- The left atrium also becomes overloaded, then dilates and hypertrophies to compensate.

- With left ventricular and atrial decompensation, blood backs up into the pulmonary circulation causing pulmonary congestion and hypertension.
- If the left atrium fails, pulmonary edema results.
- The right ventricle may then fail.

CAUSES

Mitral Stenosis
- Rheumatic heart disease
- Congenital anomaly
- Atrial myxoma
- Calcification
- Thrombus

Mitral Insufficiency (Regurgitation)
- Rheumatic heart disease
- Congenital anomaly
- Endocarditis
- Papillary muscle rupture
- Secondary to aortic valve disease

Mitral Valve Prolapse
- Intrinsic weakness
- Accompanies: endocarditis; myocarditis; atherosclerosis, systemic lupus erythematosus, acromegaly, muscular dystrophy, sarcoidosis

Aortic Stenosis
- Rheumatic heart disease
- Congenital anomaly
- Calcification
- Atherosclerosis

Aortic Insufficiency (Regurgitation)
- Rheumatic heart disease
- Congenital anomaly
- Connective tissue disease: Marfan's syndrome, myxoma
- Hypertension
- Syphilis

V

Signs & Symptoms

Mitral Stenosis

- Gradual onset of S/S
- Exertional dyspnea/fatigue
- Palpitations
- Murmur: loud S_1 followed by a snap, then a low pitched rumble; at apex
- S/S of left ventricular congestive heart failure/ pulmonary edema: cough; dyspnea, dyspnea on exertion; orthopnea; paroxysmal nocturnal dyspnea; frothy expectoration; hemoptysis; wet rales
- S/S right ventricular congestive heart failure: peripheral edema, ascites; jugular vein distention; hepatomegaly; weight gain; abdominal distress; increased central venous pressure
- S/S of atrial fibrillation: irregular rate and magnitude of pulse; faint feeling, weakness
- S/S of left embolus to brain or any visceral or peripheral artery

Mitral Insufficiency (Regurgitation)

- Usually asymptomatic or less severe S/S than mitral stenosis
- Murmur: best heard at apex; systolic; S_1 soft; S_2 split; may be S_3; high-pitched; blowing; radiates to left axilla
- If cardiac output falls: hypotension, weakness, fainting
- S/S of left ventricular congestive heart failure/ pulmonary edema
- S/S of right ventricular congestive heart failure

Mitral Valve Prolapse

- Most are asymptomatic
- May be dysrhythmias: premature ventricular contraction, supraventricular tachycardia, ventricular tachycardia
- S/S, if dysrhythmias: palpitations, chest pain, dyspnea, dizziness
- Murmur: mid-systolic click; then high-pitched late systolic murmur

Aortic Stenosis

- Exertional dyspnea/fatigue
- Chest pain, especially with exercise
- Dysrhythmia
- Syncope/confusion: indicate inadequate cerebral perfusion
- Murmur: best heard over aortic area; harsh; mid-systolic; may be split S_2
- S/S of left ventricular congestive heart failure/pulmonary edema
- S/S of right ventricular congestive heart failure

Aortic Insufficiency (Regurgitation)

- Murmur: best heard at second intercostal space on right; high-pitched, blowing, decrescendo type
- High magnitude apical and carotid pulsations
- Positive DeMusset's sign: head bobs with pulse
- Positive Corrigan's water hammer pulse: sharply rising pulse amplitude, falls away very quickly
- Palpitations: especially when in left recumbent position
- Dysrhythmias: premature ventricular contractions; supraventricular tachycardia
- Exertional dyspnea/fatigue
- S/S of left ventricular congestive heart failure/pulmonary edema
- S/S of right ventricular congestive heart failure

Diagnostics

- Chest x-ray will show enlarged cardiac shadow, pulmonary congestion, calcifications.
- EKG will define any dysrhythmias present.
- Echocardiogram will show altered valve leaflet motion, wall hypertrophy, abnormal wall motion.
- Cardiac catherization will measure increased cardiopulmonary pressures and measure cardiac output.

MEDICAL INTERVENTIONS

- Pharmacologic agents such as diuretics, vasodilators, anticoagulants, and cardiac glycosides are used to maintain cardiac output and prevent clot formation. Antibiotics are used to prevent infection.

V

- Clients whose stenotic valve disease cannot be managed with medical therapy may be treated with percutaneous balloon valvuloplasty.
- Surgery to repair or replace the diseased valve provides definitive treatment.

SELECTED NURSING DIAGNOSES WITH INTERVENTIONS

Decreased Cardiac Output

- Monitor and record vital signs and hemodynamic parameters, reporting alterations from the baseline.
- Assess for clinical manifestations of decreased cardiac output every shift, or more frequently if indicated. Be alert for the following: changes in level of consciousness; jugular venous distention; respiratory crackles and dyspnea; decreased urine output; cool, clammy, mottled skin; peripheral edema; and decreased peripheral pulses and capillary refill. Notify the physician of significant changes.
- Monitor intake and output; weigh the client daily, reporting any gain of 3 to 5 pounds within 24 hours.
- Maintain fluid restriction as prescribed.
- Elevate the head of the bed, and administer supplemental oxygen as prescribed.
- Monitor pulse oximetry continually and arterial blood gases as prescribed.
- Ensure the client's physical, emotional, and mental rest.
- Administer prescribed medications aimed at reducing cardiac workload.

Activity Intolerance

- Obtain vital signs before and during activities.
- Encourage the client to increase the amount of activity and self-care gradually, as tolerated. Ensure adequate rest periods, uninterrupted sleep cycles, and adequate nutrition.
- Provide assistance as needed. Suggest the client use a shower chair, sit down while brushing teeth, and so on.
- Consult with a physical therapist for in-bed exercises and a progressive activity plan of care.
- Discuss with the client and significant others methods to decrease energy requirements at home.

Risk for Infection

- Maintain aseptic technique for all invasive procedures.
- Monitor temperature every 4 hours. Notify physician if the client's temperature exceeds 100.5F (38.5C).
- Assess wounds and catheter sites for redness, swelling, warmth, pain, or evidence of drainage.
- Administer antibiotics as prescribed. Ensure that the client receives the full course.
- Monitor white blood cell counts and notify the physician of counts below $5000/\mu L$ or above $10,000/\mu L$.

CLIENT TEACHING

- Explain the disease process and all tests and procedures, including surgery.
- Discuss management of the client's manifestations, including activity restrictions, diet restrictions, and medication regimen.
- Teach the client about the importance of notifying all health care providers about the valve disorder or surgery so that antibiotics can be initiated prophylactically before any procedure that might allow bacterial invasion, including dental procedures.

HOME CARE CONSIDERATIONS

- Provide referrals to community resources and the address and phone number of the American Heart Association prior to discharge.
- Alert the client and significant others to manifestations that should be reported immediately to the physician.

For more information, see the following pages in Medical-Surgical Nursing *by LeMone and Burke:*
Mitral Stenosis, p. 1141
Mitral Insufficiency, p. 1142
Mitral Valve Prolapse, p. 1142
Aortic Stenosis, p. 1143
Aortic Insufficiency, p. 1144

V

Varicella Zoster Virus (VZV) Infection

Chickenpox
Herpes Zoster (Shingles)

OVERVIEW

- VZV causes two discrete clinical diseases: chickenpox and herpes zoster, also called shingles.
- *Chickenpox* is a primary infection with the highly contagious VZV that most commonly is acquired during childhood, between 5 and 9 years of age.
- The incubation period is 10 to 21 days; the infectious period is from 48 hours prior to onset of rash until all lesions are crusted over.
- The primary VZV infection is acquired via the respiratory system, and produces a systemic viremia; vesicular lesions form in a disseminated pattern.
- *Herpes zoster* is a reinfection that usually reappears after age 60, or in immunocompromised individuals; it presents as painful vesicles in a dermatomal pattern.
- The virus remains latent in the dorsal root ganglia of cranial or peripheral nerves.
- A disseminated form, usually involving the lung and/or brain, can also occur in neonates or in the immunocompromised.

CAUSES

- Infection with the varicella zoster virus (VZV), a DNA-containing herpesvirus.

Signs & Symptoms

Primary Infection

- A prodrome may precede rash; consists of headache, anorexia, malaise
- Rash: the early lesions are erythematous maculopapules, then vesicles form, then crusts. The evolution of the lesions can occur over hours to days with successive groups of lesions forming at

different times. They usually appear first on the trunk and face, then spread rapidly to other areas, including the mucous membranes of the mouth, pharynx, and vagina. The total number of lesions varies widely between individuals and can range from several to a few thousand; young children have fewer lesions than older children or adults. Immunocompromised patients have the most lesions.

- Pruritis at lesion sites
- Fever 37.8 to 39.4C (100–103F)
- Malaise
- Anorexia

Complications of Primary VZV

- Secondary infection of lesions may occur and is usually due to *Streptococcus pyogens* or *Staphylococcus aureus*
- CNS infection can occur about 3 weeks after the onset of rash and manifests as an acute cerebellar ataxia and meningeal irritation (see Meningitis)
- VZV pneumonia is the most serious complication of chickenpox; usually affects adult or immunocompromised individuals; hemorrhagic type
- Other complications include myocarditis, ulcerative keratitis, nephritis, arthritis, hepatitis, Reye's syndrome

Herpes zoster (Shingles)

- Pain: severe, deep; continuous; often debilitating; usually precedes rash by 48 to 72 hours
- Rash: unilateral, confluent, erythematous, vesicles; dermatomal pattern; most common at T3 to L3; crust over after 10 days
- Fever
- Malaise
- Complications of herpes zoster include post-herpetic neuralgia, CNS infection, disseminated infection

V

Diagnostics

- Viral culture can identify the VZV.
- Immunofluorescent methods can identify varicella in skin cells.

MEDICAL INTERVENTIONS

- The antiviral medication acyclovir is the drug of choice for herpes zoster infections. Although it does not cure the infection, it decreases the severity and the pain.
- Corticosteroids may be used to decrease inflammation; however, they also slow healing and suppress the immune response.
- Narcotic and nonnarcotic analgesics are prescribed for pain management.

SELECTED NURSING DIAGNOSES WITH INTERVENTIONS

Pain

- Assess and monitor the location, duration, and intensity of the pain.
- Administer prescribed medications regularly and evaluate their effectiveness.
- Use measures to relieve pruritis: administer prescribed medications; apply calamine lotion or wet compresses as prescribed; keep the room temperature cool; use a bed cradle to keep sheets off affected areas.
- Encourage the use of distraction and relaxation techniques.

Sleep Pattern Disturbance

- Provide appropriate interventions to relieve pain and pruritis.
- Maintain a cool environment and avoid heavy bed coverings.

Risk for Infection

- Monitor the client for signs of infection: take and record vital signs every 4 hours; assess skin lesions for erythema, pustules, discharge; monitor white cell count; assess for lymph gland enlargement.
- Use interventions to decrease the itch-scratch-itch cycle, thereby decreasing the possibility of excoriation.
- Institute infection control procedures.

CLIENT TEACHING

- Teach the client about the disease process, medications, dosage, effects and side effects, and prognosis. Tell the client that the disease is self-limiting and typically heals completely. Second occurrences of herpes zoster are rare.
- Tell the client to avoid contact with children or pregnant women until crusts have formed over the blisters. The disease is contagious to those who have not had chickenpox.
- Encourage the client to follow the suggestions listed above to help control pain and itching.

HOME CARE CONSIDERATIONS

- Tell the client to report to the physician any increase in pain, fever, chills, drainage that smells bad or has pus, or a spread in the blisters.

For more information on Varicella Zoster Virus (VZV) Infection, see Medical-Surgical Nursing *by LeMone and Burke, p. 584.*

Varicose Veins

OVERVIEW

- Varicose veins are weak, dilated veins that become tortuous and lead to valve incompetence and venous insufficiency, all of which increase the risk of forming venous thrombi.
- They may be located in peripheral vessels such as the saphenous veins in the leg or in mucosal tissues such as the esophagus (varices), scrotum (varicocele), or rectum (hemorrhoids).
- They are more common in females and are associated with occupations in which long periods of standing are required.

V

CAUSES

Leg

- Inherent vein weakness (genetic predisposition)
- Obesity
- Pregnancy
- Long periods of standing
- Heart failure

Varices

- Cirrhosis: hepatic

Hemorrhoids

- Pregnancy
- Cirrhosis
- Constipation

Signs & Symptoms

Leg

- Visible dilated, tortuous veins
- Leg heaviness/fatigue
- S/S of thrombophlebitis: warm, red, swollen leg; tender veins; positive Homan's sign
- S/S of pulmonary embolism, which develops rapidly
- Long term: venous leg ulcers

Varices

- Bleeding: hematemesis; melena
- S/S of shock: rapid, thready pulse; hypotension; cold, clammy, pale, skin

Hemorrhoids

- External hemorrhoids may be visible
- Pain
- Itching
- Bleeding

Diagnostics

- Doppler flow studies show retrograde flow in leg veins.
- Phlebography outlines vein and shows the condition of valves.

- Esophagoscopy is used to locate and visualize varices.
- Stool for occult blood will signify bleeding due to varices or hemorrhoids.
- Sigmoidoscopy to confirm internal hemorrhoids and rule out carcinoma.

MEDICAL INTERVENTIONS

- Conservative measures include antiembolism stockings and regular, daily walking and leg elevation.
- Mild analgesics may relieve the pain associated with varicose veins.
- Compression sclerotherapy and vein stripping are surgical techniques that may alleviate the major symptoms of varicose veins; however, there is no real cure.

SELECTED NURSING DIAGNOSES WITH INTERVENTIONS

Pain

- Assess the client's pain.
- Teach and reinforce methods for relieving pain that do not involve the use of analgesic agents.
- Encourage the client to discuss possible relationships between episodes of pain and life stressors.
- Collaborate with the client to establish a plan of pain control.
- Regularly evaluate the effectiveness of interventions used to minimize pain.

Altered Tissue Perfusion: Peripheral

- Assess peripheral pulses, capillary refill time, skin temperature, and degree of edema.
- Teach the client to apply properly fitted supportive or antiembolic stockings and to remove them each day for 30 to 60 minutes.
- Teach the client to exercise the extremities at regular intervals.
- Teach the client how to position the legs to promote tissue perfusion.

Risk for Impaired Skin Integrity

- Assess the skin on the lower extremities for warmth, erythema, moisture, and signs of breakdown as part of an initial examination.

V

- Teach clients about daily skin hygiene.
- Teach the client to protect the extremities from external forces that may cause skin breakdown.
- Encourage adequate nutrition and fluid intake.

CLIENT TEACHING

- Teach the clients about the disease process, management of symptoms, pain relief measures, and the importance of avoiding injury to the extremities.
- Teach the client to report any signs of neurovascular dysfunction, including numbness, coldness, pain, or tingling of an extremity.
- Teach clients the importance of daily walks, the correct technique for applying antiembolism stockings, and the necessity of elevating the legs and avoiding standing or sitting in one place for prolonged periods.

HOME CARE CONSIDERATIONS

- Stress the importance of follow-up care with the physician or surgeon as recommended.
- For the client suffering from a body image disturbance related to varicose veins, a referral to a psychologic counselor or support group may be appropriate.

For more information on Varicose Veins, see Medical-Surgical Nursing *by LeMone and Burke, p. 1250.*

Vitiligo

OVERVIEW

- Vitiligo is a skin disorder characterized by large patches of depigmentation.
- It affects a small portion of the U.S. population; mostly seen in people ages 10 to 30; the peak age is 20.

- It affects both sexes in equal proportions.
- Vitiligo is cosmetically a concern.

CAUSES

- Unknown
- Suspected: autoimmune

Signs & Symptoms

- Depigmentation: symmetric areas of complete color loss; skin as white as chalk.
- Areas: face, extremities, hands, nipples, anus

Diagnostics

- Skin biopsy shows complete lack of melanocytes; no inflammation

MEDICAL INTERVENTIONS

- Phototherapy provides significant repigmentation in about 50% of cases.
- Pharmacologic therapy includes corticosteroid creams.

SELECTED NURSING DIAGNOSES

- Body Image Disturbance
- Risk for Chronic Low Self-Esteem

SELECTED NURSING INTERVENTIONS

- Assess and document the client's verbal and nonverbal responses to the condition.
- Actively listen to the client and acknowledge the reality of concerns about treatment, progress, and prognosis.
- Encourage the client to share feelings about the skin changes and to grieve.
- Encourage the client to discuss how the skin change has affected self-concept.
- Assist the client to identify ways to cover the depigmented areas to make them less obvious and to choose clothing, makeup, and hair styles to enhance self-esteem.

V

- Encourage the client to focus on strengths, positive personal traits, and accomplishments, and not on physical changes.

CLIENT TEACHING

- Teach the client about the disease process, treatment options, effects and side effects, and prognosis.
- Teach positive behavior skills through role play, role model, discussion, and so on.

HOME CARE CONSIDERATIONS

- Offer the client a referral to a psychologist for assistance with adjustment to physical changes and associated self-esteem changes. Provide information about the value of counseling and other available community resources.

For more information on Vitiligo, see Medical-Surgical Nursing *by LeMone and Burke, p. 560.*

Table 1 Normal ABG Values

	Range	Average
pH	7.35–7.45	7.4
$Paco_2$	35–45 mm Hg	40 mm Hg
HCO_3	22–26 mEq/L	24 mEq/L
Pao_2	80–100 mm Hg	95 mm Hg
Sao_2*	94–100%	96%
O_2 Content	15–25 mL%	19 mL% (Hg = 15 g)

*Percent hemoglobin saturated with O_2

Table 2 ABG Changes in Acid-Base Disorders

	pH	$Paco_2$	HCO_3
Respiratory acidosis			
Uncompensated	**decreased**	increased	normal
Compensated	normal	increased	increased
Respiratory alkalosis			
Uncompensated	increased	**decreased**	normal
Compensated	normal	**decreased**	**decreased**
Metabolic acidosis			
Uncompensated	**decreased**	normal	**decreased**
Compensated	normal	**decreased**	**decreased**
Metabolic alkalosis			
Uncompensated	**increased**	normal	**increased**
Compensated	normal	**increased** (limited)	**increased**

Table 3	Types of Anemia		
Name	Mechanism	Laboratory Indicators	Specific S/S
	Hypoproliferative		
Pernicious	↓Serum B_{12}	Macrocytic RBCs ($↓MCV$) Negative Schilling test	Dyspepsia, glossitis, stomatitis, numbness, tingling, clumsiness
Folate deficiency	↓Serum folic acid	Macrocytic RBCs ($↓ MCV$) ↓Serum folate	Similar to pernicious anemia
Iron deficiency	↓Serum iron (Fe) Chronic bleeding	↓RBCs, ↓[Hgb], ↓HCT Microcytic/hypochromic RBCs ↓MCV, ↓MCHC, ↓Serum Fe, ↓TIBC	Stomatitis, brittle hair/nails, koilonychia, pica, heart murmurs
Aplastic	Bone marrow damage •radiation •chemotherapy •infection	↓RBCs, ↓ [Hgb], ↓ HCT normocytic RBCs ↓WBCs, ↓platelets	S/S of anemia, frequent infection, bleeding disorders

Hemorrhagic

Acute	Blood loss/short time course (i.e., minutes, hours, days)	↓RBC, ↓[Hgb], ↓HCT Normocytic/chromic RBCs ↓Reticulocytes, ↓nucleated RBCs	Hypotension, dizziness, vertigo, restlessness, thirst, rapid/thready pulse, may progress to shock, coma, and death
Chronic	Blood loss/long course (i.e., weeks, months, years)	Similar to iron-deficiency anemia	Similar to iron-deficiency anemia

Hemolytic

G6PD deficiency	Genetic, autosomal-recessive	↓G6PD enzyme in RBCs ↓G6PD, ↓HCT, ↓bilirubin Positive for Heinz bodies	S/S anemia and jaundice
Sickle cell disease	Genetic, autosomal-recessive, defective Hgb molecule	Positive for sickle cells, target cells RBC count/morphology depend on stage	Multiple organ-system ischemia, pain and dysfunction
Transfusion reaction	Acquired, immune-mediated RBC destruction	Varying degrees of anemia, ↓bilirubin	Fever, S/S hypersensitivity, S/S shock, jaundice

Key: ↓ = decreased; G6PD = glucose-6-phosphatase deficiency; RBC = red blood cell; Hgb = hemoglobin; [Hgb] = hemoglobin concentration; HCT = hematocrit; MCHC = mean corpuscular hemoglobin concentration; MCV = mean corpuscular volume; TIBC = total iron binding capacity; WBC = white blood cell.

Tables

Community Resource Directory

RESOURCES BY TOPIC

NURSING ORGANIZATIONS

**American Association of
Critical-Care Nurses**
Aliso Viejo, CA
(800) 899-2226
www.aacn.com

**American Association of
Neuroscience Nurses**
Chicago, IL
(312) 993-0043
www.aann.org

**American Association of
Nurse Attorneys**
Pensacola, FL
(850) 484-9987

**American Association of
Occupational Health Nurses**
Atlanta, GA
(800) 241-8014
www.aaohn.org

**American Association of
Spinal Cord Injury Nurses**
Flushing, NY
(718) 803-3782
www.aascin.org

**American College of
Nurse-Midwives**
Washington DC
(202) 289-0171
www.acnm.org

**American Holistic Nurses
Association**
Flagstaff, AZ
(800) 278-AHNA
www.ahna.org

**American Nephrology Nurses
Association**
Pitman, NY
(888) 600-2662
anna.inurse.com

**American Nurses
Association**
Washington DC
(800) 274-4ANA
www.nursingworld.org

**American Society of
Ophthalmic Registered
Nurses**
San Francisco, CA
(415) 561-8513
webeye.ophth.uiowa.edu/
asorn

**American Society of
Plastic and Reconstructive
Surgical Nurses**
Box 56, N. Woodbury Road
Pitman, NJ
(609) 256-2340

**Association of
Nurses in AIDS Care**
704 Stony Hill Road
Suite M106
Yardley, PA 19067
(215) 321-2371

**Association of
Operating Room Nurses**
Denver, CO
(800) 755-2676
www.aorn.org

**Association of
Rehabilitation Nurses**
Glenview, IL
(800) 229-7530
www.rehabnurse.org

**Association of Rheumatology
Health Professionals**
Atlanta, GA
(404) 633-3777
www.rheumatology.org/arhp/

Canadian Nurses Association
Ottawa, Ontario
Canada
(613) 237-2133
www.cna_nurses.ca

**Dermatology Nurses
Association**
Pitman, NJ
(609) 256-2330
dna.inurse.com

**Emergency Nurses
Association**
Park Ridge, IL
(800) 243-8362
www.ena.org

Intravenous Nurses Society
Belmont, MA
(617) 489-5205
www.ins1.org

**National Association of
Orthopedic Nurses**
Pitman, NJ
(609) 256-2310
naon.inurse.com

National League for Nursing
New York, NY
(212) 989-9393
www.nln.org

**National Organization for
the Advancement of
Associate Degree Nursing**
1730 North Lynn Street
Suite 502
Arlington, VA 22209
(703) 525-1191

**National Student Nurses
Association**
New York, NY
(212) 581-2211
www.thomson.com/nsna

**North American Nursing
Diagnosis Association**
Philadelphia, PA
(215) 545-8105
www.nanda.org

Oncology Nursing Society
Pittsburgh, PA
(412) 921-7373
www.ons.org

**Society of Otorhinolaryngol-
ogy and Head/Neck Nurses**
116 Canal Street, Suite A
New Smyrna Beach, FL 32618
(904) 428-1695

**Wound, Osotomy, and
Continence Nurses**
Costa Mesa, CA
(714) 476-0268
www.wocn.org

RESOURCES BY TOPIC

Aging

Alzheimer's Association
Chicago, IL
(800) 272-3900
www.alz.org

The American Association for International Aging
1133 20th Street NW
Suite 330
Washington DC
(202) 833-8893

American Association of Home for the Aging
Washington DC
(202) 783-2242
www.aahsa.org

American Association of Retired Persons (AARP)
Washington DC
(800) 424-3410
www.aarp.org
(Provides informational material related to retirement and aging)

American College of Health Care Administrators
Alexandria, VA
(703) 549-5822
www.achca.org

American Council of the Blind
Washington DC
(202) 467-5081
www.acb.org

American Federation for Aging Research (AFAR)
New York, NY
(212) 752-2327
www.afar.org

American Foundation for the Blind
New York, NY
(212) 752-2327
www.ige.apc.org/afb

American Geriatrics Society, Inc.
New York, NY
(212) 308-1414
www.americangeriatrics.org

American Health Care Association
Washington DC
(202) 842-8444
www.ahca.org

American Society on Aging
San Francisco, CA
(415) 543-2617
www.asaging.org

Gerontological Society of America
Washington DC
(202) 842-1150
www.geron.org

Gray Panthers
Washington DC
(800) 280-5362
www.graypanthers.org

National Council on the Aging, Inc.
Washington DC
(202) 479-1200
www.ncoa.org
(See white or yellow pages of telephone directory for listing of local chapter)

AIDS (Acquired Immune Deficiency Syndrome)

AIDS Clinical Trials Information Service
Bethesda, MD
(301) 496-8210
www.actis.org

American Foundation for AIDS Research
Los Angeles, CA
(213) 857-5900
www.amfar.org
(Publishes AIDS/HIV Treatment Directory)

Canadian AIDS Society
Ottawa, Ontario
Canada
(613) 230-3580
www.web.net/~casinfo/index_
e.html

**Gay Men's Health Crisis
Network**
New York, NY
(212) 807-6664
www.gmhc.org

**National Association of
People with AIDS**
Washington DC
(202) 898-0414
www.napwa.org

National Gay Task Force Crisis Line
(800) 221-7044
www.ngltf.org

**San Francisco AIDS
Foundation**
San Francisco, CA
(800) 367-2437
www.sfaf.org

Shanti Project
San Francisco, CA
(415) 864-2273
www.emf.net/%7Echetham/
gshpct-1.html

Alcohol Abuse

Al-Anon Family Group Headquarters
New York, NY
(800) 344-2666
www.al-anon-alateen.org

**Al-Anon Family Groups
National Public Information**
P.O. Box 6433, Station "J"
Ottawa, Ontario K2A 3Y6
Canada
(613) 722-1830

**Alcohol and Drug Problems
Association of North
America**
1101 15th Street, NW
Suite 204
Washington DC 20005

Alcoholics Anonymous
New York, NY
(212) 870-3400
www.alcoholics.anonymous.
org

Alcoholics Anonymous
234 Eglington Avenue E
Toronto, Ontario M4P 1K5
Canada
(416) 487-5591

American Liver Foundation
Cedar Grove, NJ
(201) 256-2550
gi.ucsf.edu/alf.html

**Drug Information
Association, Inc.**
Fort Washington, PA
(215) 628-2288
www.diahome.org

**National Council on
Alcoholism, Inc.**
New York, NY
(212) 206-6770
www.ncadd.org

Allergies

**American Academy of
Allergy and Immunology**
Milwaukee, WI
(800) 822-ASMA
www.aaaai.org

**The Asthma and Allergy
Foundation of America**
Washington DC
(800) 7-ASTHMA
www.aafa.org
*(See also Asthma; Lung
Disease)*

Alzheimer's Disease

Alzheimer's Association
Chicago, IL
(800) 272-3900
In Illinois: (800) 572-6037
www.alz.org

Alzheimer's Society of Canada
Toronto, Ontario
Canada
(416) 488-8772
www.alzheimer.ca
(See also Neurologic Disorders)

Amputees

American Amputee Foundation
P.O. Box 250218
Hillcrest Station
Little Rock, AR 72225
(501) 666-2523

Amputees in Motion
P.O. Box 2703
Escondido, CA 92025
(619) 454-9300

Amputee Shoe and Glove Exchange
P.O. Box 27067
Houston, TX 77227

Disabled Sports USA
Rockville, MD
(301) 217-0960
www.nas.com/~dsusa

National Amputation Foundation
73 Church Street
Malverne, NY 11565
(516) 887-3600

National Easter Seals Society
Chicago, IL
(312) 726-6200
www.seals.com

National Odd Shoe Exchange
7102 North 35th Avenue
Suite 2
Phoenix, AZ 85051
(602) 841-6691

Amyotrophic Lateral Sclerosis (ALS)

Amyotrophic Lateral Sclerosis Association
Woodland Hills, CA
(818) 340-7500
www.ALSA.org

Anesthesiologists

American Society of Anesthesiologists
Park Ridge, IL
(847) 825-5586
www.asahq.org

Malignant Hyperthermia Association of the United States (MHAUS)
Sherburne, NY
(800) 98-MHAUS
www.mhaus.org/index.html

Anorexia

(See Eating Disorders)

Arthritis and Connective Tissue Disorders

Arthritis Foundation
Atlanta, GA
(800) 283-7800
www.arthritis.org

Arthritis Society
Toronto, Ontario
Canada
(416) 967-1414
www.arthritis.ca/cra.html

Fibromyalgia Network
Tuscon, AZ
(800) 853-2929
www.fmnetnews.com/pages/basics.html

Lupus Foundation of America, Inc.
Rockville, MD
(800) 558-0121
www.lupus.org

Lyme Disease Foundation
Hartford, CT
(800) 525-2000
www.lyme.org

*National Institute of
Arthritis and Musculoskeletal
and Skin Diseases*
National Institute of Health
Bethesda, MD
(301) 396-4000

Scleroderma Foundation
Danvers, MA
(978) 750-4499
www.scleroderma.org

*Sjogren's Syndrome
Foundation, Inc.*
Port Washington, NY
(516) 767-2866
www.sjogrens.com

Spondylitis Association
Sherman Oaks, CA
(800) 777-8189
www.spondylitis.org

*United Scleroderma
Foundation, Inc.*
Watsonville, CA
(408) 728-2202
www.scleroderma.com

Asthma

*Allergy Foundation of
Canada*
Saskatoon, SK
Canada
(306) 373-7591
www.mediconsult.com/
allergies/shareware/life/afoc.
html

American Lung Association
New York, NY
(800) 586-4872
www.lungusa.org

*Asthma and Allergy
Foundation of America*
Washington DC
(800) 7-ASTHMA
www.aafa.org
(See also Lung Disease)

*National Jewish Center for
Immunology and Respiratory
Medicine*
Denver, CO
(800) 222-5864
www.njc.org

Birth Control

*Association for Voluntary
Surgical Contraception*
New York, NY
(212) 561-8095
www.avsc.org
*(Provides information and
referrals to individuals
considering tubal ligation or
vasectomy)*

*Planned Parenthood
Federation of America*
New York, NY
(800) 829-7732
www.plannedparenthood.org

Birth Defects

Cystic Fibrosis Foundation
Bethesda, MD
(301) 951-4422
www.cff.org

*March of Dimes Birth
Defects Foundation
Public Health Education
Foundation*
White Plains, NY
(914) 428-7100
www.modimes.org

Blindness

*American Foundation for
the Blind*
New York, NY
(212) 620-2000
(800) 232-5463
www.ige.apc.org/afb/

Braille Institute
Los Angeles, CA
www.brailleinstitute.org

**Canadian Council of
the Blind**
P.O. Box 2310, Station "D"
Ottawa, Ontario K1P 5W5
Canada
(613) 567-0311

Guide Dogs for the Blind
San Rafael, CA
(510) 479-4000
www.guidedogs.com

**National Eye Institute
Information Officer**
Bethesda, MD
(301) 496-5248
www.nei.nih.gov

**National Federation of
the Blind**
Baltimore, MD
(410) 659-9314
www.nfb.org

Recording for the Blind, Inc.
Princeton, NJ
(800) 803-7201
www.rfbd.org

Blood Banks

American Red Cross
Washington DC
(202) 737-8300
www.crossnet.org
*(See white or yellow pages of
telephone directory for listing of
local chapter)*

Breast Cancer

American Cancer Society
Atlanta, GA
(800) ACS-2345
www.cancer.org

Breast Cancer Advisory
P.O. Box 224
Kensington, MD 20895

Look Good, Feel Better
c/o American Cancer Society
Atlanta, GA
(404) 320-3333
www.lgfb.ca/
*(Program that teaches skills to
cope with appearance changes
from chemotherapy)*

**National Alliance of Breast
Cancer Organizations**
New York, NY
(212) 719-0154
www.nabco.org

**National Breast Cancer
Coalition**
Washington DC
(202) 296-7477
www.natlbcc.org
*(A national grass-roots advocacy
network of more than 300 local
breast cancer organizations,
committed to increase federal
funding for breast cancer
research)*

**National Cancer Institute
Public Inquiry Section
Office of Cancer
Communications**
National Cancer Institute
Bethesda, MD
www.nci.nih.gov

**National Women's
Health Network**
(202) 347-1140
*(A national consumer organiza-
tion offering information on a
variety of women's health
issues including breast cancer;
bi-monthly newsletter and specialized information packets)*

Reach to Recovery
American Cancer Society
Atlanta, GA
(800) ASC-2345
www.cancer.org
*(Support program for women
who have undergone
mastectomies as a result
of breast cancer)*

Y-ME Breast Cancer Support Program
Homewood, IL
(800) 221-2141
www.y-me.org
(See also Cancer)

Bulimia

(See Eating Disorders)

Burn Injuries

American Burn Association
Chicago, IL
www.ameriburn.org

National Burn Victim Foundation
Basking Ridge, NJ
(908) 953-9091
www.nbrf.org

Phoenix Society National Organization for Burn Victims
11 Rust Hill Road
Levittown, PA 19056
(215) 946-4788
(Self-help organization for burn victims and their families)

Cancer

American Cancer Society
Atlanta, GA
(800) 227-2345
www.cancer.org
(See white pages of telephone directory for listing of local chapter)

American Lung Association
New York, NY
(212) 315-8700
www.lungusa.org

Breast Cancer Advisory Center
P.O. Box 224
Kensington, MD 20895

Canadian Cancer Society
Toronto, Ontario
Canada
(416) 480-7580
www.ontario,cancer.ca

Cancer Connection
Kansas City, MO
(816) 932-8453
www.cancer-connection.com
(Support group that matches cancer patients with volunteers who are cured, in remission, or being treated for same type of cancer)

CANCERFAX:
(301) 402-5874
(Up-to-date information on many cancers, delivered via FAX to physicians and patients; physicians' information includes many references to the cancer literature)

Cancer Information Service
National Cancer Institute
Bethesda, MD
(800) 4-CANCER
www.nci.hih.gov
(Supplies cancer information to the general public)

DES Action, USA
Oakland, CA
(510) 465-4011
(800) DES-9288

Food and Drug Administration
Rockville, MD
(800) FDA-1078
www.fda.gov
(Information on adverse reactions to drug therapy)

I Can Cope
American Cancer Society, Inc.
Atlanta, GA
(800) 227-2345
www.cancer.org
(Group education and support program offered by health professionals over several weeks)

Leukemia Society of America, Inc.
New York, NY
(212) 573-8484
www.leukemia.org

Look Good, Feel Better
American Cancer Society, Inc.
Atlanta, GA
(404) 320-3333
www.lgfb.ca
(Program that teaches skills to cope with appearance changes from chemotherapy)

Make Today Count
P.O. Box 6063
Kansas City, KS 66106
(913) 362-2866

National Cancer Information Clearinghouse
Bethesda, MD
(301) 496-4070
www.nci.nih.gov

National Coalition for Cancer Survivorship
Silver Springs, MD
(301) 650-8868
www.cansearch.org

National Council of Independent Living
2111 Wilson Boulevard
Suite 405
Arlington, VA 22201
(703) 525-3406

National Hospice Organization
Arlington, VA
(703) 243-5900
www.nho.org

National Lymphederma Network
San Francisco, CA
(800) 541-3259
www.lymphnet.org
(A network of specialized clinics devoted to the management of lymphedema)

Ostomy Rehabilitation
(One-on-one support by trained ostomy volunteers in conjunction with enterostomal therapists)

Reach to Recovery
American Cancer Society
Atlanta, GA
(404) 320-3333
www.cancer.org
(A program that provides support for breast cancer clients and families)

United Ostomy Association, Inc.
Irvine, CA
(800) 826-0826
www.uoa.org
(See also Breast Cancer; Lung Cancer; Smoking and Tobacco; Terminal Illness)

Vital Options
Los Angeles, CA
(818) 508-5657
www.vitaloptions.org
(An organization offering support and education to young people with cancer)

Chiropractic

American Chiropractic Association
Arlington, VA
(800) 368-3083
www.amerchiro.org

Colitis

Crohn's and Colitis Foundation of Canada
Toronto, Ontario
Canada
(416) 920-5035
www.ccfc.ca

Crohn's and Colitis Foundation
New York, NY
(800) 932-2423
www.ccfa.org

United Ostomy Association, Inc.
Irvine, CA
(800) 826-0826
www.uoa.org

Counseling Services

Family Service Association of America
Milwaukee, WI
(414) 359-2111
www.nahsc.org
(Organization of local family counseling agencies throughout North America)

Deafness

(See Hearing Impairment)

Death and Grieving

American Association of Retired Persons
Widowed Persons Service
Washington DC
(800) 424-3410
www.aarp.org

The Candlelighters Foundation
Bethesda, MD
(800) 366-2223
www.candlelighters.org

Choice in Dying, Inc.
New York, NY
(212) 366-5540
www.choices.org/index.html

The Compassionate Friends
Oak Brook, IL
(708) 990-0010
www.compasionatefriends.com

Dying With Dignity
Toronto, Ontario
Canada
(416) 486-3998
www.web.apc.org/dwd

The Hemlock Society
Eugene, OR
(503) 342-5738
www.irsociety.com/hemlock.htm

Make-A-Wish Foundation
Phoenix, AZ
(800) 722-9474
www.makeawish.org

National Council on Aging, Inc.
Washington DC
(202) 479-1200
www.ncoa.org

National Hospice Organization
Arlington, VA
(703) 243-5900
www.nho.org

National SIDS Resource Center
Mclean, VA
(703) 821-8955
www.circsol.com/sids

Parents Without Partners, Inc.
Chicago, IL
(312) 644-6610
www.parentswithoutpartners.org
(See also AIDS; Hospices; Terminal Illness)

Dental Health

American Dental Association
Chicago, IL
(312) 440-2500
www.ada.org

National Institute of Dental Research
Bethesda, MD
(301) 496-4261
www.nidr.nih.gov

Diabetes

American Diabetes Association
Alexandria, VA
(703) 549-1500
www.diabetes.org

American Dietetic Association
Chicago, IL
(312) 899-0400
www.eatright.org

American Foundation for the Blind
New York, NY
(212) 620-2000
www.ige.apc.org/afb

Canadian Diabetes Association
Toronto, Ontario
Canada
(416) 382-4440
www.diabetes.ca/index.htm

Juvenile Diabetes Foundation
New York, NY
(800) 223-1138
www.jofcure.org

MedicAlert Foundation
Turlock, CA
(800) 344-3226
www.medicalert.org

Digestive Diseases

American Gastroenterological Association
Bethesda, MD
(301) 654-2055
www.gastro.org

American Society of Nutritional Science
Bethesda, MD
(301) 530-7050
www.faseb.org/asns

American Society for Gastrointestinal Endoscopy
Manchester, MA
(508) 526-8330
www.hsc.missouri.edu/ASGE/
docs/asge.html

National Digestive Diseases and Education and Information Clearinghouse
Bethesda, MD
(301) 654-3810
www.niddk.nih.gov/health/
digest/nddic.htm
(See also Colitis)

Disabled

(See Handicapped and Disabled)

Drug Abuse

Cocaine Anonymous
(See white pages of telephone directory for local chapter)

CokEnders
(See white pages of telephone directory for local chapter)

Ear and Hearing Disorders

Alexander Graham Bell Association for the Deaf, Inc.
Washington DC
(202) 337-5220
www.agbell.org

American Academy of Facial and Reconstructive Surgery
Washington DC
(703) 299-9291
www.aafprs.org

American Academy of Otolaryngology—Head and Neck Surgery
Alexandria, VA
(703) 836-4444
www.entnet.org

American Speech-Language-Hearing Association
Rockville, MD
(301) 987-5700
www.asha.org

American Tinnitus Association
Portland, OR
(503) 248-9985
www.ata.org

International Hearing Dog, Inc.
Henderson, CO
(303) 287-EARS
members.aol.com/IHDI/IHDI.
html

International Hearing Society
Livonia, MI
(800) 521-5247
www.co.merced.ca.us/pitd/be.
htm

National Association for Hearing and Speech Action
10801 Rockville Pike
Rockville, MD 20852
(800) 638-8255

National Association for the Deaf
Silver Spring, MD
(301) 587-1788
www.nad.org

Self-Help for Hard of Hearing People
Bethesda, MD
(301) 657-2248
www.shhh.org

The National Hearing Conservation Association
Des Moines, IA
(515) 243-1558
www.hearingconservation.org

Eating Disorders

American Anorexia/Bulimia Association, Inc. (AABA)
New York, NY
(212) 734-1114
members.aol.com/amanbu
(Self-help group that provides information and referrals to physician and therapists)

Anorexia Nervosa and Related Eating Disorders, Inc.
Eugene, OR
(503) 344-1144
www.anred.com

National Anorexic Aid Society, Inc.
1925 E. Dublin-Granville Road
Columbus, OH
(614) 436-1112

Endometriosis

Endometriosis Association
8585 N. 76th Place
Milwaukee, WI
(800) 992-3636

Epilepsy

Epilepsy Foundation of America
Landover, MD
(800) 332-1000
www.efa.org
(See also Neurologic Disorders)

Eye Disorders

American Academy of Ophthalmology
San Francisco, CA
(415) 561-8500
www.eyenet.org

American Foundation for the Blind
New York, NY
(800) AFB-LIND
www.ige.apc.org/afb

American Optometric Association
Bethesda, MD
(301) 718-6574
www.aoanet.org

Better Vision Institute, Inc.
Arlington, VA
(209) 243-1508
(800) 424-VICA
www.visionsite.org/info.htm

Contact Lens Society of America
11735 Bowman Green Drive
Reston, VA 22090

Eye Bank Association of America
Washington DC
(202) 775-4999
www.restoresight.org/index.
html

Leader Dogs for the Blind
Rochester, MI
(313) 651-9011
www.leaderdog.com

National Braille Association
Rochester, NY
(716) 473-0900
www.nbp.org

**National Federation of
the Blind**
Baltimore, MD
(410) 659-9314
www.nfb.org

**National Society to Prevent
Blindness**
500 East Remington Road
Schaumburg, IL 60173

Recording for the Blind, Inc.
Princeton, NJ
(800) 803-7201
www.rfbd.org

Seeing Eye
Morristown, NJ
(973) 539-4425
www.seeingeye.org

Taping for the Blind
3935 Essex Lane
Houston, TX 77027
(713) 622-2767

Fibromyalgia

Fibromyalgia Network
Tuscon, AZ
(800) 853-2929
www.fmnetnews.com/pages/
basics.html

Genetic Disorders

**Hereditary Disease
Foundation**
Santa Monica, CA
(310) 458-4183
www.hdfoundation.org/index.
html

**National Clearinghouse for
Human Genetic Diseases**
2000 15th Street N
Suite 701
Arlington, VA 22201-2617
(713) 524-7802
*(Provides information about
inherited diseases; see also
Birth Defects)*

Handicapped and Disabled

**American Alliance for
Health, Physical Education,
Recreation, and Dance**
Reston, VA
(703) 476-3400
www.aahperd.org
*(Provides information about
recreation and fitness opportunities for the handicapped)*

**National Council of
Independent Living**
2111 Wilson Boulevard
Suite 405
Arlington, VA
(703) 525-3406

**National Rehabilitation
Information Center**
Silver Springs, MD
(800) 227-0216
(800) 34-NARIC
www.naric.com

Special Olympics
Washington DC
(202) 628-3630
www.specialolympics.org

Health Care

**American Medical
Association**
Chicago, IL
(312) 464-4470
www.ama.assn.org
*(See also Chiropractic; Dental
Health; Holistic Medicine;
Mental Health; Osteopathic
Medicine)*

Heart Disease

American Heart Association
Dallas, TX
(214) 373-6300
www.amhrt.org

Coronary Club
9500 Euclid Avenue
Cleveland, OH 44106

Heart and Stroke Foundation of Canada
Ottawa, Ontario
Canada
(613) 237-4381
www.hsf.ca

Heart Information Center
National Heart Institute
U.S. Public Health Service
9000 Rockville Pike
Bldg. 31, Room 4A21
Bethesda, MD 20892

International Society for Cardiovascular Surgery
13 Elm Street
P.O. Box 1565
Manchester, MA 01944

Mended Hearts
Dallas, TX
(214) 706-1442
www.mendedhearts.org
(Support group for persons who have undergone heart surgery, and their families; see also Hypertension; Stroke)

Hemophilia

Hemophilia Foundation
New York, NY
(212) 219-8180
www.hemophilia.org
(See also Genetic Disorders)

High Blood Pressure

(See Hypertension)

Holistic Medicine

American Holistic Nurses Association
Flagstaff, AZ
(800) 278-AHNA
www.ahna.org

Hospices

National Hospice Organization
Arlington, VA
(703) 243-5900
www.nho.org

Huntington's Disease

Huntington's Disease Foundation of America
140 West 22nd Street
6th Floor
New York, NY 10011
(212) 242-1968
(800) 345-4372

Incest

(See Sexual Abuse and Assault)

Infectious Diseases

American Lung Association
New York, NY
(212) 315-8700
www.lungusa.org

American Public Health Association
1015 15th Street NW
Washington DC 20005
(202) 789-5600

American Social Health Association
Raleigh, NC
(919) 361-8400
www.ashastd.org

American Venereal Disease Association
Box 1753
Baltimore, MD 21203-1753

Centers for Disease Control
Atlanta, GA
(404) 639-3634
www.cdc.gov

National Foundation for Infectious Diseases
Bethesda, MD
(301) 656-0003
www.nfid.org

National Institute of Allergy and Infectious Diseases
National Institute of Health
9000 Rockville Pike
Bethesda, MD 20892

World Health Organization
Washington DC
(202) 466-5883
www.who.org
(See also Sexually Transmitted Diseases)

Kidney Disease

American Kidney Fund
Rockville, MD
(301) 881-3052
www.arbon.com/kidney/home.htm

American Association of Kidney Patients
Tampa, FL
(800) 749-2257
www.aakp.org

Kidney Foundation of Canada
Hamilton, Ontario
Canada
(905) 574-5222
www.networx.on.ca/~kidney/index.htm

National Kidney Foundation, Inc.
New York, NY
(212) 889-2210
www.kidney.org

Learning Disorders

Learning Disabilities Association
Pittsburgh, PA
(412) 341-1515
www.ldanatl.org

Liver Disease

American Liver Foundation
Cedar Grove, NJ
(800) 223-0179
www.sadieo.ucsf.edu/ALF/ALFfinal/homepagealf.html

Canadian Liver Foundation
Toronto, Ontario
Canada
(416) 964-1953
is.dal.ca/~stanet/database/liver.html

Lung Disease

American Lung Association
New York, NY
(800) 586-4872
www.lungusa.org

American Thoracic Society
New York, NY
(212) 315-8700
www.thoracic.org/index.html

Canadian Lung Association
Ottawa, Ontario
Canada
(613) 237-1208
www.lung.ca/cla.html
(See also Asthma; Cancer; Smoking and Tobacco)

Lupus Erythematosus

Lupus Canada
Calgary, Alberta
Canada
(800) 661-1468
www.lupuscanada.org

Lupus Foundation of America
Rockville, MD
(800) 558-0121
www.lupus.org/lupus

Medical Identification

MedicAlert Foundation International
Turlock, CA
(209) 668-3333
(800) ID-ALERT
www.medicalert.org
(Provides those with medical problems, bracelets, or neck chains with special emblems to alert medical or law enforcement personnel)

Medical Organizations

American Academy of Family Physicians
Kansas City, MO
(816) 333-9700
home.aafp.org/aafpf/index.html

American Academy of Pediatrics
Elk Grove, IL
(800) 433-9016
www.aap.org

American College of Obstetricians and Gynecologists
Washington DC
(202) 638-5577
www.acog.org

American Medical Association
Chicago, IL
(312) 464-5000
www.ama-assn.org

Medications (Prescription and Over-the-Counter)

Food and Drug Administration (FDA)
Office of Consumer Affairs
Public Inquiries
Rockville, MD
(301) 443-3170
www.fda.gov

Mental Health

American Psychiatric Association
Washington DC
(202) 682-6000
www.thebody.com/apa/apapage.html

American Psychologist Association
Washington DC
(202) 336-5500
www.apa.org

Mental Retardation

The ARC
Arlington, TX
(817) 261-6003
www.THEARC.org

Multiple Sclerosis

National Multiple Sclerosis Society
New York, NY
(212) 986-3240
(800) 624-8236
www.nmss.org

Muscular Dystrophy

Muscular Dystrophy Association
Tuscon, AZ
(602) 529-2000
www.mda.org.au

Myasthenia Gravis

Myasthenia Gravis Foundation
Chicago, IL
(312) 427-6252
(800) 541-5454
www.myasthenia.org

Neurologic Disorders

Alzheimer's Association
Chicago, IL
(800) 272-3900
www.alz.org

Alzheimer's Society of Canada
Toronto, Ontario
Canada
(416) 925-3552
www.alzheimers.ca

American Lateral Sclerosis Association
15300 Ventura Boulevard
Suite 315
Sherman Oaks, CA 91403

American Parkinson Disease Association
New York, NY
(212) 732-9550
www.apda.qpg.com

American Speech-Language Hearing Association
Rockville, MD
(301) 897-5700
www.asha.org

Amyotrophic Lateral Sclerosis Association
Woodland Hills, CA
(818) 880-9007
www.alsa.org

Epilepsy Foundation of America
Landover, MD
(301) 459-3700
(800) EFA-1000
www.efa.org

Guillain-Barré Syndrome Foundation International
Wynnewood, PA
(215) 667-0131
www.adsnet.com/jsteeinhi/html/gbs/gbsfi.html

Hereditary Disease Foundation
Santa Monica, CA
(310) 458-4183
www.hdfoundation.org

Huntington's Disease Foundation of America
140 West 22nd Street
6th Floor
New York, NY 10011
(212) 242-1968
(800) 345-4372

Independent Living for the Handicapped
1301 Belmont Street NW
Washington DC 20009
(202) 797-9803

Information Center for Individuals with Disabilities
Fort Point Place, 1st Floor
27-43 Wormwood Street
Boston, MA 02210-1606

MedicAlert
Turlock, CA
(800) 344-3226
www.medicalert.org

Muscular Dystrophy Association
Tuscon, AZ
(602) 529-2000
www.mda.org.au

Myasthenia Gravis Foundation
Chicago, IL
(312) 427-6252
(800) 541-5454
www.myasthenia.org

National Easter Seal Society
Chicago, IL
(312) 726-6200
www.seals.com

National Headache Foundation
Chicago, IL
(312) 878-7715
www.headaches.org

National Institute of
Neurological and
Communicative Disorders
and Stroke
National Institutes of Health
Bethesda, MD
(301) 496-4000
www.ninds.nih.gov

National Multiple Sclerosis
Society
New York, NY
(800) 624-8236
www.nmss.org

National Parkinson
Foundation
Miami, FL
(305) 547-6666
www.parkinson.org

National Spinal Cord Injury
Association
Woburn, MA
(617) 935-2722
www.spinalcord.org

Paralyzed Veterans of
America
Washington DC
(202) 872-1300
www.pva.org

Parkinson's Disease
Foundation
Columbia Presbyterian Medical Center
640 West 168th Street
New York, NY 10032
(212) 923-4700
(See also Alzheimer's Disease;
Mental Health; Stroke)

Nutrition

American Society for
Nutritional Sciences
Bethesda, MD
(301) 530-7050
www.nutrition.org

American Dietetic
Association Foundation
Chicago, IL
(312) 899-0040
www.eatright.org/foundation.
html

Food and Drug
Administration (FDA)
Office of Consumer Affairs
Public Inquiries
Rockville, MD
(301) 443-3170
www.fda.gov

Food and Nutrition Board
National Academy of Science
Institute of Medicine
2101 Constitution Avenue
NW
Washington DC 20418
(202) 334-2238
(See goverment pages of
telephone directory for state or
local departments of agriculture
extension services)

Obesity

(See Nutrition; Weight Control)

Organ Donations

Canadian Coalition on
Organ Donor Awareness
c/o Pharmaceutical Manufacturer's Association of Canada
1111 Prince of Wales Drive
Suite 302
Ottawa, Ontario
Canada
(613) 727-1380

Living Bank
Houston, TX
(713) 961-9431 in Texas
(800) 528-2971
www.livingbank.org
(Provides information and acts
as registry and referral service
for people wanting to donate
organs for research or
transplantation)

MedicAlert Organ Donor Program
Turlock, CA
(209) 668-3333
(800) ID-ALERT
www.medicalert

Osteopathic Medicine

American Osteopathic Association
Chicago, IL
(312) 280-5800
www.am-osteo.assn.org

Pain

American Pain Society
Skokie, IL
(708) 966-5595
www.ampainsoc.org

Canadian Pain Society
London, Ontario
Canada
(519) 455-5110
www.medicine.dal.ca/cps/index.html

International Pain Foundation
Seattle, WA
(206) 547-2157
www.halcyon.com/iasp

National Osteoporosis Foundation
Washington DC
(202) 223-2226
www.nof.org

Osteogenesis Imperfecta Foundation, Inc.
5005 W. Laurel Avenue
Suite 210
Tampa, FL 33607-3836

Pancreatitis

(See Digestive Diseases)

Parkinson's Disease

American Parkinson Disease Association
New York, NY
(212) 732-9550
www.apda.qpg.com

National Parkinson Foundation
Miami, FL
(305) 547-6666
www.parkinson.org

Parkinson's Disease Foundation
Columbia Presbyterian
Medical Center
640 West 168th Street
New York, NY 10032
(212) 923-4700
(See also Neurologic Disorders)

Physical Fitness

American Physical Fitness Research Institute
654 North Sepulveda
Boulevard
Los Angeles, CA 90049

Poison/Toxic Substances

National Pesticide Information Clearing House
(800) 858-7378
www.ace.orst.edu/info/nptn

Poison Control Branch
Food and Drug Administration
Rockville, MD
(888) 463-6332
www.fda.gov

Rape

National Clearinghouse on Marital and Date Rape
Berkeley, CA
(510) 524-1582
members.aol.com/ncmdr/index.html
(For-profit referral service)

National Coalition Against Sexual Assault (NCASA)
Enola, PA
(717) 728-9764
www.ncasa.org

Rehabilitation

Rehabilitation Services Administration
Office of Special Education and Rehabilitation Services
Department of Education
Washington DC
(202) 401-0689
www.ed.gov/offices/OSERS/RSA/rsa.html

Reye's Syndrome

Reye's Syndrome Foundation of Canada
c/o Children's Hospital of Western Ontario
Department of Pediatrics
800 Commissioners Road E
London, Ontario N6C 2V5
Canada

National Reye's Syndrome Foundation
P.O. Box 829
426 North Lewis
Bryan, OH 43506
(419) 636-2679
(800) 233-7393
www.bright.net/~reyessyn

Rural Health

National Rural Health Association
Kansas City, MO
(816) 756-3140
www.nrharural.org

Self-Care/Self-Help

National Self-Help Clearinghouse
New York, NY
(212) 354-8525
www.selfhelpweb.org
(Provides information about self-help support)

Sexual Abuse and Assault

National Committee for Prevention of Child Abuse
Chicago, IL
(800) 556-2722
www.childabuse.org

Sex Education

American Association of Sex Educators, Counselors, and Therapists
Chicago, IL
(312) 644-0828
www.aasect.org

Sexual Difficulties

Sexaholics Anonymous
Nashville, TN
(615) 331-6230
www.sa.org
(Self-help group for sex addicts)

Sexually Transmitted Diseases

Herpes Resource Center
13827 Research Triangle Park
Raleigh, NC 27709
(919) 361-8400

National Institute of Allergy and Infectious Diseases
National Institute of Health
Bethesda, MD
National STS Hotline
(800) 227-8922
www.ashastd.org

Sickle Cell Anemia

National Association for Sickle Cell Disease (NASCD)
Los Angeles, CA
(800) 421-8453
www.sicklecelldisease.org

Skin Cancer

American Cancer Society,
Atlanta, GA
(800) 227-2345
www.cancer.org

Skin Cancer Foundation
245 Fifth Avenue
New York, NY 10016
(212) 725-5176

Skin Disease

American Cancer Society
Atlanta, GA
(800) 227-2345
www.cancer.org

**National Psoriasis
Foundation**
Portland, OR
(503) 244-7404
www.psoriasis.org

Skin Cancer Foundation
245 Fifth Avenue
New York, NY 10016
(212) 725-5176

Sleep Disorders

**American Sleep Disorders
Association**
Rochester, MN
(507) 287-6006
www.asda.org

Smoking and Tobacco

**Action on Smoking and
Health (ASH)**
Washington DC
(202) 659-4310
www.ash.org

American Cancer Society
Atlanta, GA
(404) 320-3333
(800) 227-2345
www.cancer.org
*(Provides information about
quitting smoking and smoking
cessation programs)*

American Heart Association
Dallas, TX
(214) 373-6300
www.amhrt.org
*(Provides information about
quitting smoking and smoking
cessation programs; see white
pages of telephone directory for
listing of local chapters)*

American Lung Association
New York, NY
(212) 315-8700
www.lungusa.org
*(Provides information about
quitting smoking and smoking
cessation programs; see white
pages of telephone directory for
local chapters)*

**Association of Community
Cancer Centers**
Rockville, MD
(301) 984-9496
www.accc-cancer.org

**Cancer Information Service
(CIS)**
Bethesda, MD
(800) 4-CANCER
www.nci.hih.gov
*(Program of the National Cancer
Institute (NCI), this service provides information about cancer,
answers questions, disseminates
literature, and provides up-to-
date information about new cancer treatment trials)*

**National Coalition for
Cancer Survivorship**
Silver Springs, MD
(301) 650-8868
www.cansearch.org

**National Hospice
Organization**
Arlington, VA
(703) 243-5900
www.nho.org

Stress Reduction

*(See white or yellow pages of
telephone directory for listings on
Biofeedback Therapy and Training; Crisis Centers; Medication)*

Stroke

Council on Stroke
American Heart Association
Dallas, TX
(214) 373-6300
www.amhrt.org

Terminal Illness

The Hemlock Society
Eugene, OR
(503) 342-5748
www.irsociety.com/hemlock.
htm
(Promotes tolerance of the right of terminally ill persons to end their lives in a planned manner)

Make-A-Wish Foundation
Phoenix, AZ
(800) 722-9474
www.makeawish.org
(Dedicated to granting the special wishes of terminally ill children)

Weight Control

American Dietetic Association
Chicago, IL
(312) 899-0040
www.eatright.org

Canadian Dietetic Association
480 University Avenue
Suite 601
Toronto, Ontario M3G 1V2
Canada

Overeaters Anonymous
Rio Rancho, NM
(505) 891-2662
www.overeatersanonymous.org
(See white pages of telephone directory for listing of local chapters)

TOPS (Take Off Pounds Sensibly)
Milwaukee, WI
(414) 482-4620
www.tops.org
(See white pages of telephone directory for listing of local chapter)

Weight Watchers International, Inc.
Jericho, NY
(800) 651-6000
www.weightwatchers.com
(See white pages of telephone directory for listing of local chapter)

Woman's Health

Boston Women's Health Book Collective
Somerville, MA
(617) 625-0271
www.feminist.com/ourbodies.
htm
(Publishes Our Bodies, Ourselves, a well-known book on women's health)

National Action Forum for Older Women and Stony Brook: A Center for the Health and Housing of Women Over 40
State University of New York
School of Allied Health
Professions
Health Sciences Center
Stony Brook, NY 11794
(Promotes an improved quality of life for women in midlife and older; publishes a newsletter, Forum)

Women's Sports Foundation
New York, NY
(800) 227-3988
www.lifetimetv.com/wosport/

Index

A

Abdominal aortic aneurysm, 26
ABG values, 571t
Acid-based disorders, 1–5, 571t
Acquired immune deficiency syndrome (AIDS), 253–259
See also Kaposi's sarcoma
Activity intolerance
CHF and, 228–229
hepatitis and, 238
occupational lung disease and, 367
pneumonia and, 428–429
valvular heart disease and, 560
Acute demyelinating polyneuropathy, 221–224
Acute gastritis, 199–202
Acute glomerulo-nephritis, 210–211
Acute infection poliomyelitis, 433–436
Acute lymphocytic leukemia (ALL), 316–321
Acute myelocytic leukemia (AML), 316–321
Acute pancreatitis, 390–394

Acute pericarditis, 405–406
Acute pyelonephritis, 464–467
Acute renal failure (ARF), 474–484
Acute respiratory acidosis, 2-3
Acute respiratory distress syndrome (ARDS), 6–9
Acute tonsillitis, 533–535
Addison's disease, 10–12
See also Adrenal insufficiency
Adrenal insufficiency, 10–12
Alcoholic cirrhosis, 113–118
Alcoholic hepatitis, 236–239
Altered cerebral tissue perfusion, 96, 297
Altered health maintenance, hypertension and, 276–277
Altered nutrition
acute renal failure and, 481–482
AIDS and, 257
cancer and, 80–81
colorectal cancer and, 120
gastritis and, 201
hepatitis and 238–239